LGVAH

BI 3569502 1

D1388222

Thieme

Color Atlas of Ultrasound Anatomy

Berthold Block, MD

Private Practice
Braunschweig
Germany

2nd edition

556 illustrations

Thieme
Stuttgart · New York

Library of Congress Cataloging-in-Publication Data

Block, Berthold, MD.
[Der Sono-Guide – Taschenatlas der sonographischen Schnittbilddiagnostik. English]
Color atlas of ultrasound anatomy / Berthold Block. – 2nd ed.
p. ; cm.
Includes index.
ISBN 978-3-13-139052-3 (alk. paper)
1. Ultrasonic imaging–Atlases. 2. Human anatomy–Atlases, Handbooks. I. Title.
[DNLM: 1. Ultrasonography–Atlases. 2. Ultrasonography–Handbooks. WI 17]
QM25.R595 2012
616.03'565–dc22 2011019360

This book is an authorized, revised new edition based on the German edition published and copyrighted 2003 by Georg Thieme Verlag, Stuttgart. Title of the German edition: Der Sono-Guide – Taschenatlas der sonographischen Schnittbilddiagnostik.

New updated parts translated by:
Terry C. Telger, Fort Worth, TX, USA

Illustrator: Gay & Sender, Bremen, Germany

1st English edition 2004

1st Chinese Edition 2008
1st Croatian Edition 2008
1st Czech Edition 2004
1st French Edition 2005
1st German Edition 2003
1st Greek Edition 2009
1st Italian Edition 2004
1st Japanese Edition 2007
1st Polish Edition 2005
1st Portuguese Edition 2005
1st Spanish Edition 2003
1st Turkish Edition 2006

© 2012 Georg Thieme Verlag,
Rüdigerstrasse 14, 70469 Stuttgart, Germany
http://www.thieme.de
Thieme New York, 333 Seventh Avenue,
New York, NY 10001, USA
http://www.thieme.com

Cover design: Thieme Publishing Group
Typesetting by Gay & Sender, Bremen, Germany
Printed in China by Everbest Printing Co, Ltd

ISBN 978-3-13-139052-3 1 2 3 4 5 6

Important note: Medicine is an ever-changing science undergoing continual development. Research and clinical experience are continually expanding our knowledge, in particular our knowledge of proper treatment and drug therapy. Insofar as this book mentions any dosage or application, readers may rest assured that the authors, editors, and publishers have made every effort to ensure that such references are in accordance with **the state of knowledge at the time of production of the book.**
Nevertheless, this does not involve, imply, or express any guarantee or responsibility on the part of the publishers in respect to any dosage instructions and forms of applications stated in the book. **Every user is requested to examine carefully** the manufacturers' leaflets accompanying each drug and to check, if necessary in consultation with a physician or specialist, whether the dosage schedules mentioned therein or the contraindications stated by the manufacturers differ from the statements made in the present book. Such examination is particularly important with drugs that are either rarely used or have been newly released on the market. Every dosage schedule or every form of application used is entirely at the user's own risk and responsibility. The authors and publishers request every user to report to the publishers any discrepancies or inaccuracies noticed. If errors in this work are found after publication, errata will be posted at www.thieme.com on the product description page.

Some of the product names, patents, and registered designs referred to in this book are in fact registered trademarks or proprietary names even though specific reference to this fact is not always made in the text. Therefore, the appearance of a name without designation as proprietary is not to be construed as a representation by the publisher that it is in the public domain.

This book, including all parts thereof, is legally protected by copyright. Any use, exploitation, or commercialization outside the narrow limits set by copyright legislation, without the publisher's consent, is illegal and liable to prosecution. This applies in particular to photostat reproduction, copying, mimeographing, preparation of microfilms, and electronic data processing and storage.

Preface

Ultrasound scanning yields a series of sectional images. The basis for interpreting the examination is the individual sectional image. At first sight, it is easy to be confused by the variable appearance of an ultrasound scan of the same region in different patients. This has numerous causes, including differences in density, body fat, age-related differences, overlying gas, and artifacts. In most cases the apparent discrepancies are not based on true anatomical differences. When a systematic scanning routine is closely followed, series of sectional images can be obtained in every patient with remarkable consistency. Even if the images themselves vary, the anatomical relationships that are demonstrated remain constant.

When the book was conceived and produced in 2003, the publisher and the author were breaking new ground. The strong international demand has shown that there was an obvious need for a complete and systematic overview of sonographic anatomy.

For the new edition, numerous illustrations were replaced by new ones and completely new series of images were added. The new images were acquired on a system that General Electric kindly loaned to us for our use. I thank Mrs. Katharina Wasser and Mrs. Jana Steding for providing the machine and technical guidance. I also thank Mr. Jan-Hendrik Hering of Hering Ultraschalltechnik/Sonoring, Germany, for mediating contact with General Electric and for his helpful support in all matters.

Many people have contributed to the success of this book. I wish to thank Dr. Hartwig Schöndube and Dr. Matthias Geist, and I extend special thanks to Dr. Waldemar Muschol and Dr. Helge Dönitz for their help with the new edition. I am also grateful to the staff at Thieme Medical Publishers who made this new edition possible, especially Mr. Stephan Konnry, Ms. Gabriele Kuhn-Giovannini and Ms. Elisabeth Kurz.

Berthold Block
Braunschweig, Germany

BIRMINGHAM CITY UNIVERSITY
Book no 35695021
Subject no. 616.07543 Blo
LIBRARY

Table of Contents

The numbers shown on the scanning paths refer to the corresponding *figure numbers*

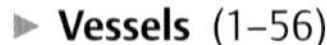

▶ **Vessels** (1–56)

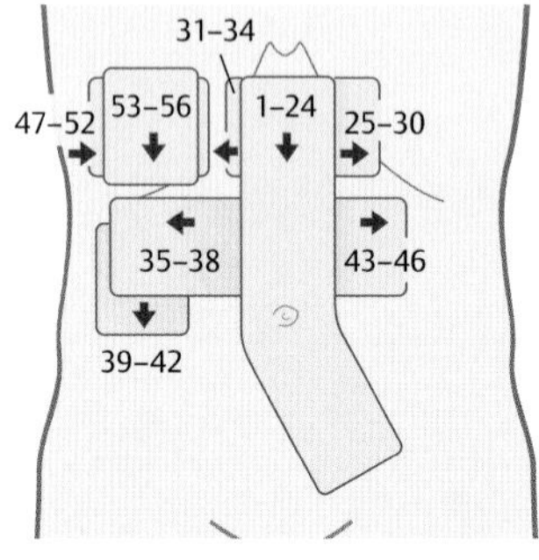

▶ **Liver** (57–100)

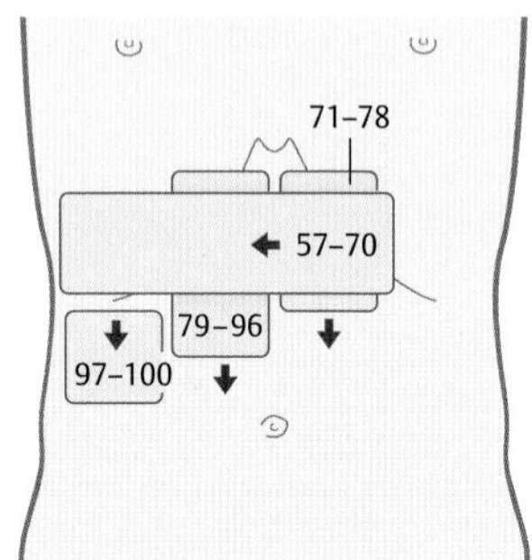

▶ **Gallbladder** (101–132)

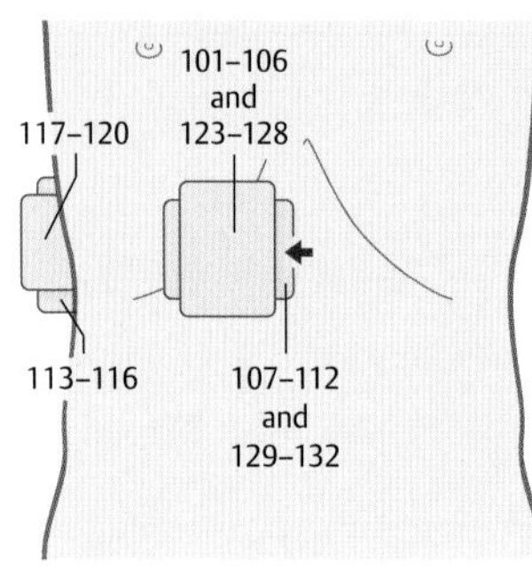

▶ **Pancreas** (133–164)

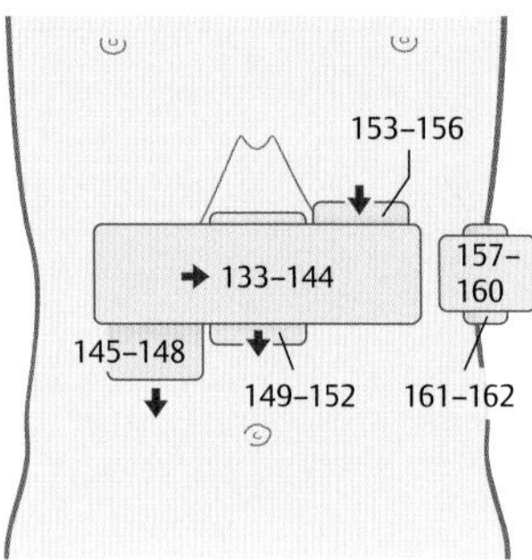

▶ **Spleen** (165–174)

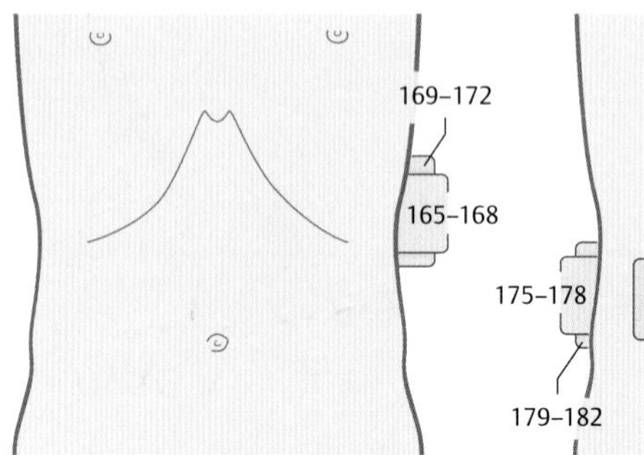

▶ **Kidney** (175–200)

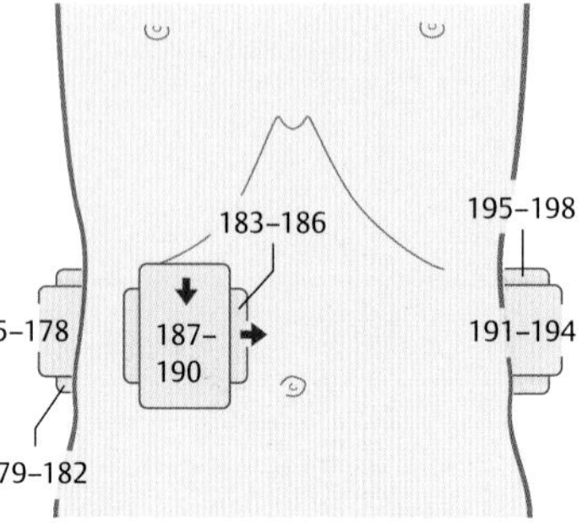

in this book.

▶ **Adrenal gland** (201–214)

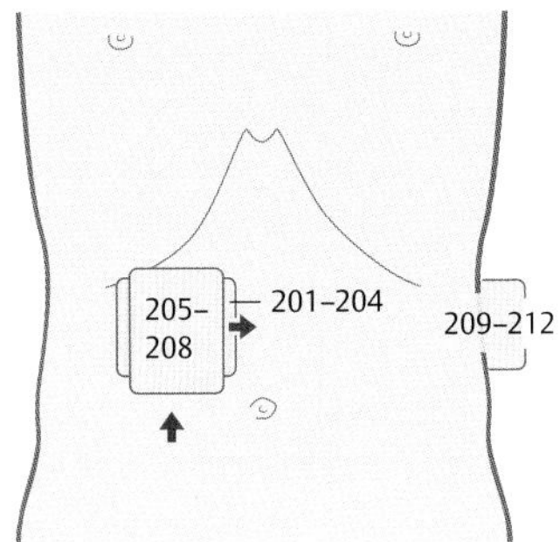

▶ **Stomach** (215–238)

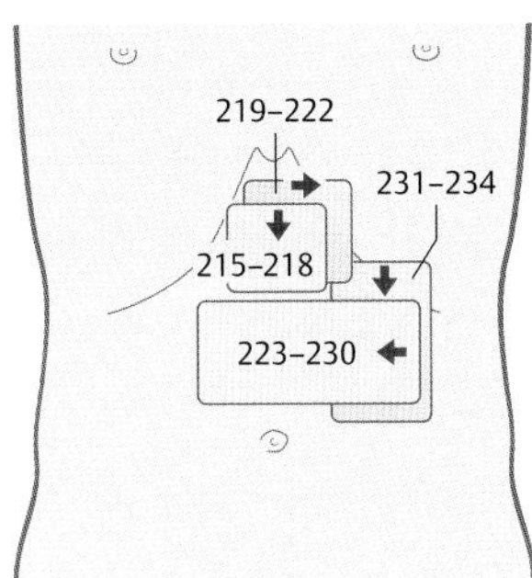

▶ **Bladder** (239–244)

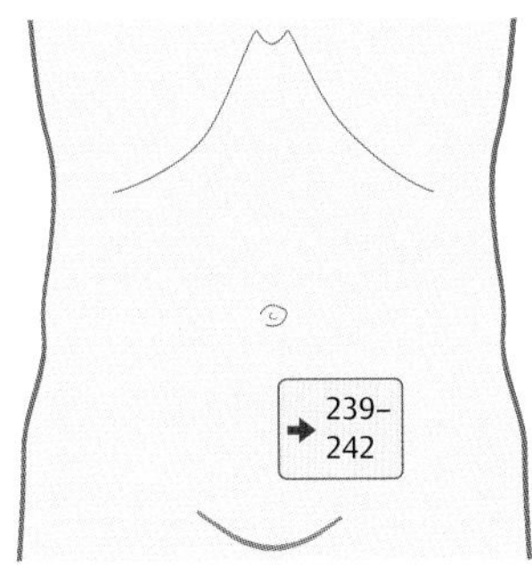

▶ **Prostate** (245–254)

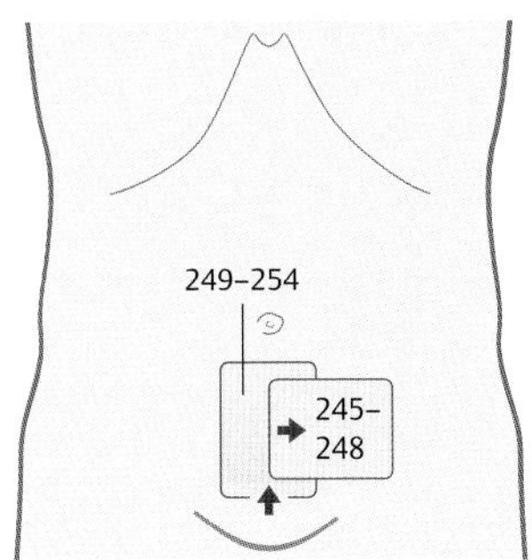

▶ **Uterus** (255–264)

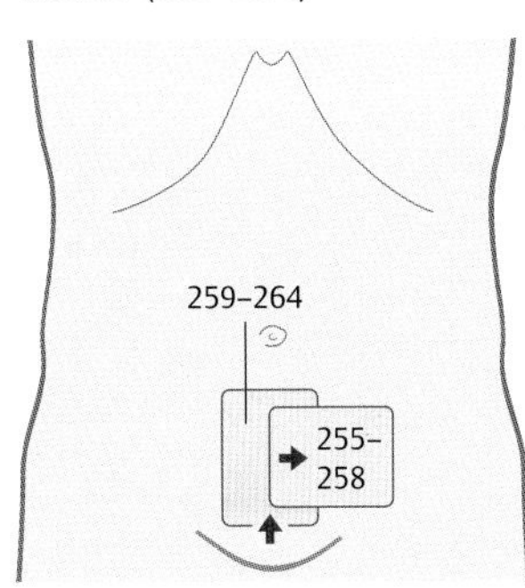

▶ **Thyroid gland** (265–278)

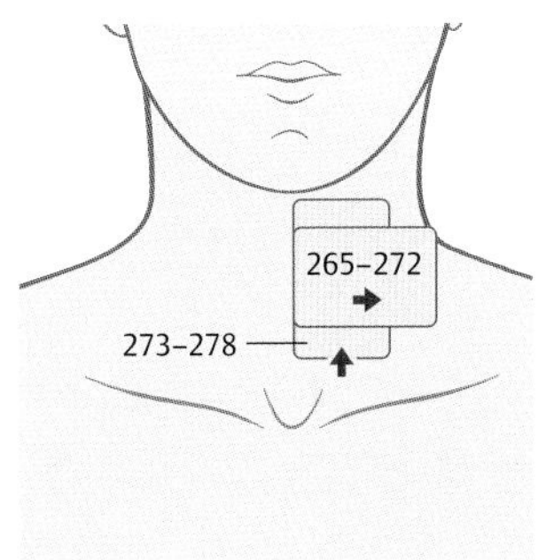

Scanning Planes

Note: *The number key for the diagrams is on the fold-out flap inside the back cover.*

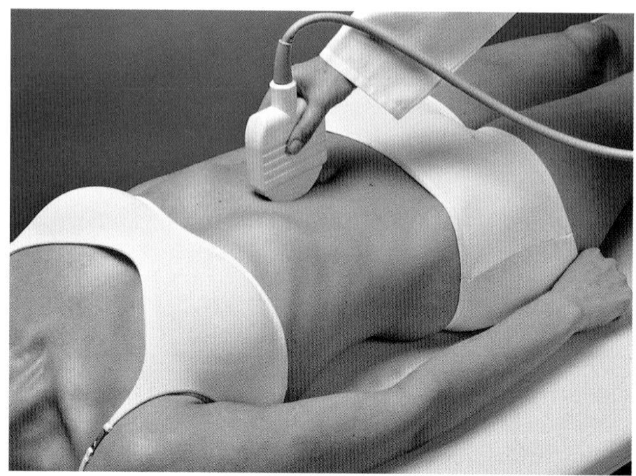

▶ **Upper abdominal longitudinal scan, center**

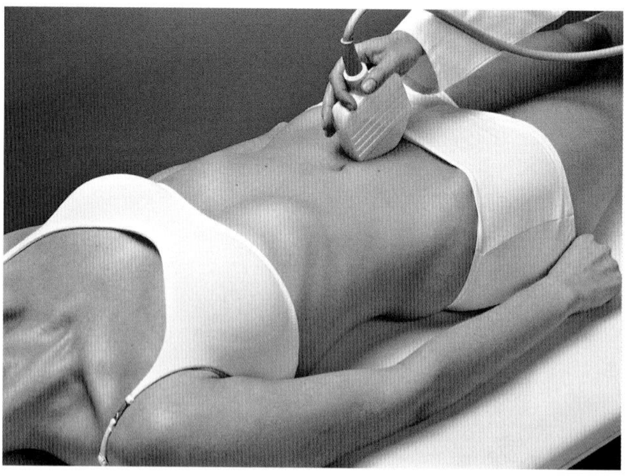

▶ **Lower abdominal longitudinal scan, center**

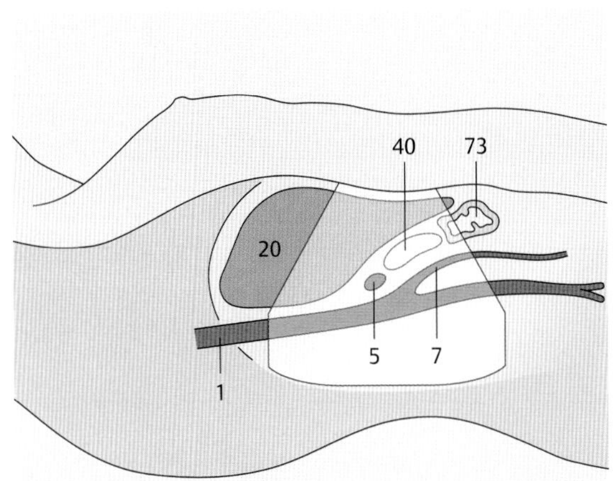
40
73
20
5
7
1

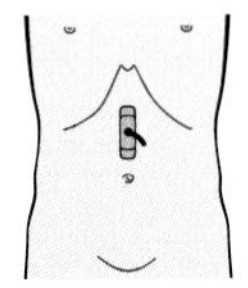

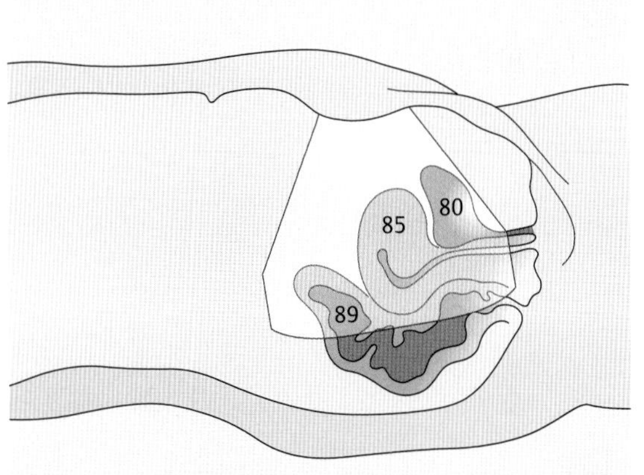
80
85
89

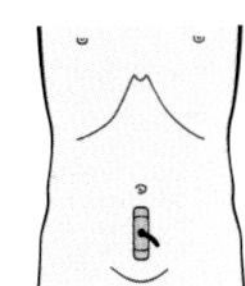

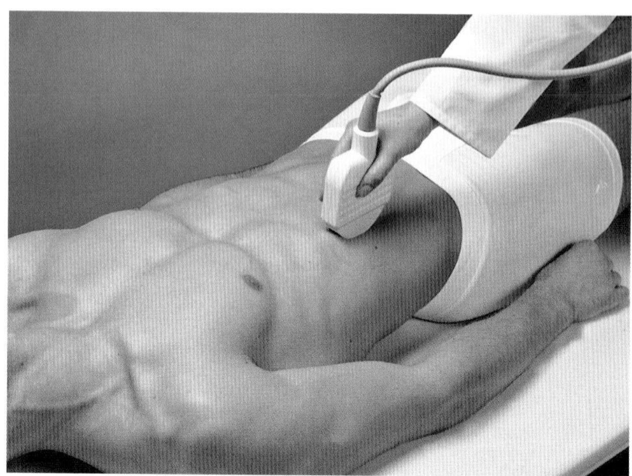

▶ Upper abdominal longitudinal scan, right side

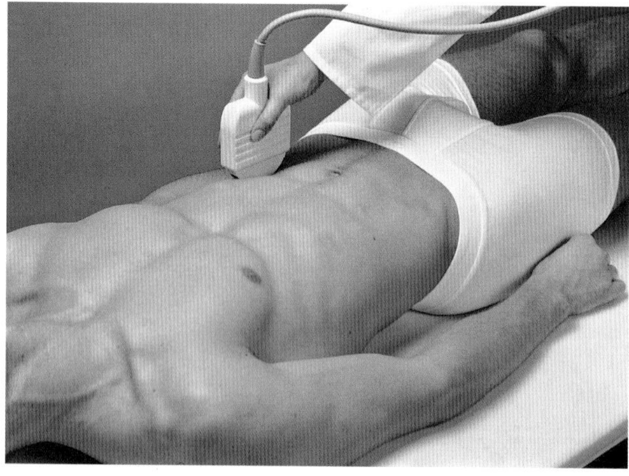

▶ Upper abdominal longitudinal scan, left side

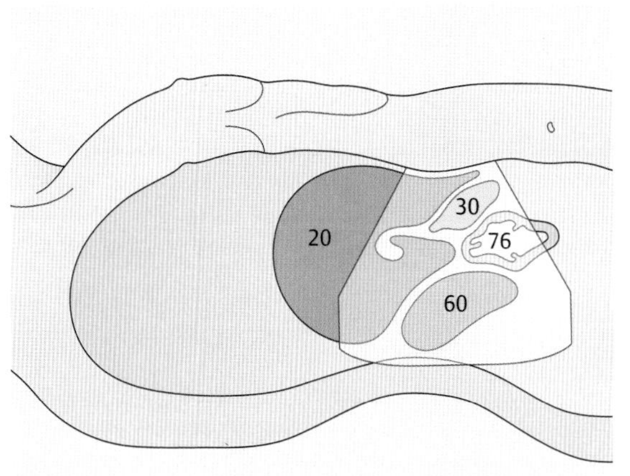
20
30
76
60

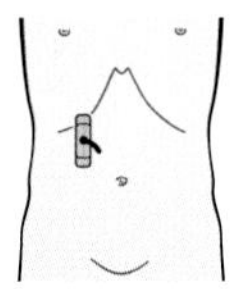

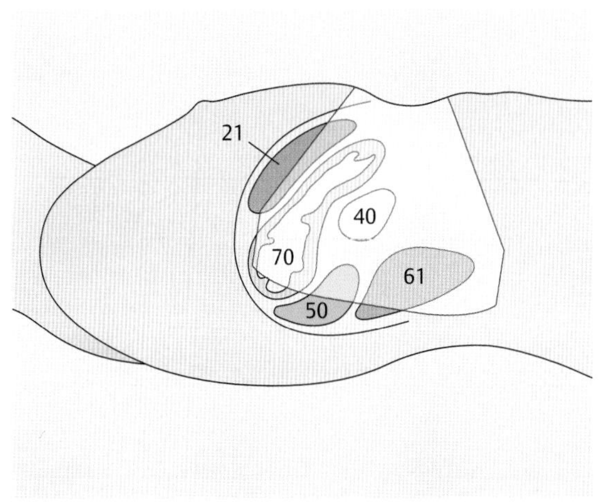
21
40
70
61
50

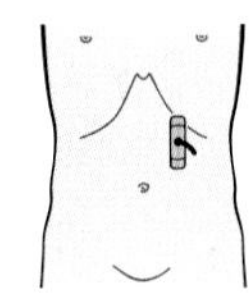

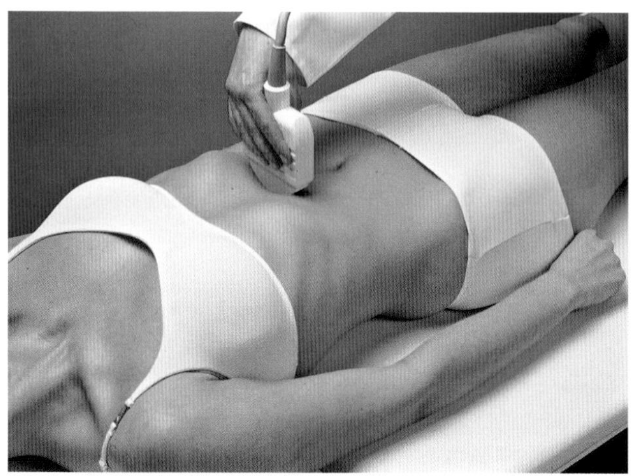

▶ **Upper abdominal transverse scan, center**

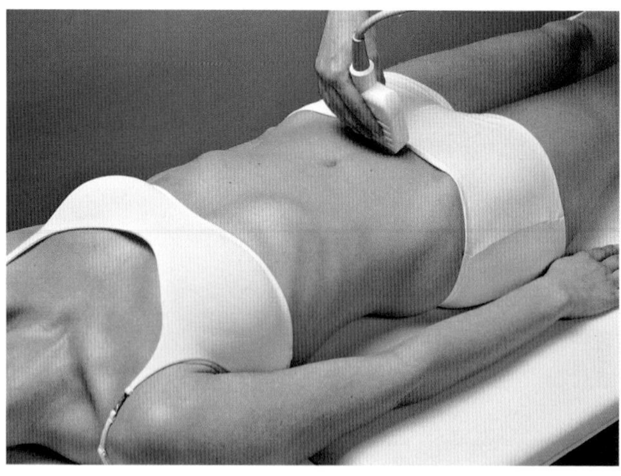

▶ **Lower abdominal transverse scan, center**

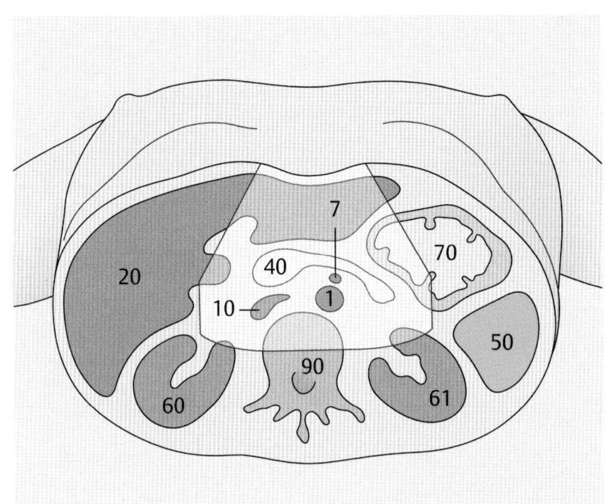
7
70
40
20
1
10
50
90
60
61

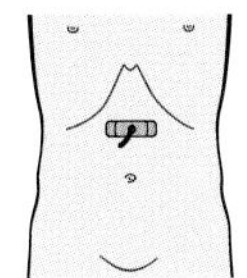

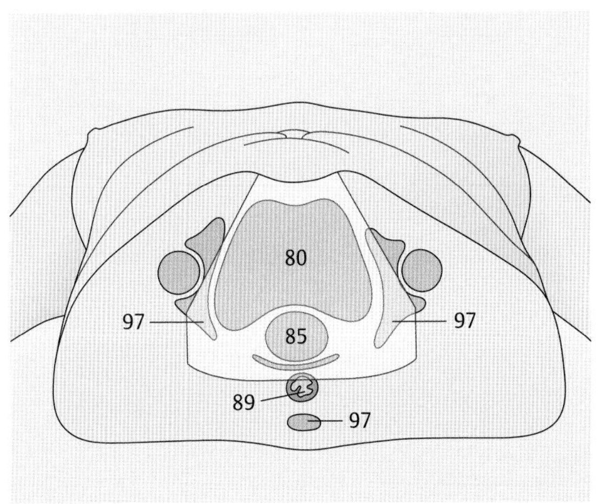
80
97
97
85
89
97

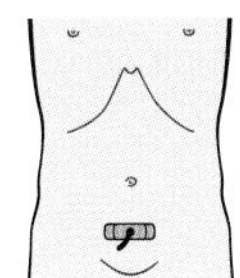

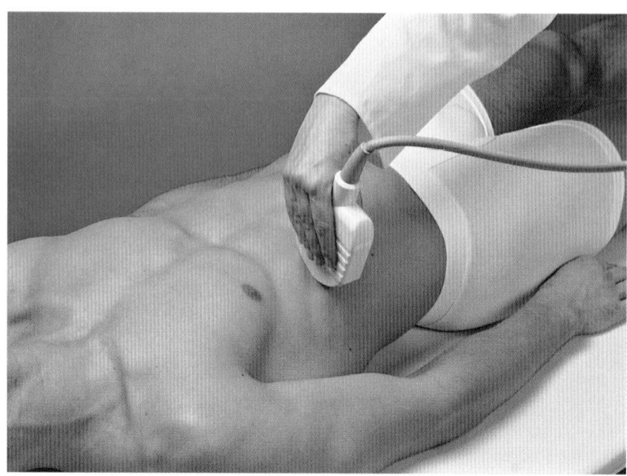

▶ **Upper abdominal transverse scan, right side**

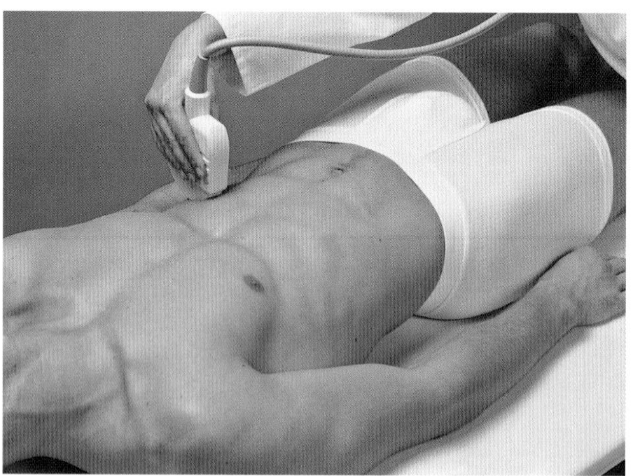

▶ **Upper abdominal transverse scan, left side**

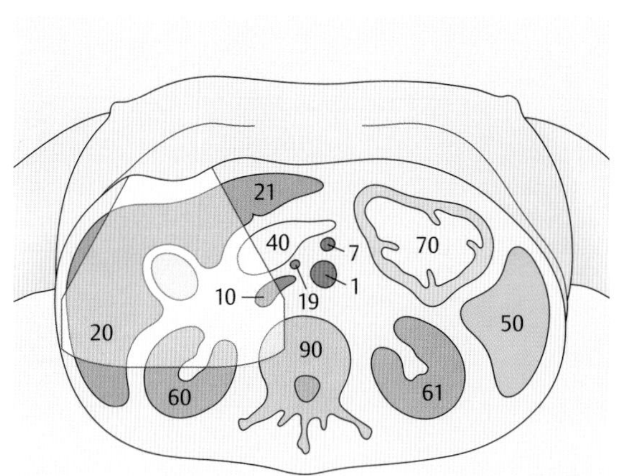
21
40
7
70
1
10
19
20
50
90
60
61

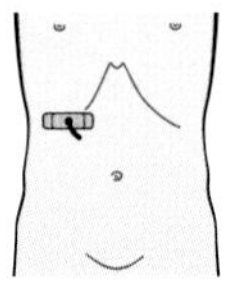

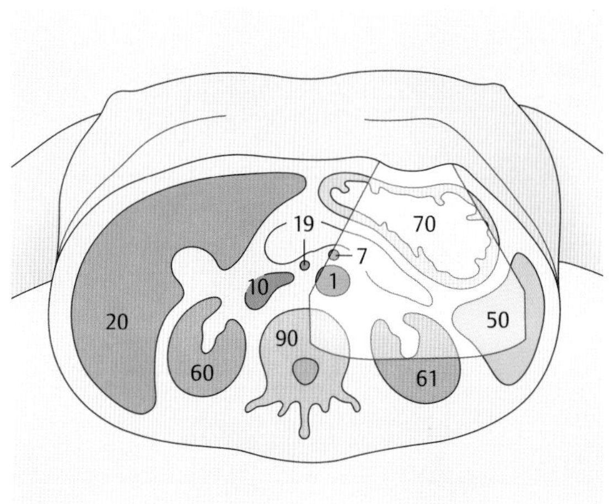
19
70
7
10
1
20
50
90
60
61

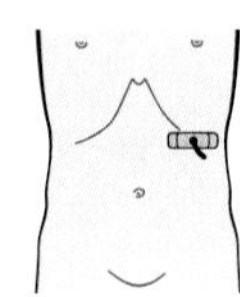

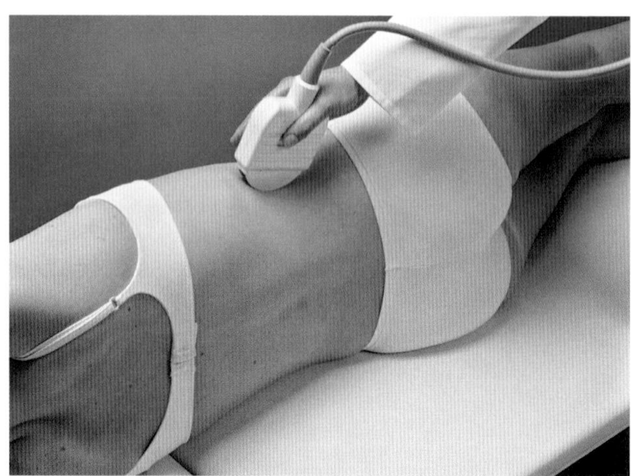

▶ **Longitudinal flank scan, right side**

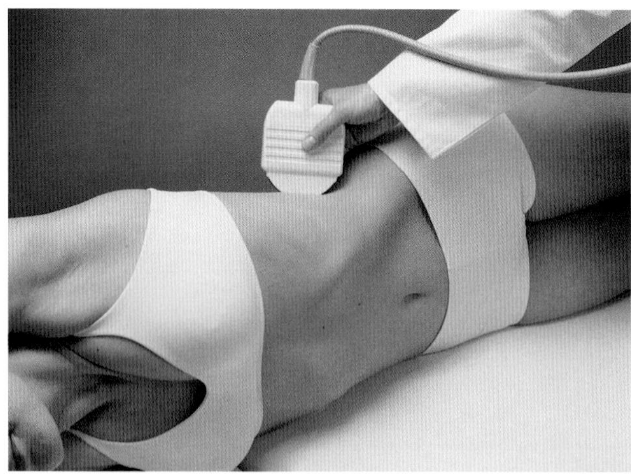

▶ **Longitudinal flank scan, left side**

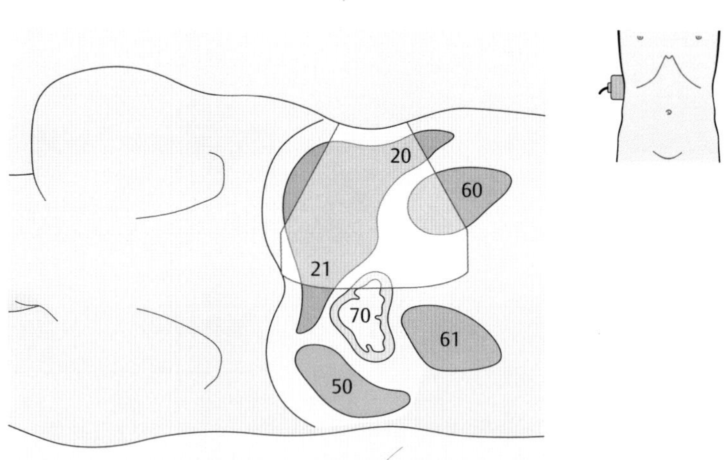
20
60
21
70
61
50

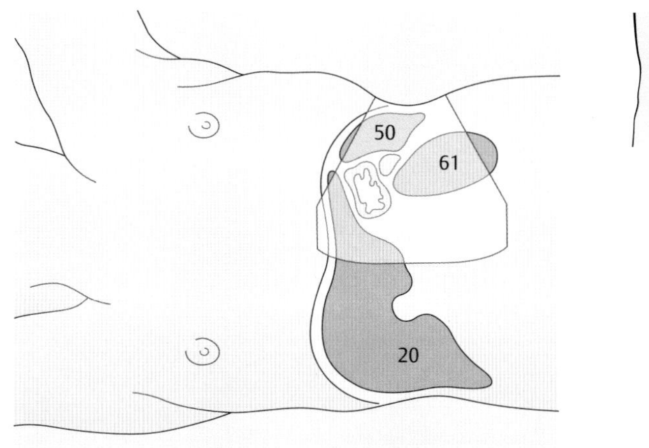
50
61
20

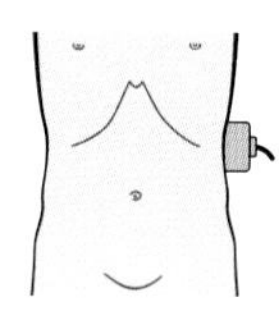

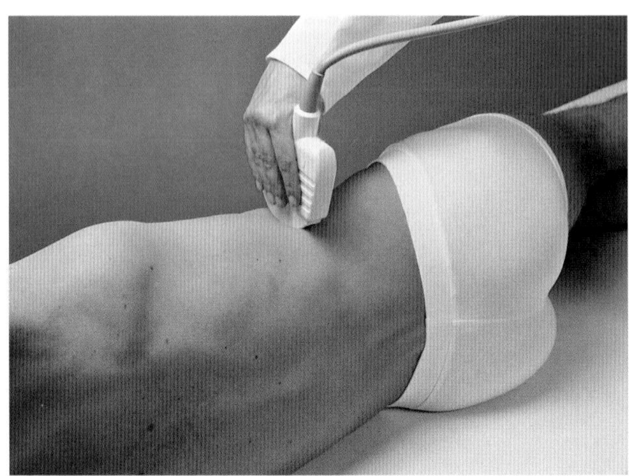

▶ **Transverse flank scan, right side**

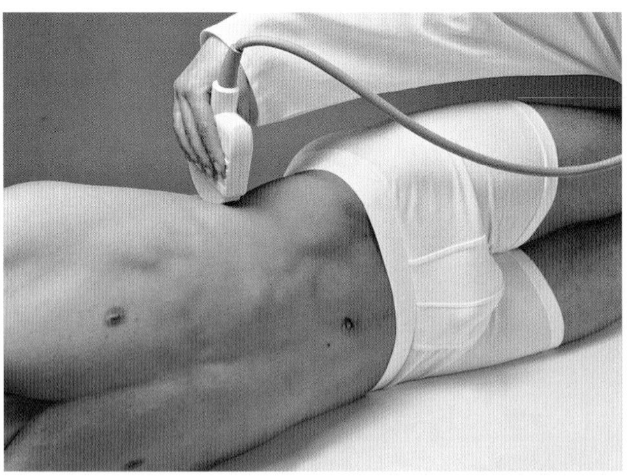

▶ **Transverse flank scan, left side**

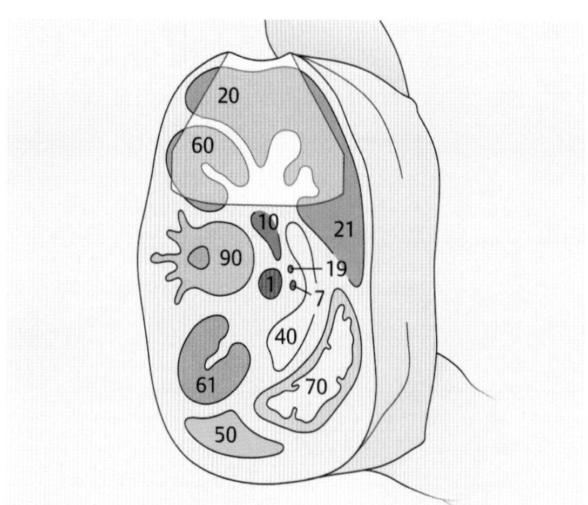
20
60
10
21
90
19
1
7
40
61
70
50

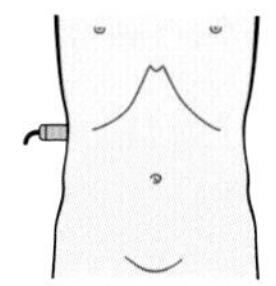

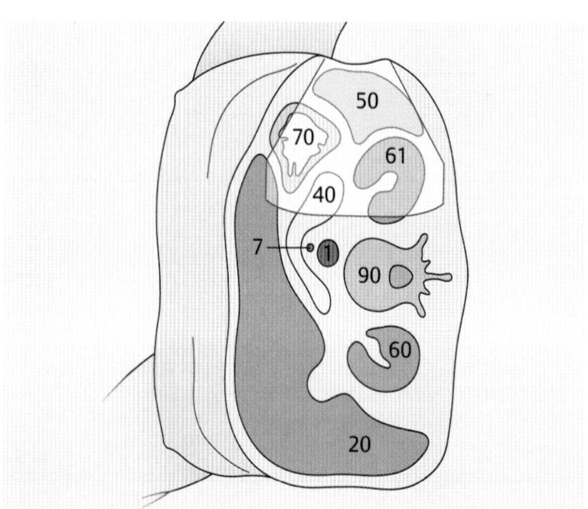
50
70
61
40
7
1
90
60
20

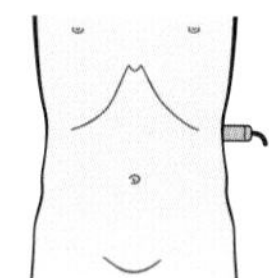

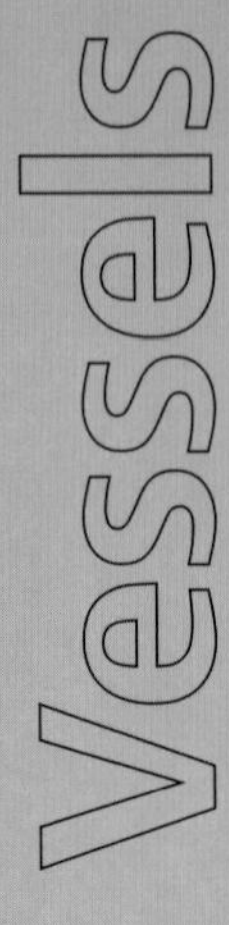
1 Vessels

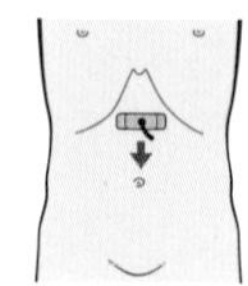

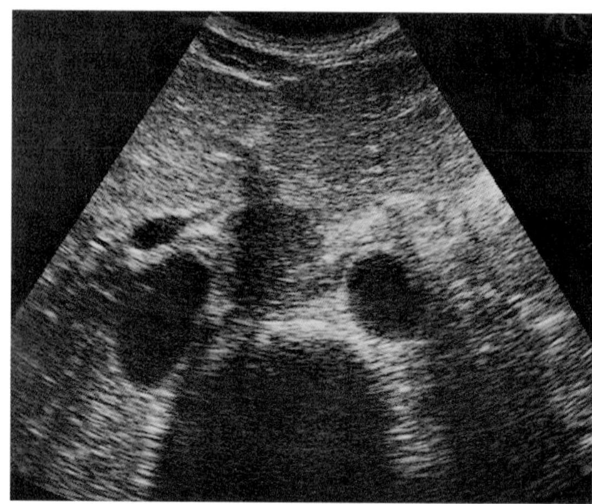

▶ **1** Passage of aorta and vena cava through diaphragm

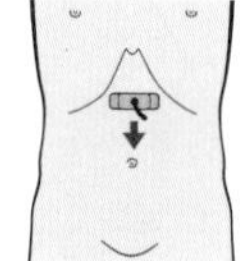

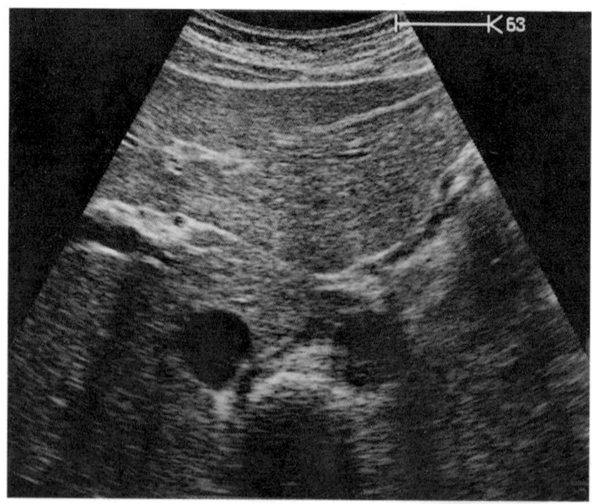

▶ **2** Left gastric artery

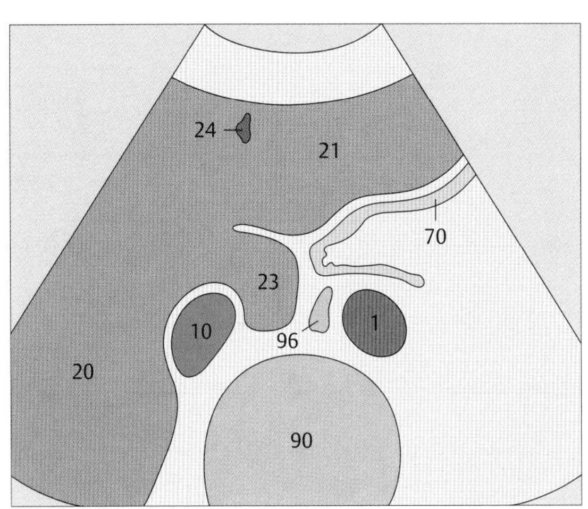

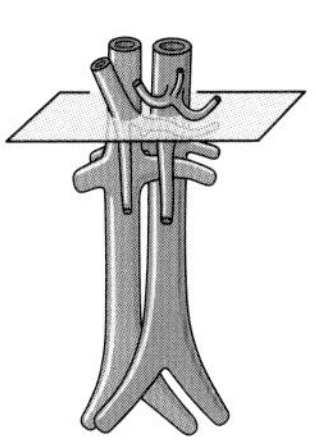

Just below the diaphragm, the vena cava is surrounded by liver tissue. The aorta lies directly behind the gastroesophageal junction, often making the vessel more difficult to scan.

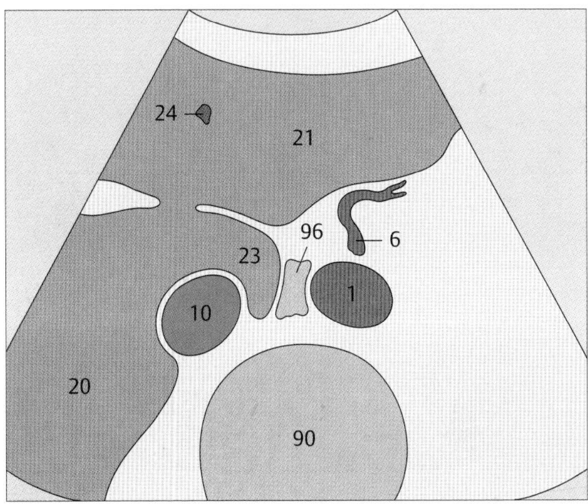

The left gastric artery is identified as a small-caliber vessel cranial to the celiac trunk.

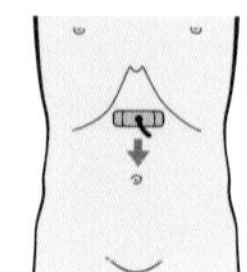

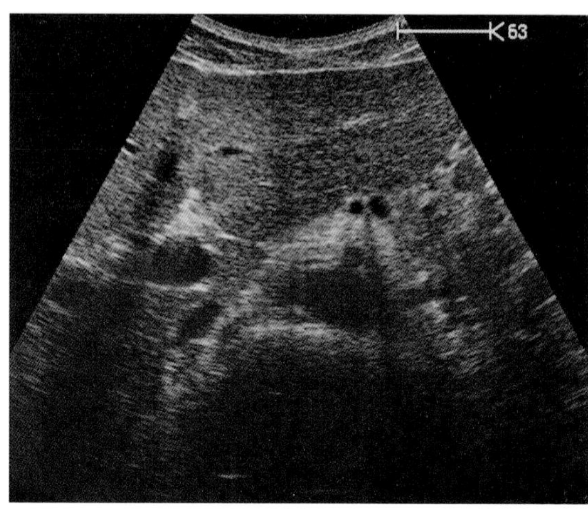

▶ **3** Celiac trunk

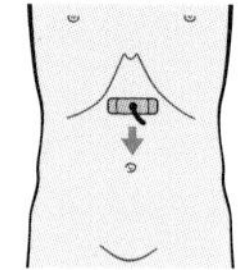

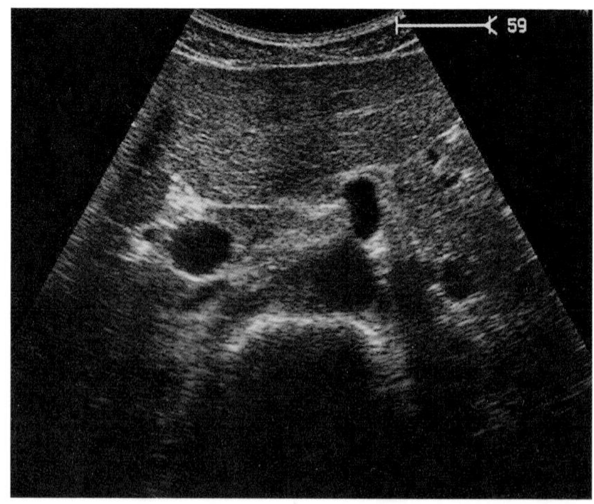

▶ **4** Celiac trunk

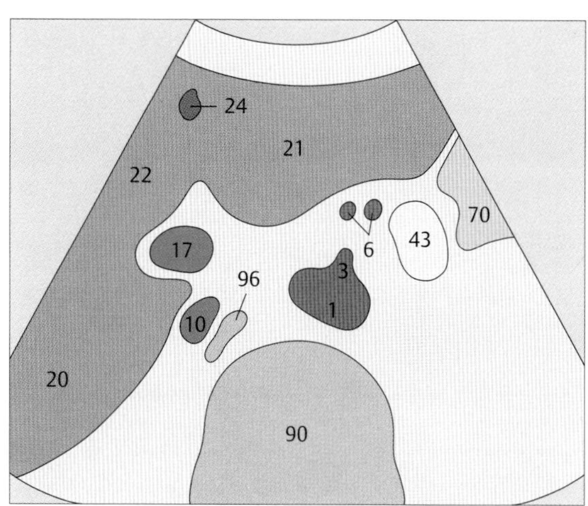

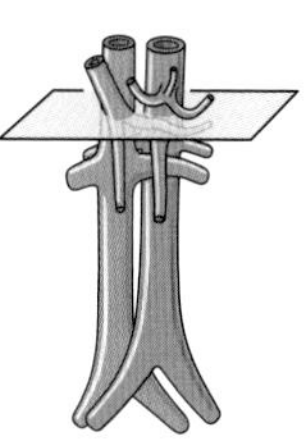

After arising from the aorta, the celiac trunk runs a short distance to the left.

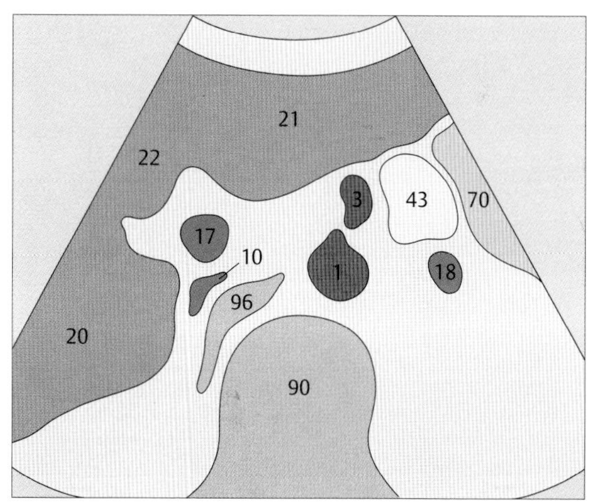

The proximal part of the celiac trunk also turns slightly downward in most cases.

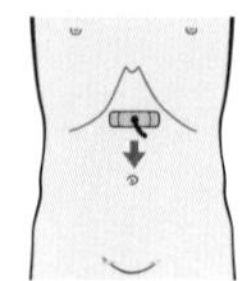

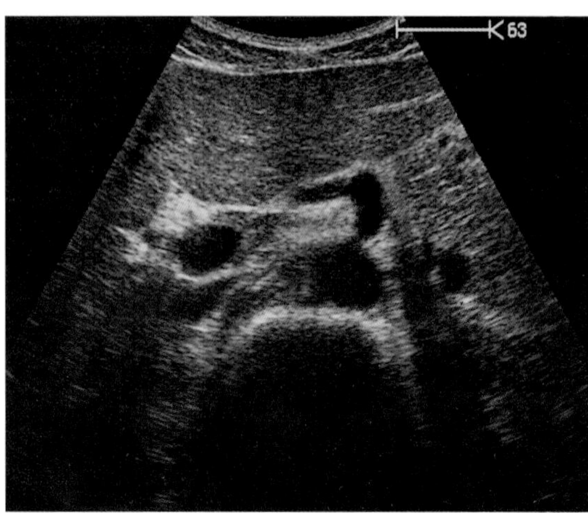

▶ **5** Hepatic artery

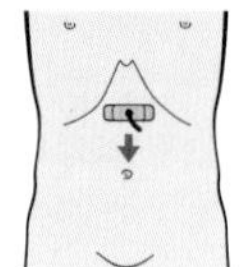

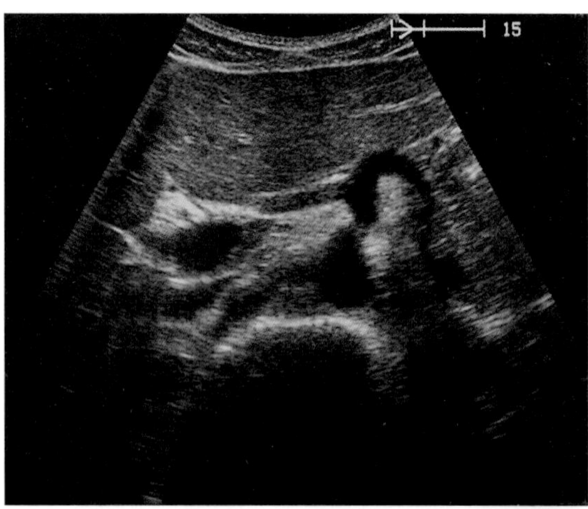

▶ **6** Splenic artery

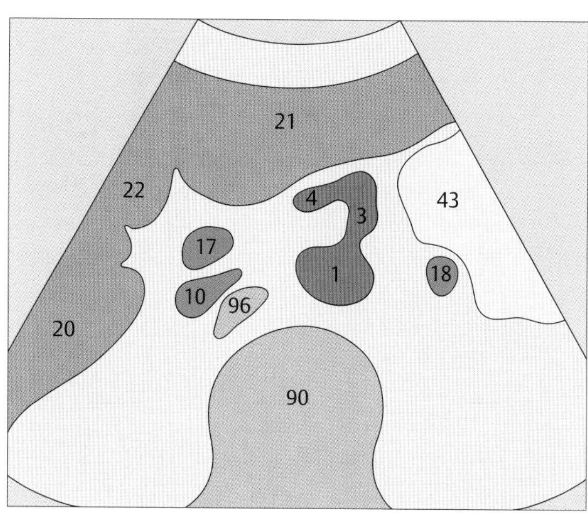

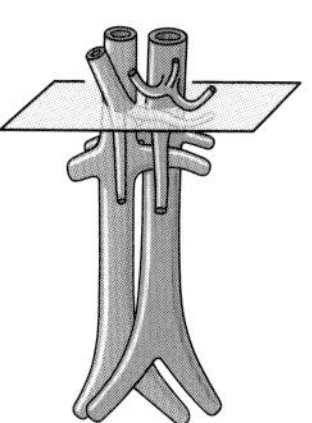

The celiac trunk runs slightly to the right, giving rise to the hepatic artery.

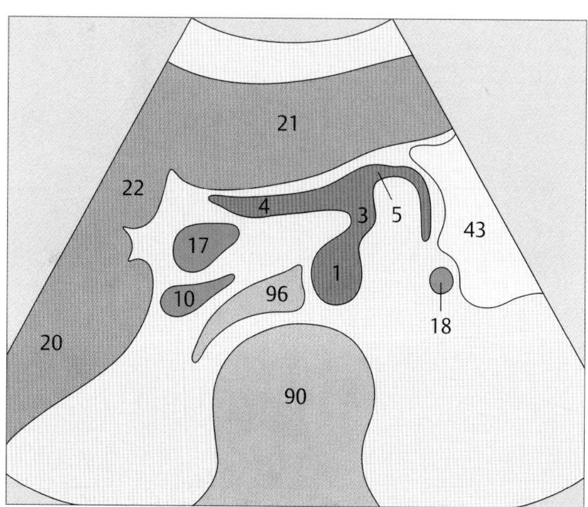

The splenic artery branches from the celiac trunk at a right angle.

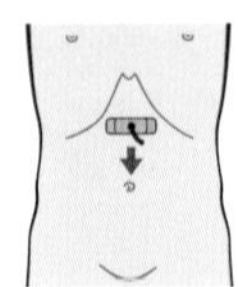

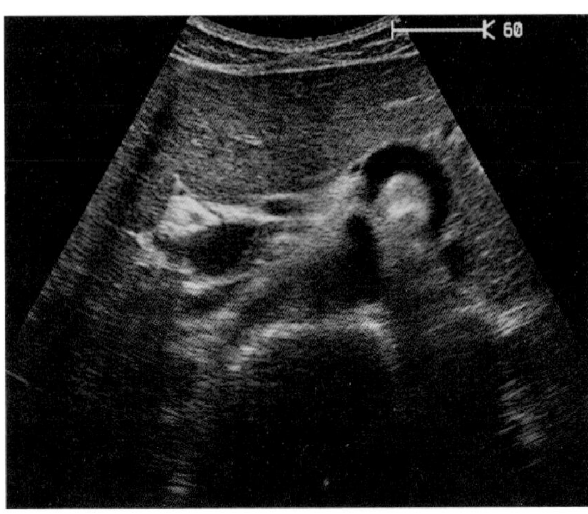

▶ **7** Superior mesenteric artery

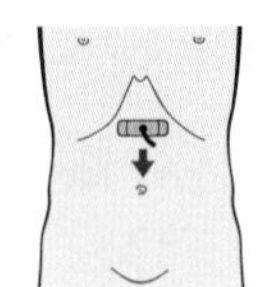

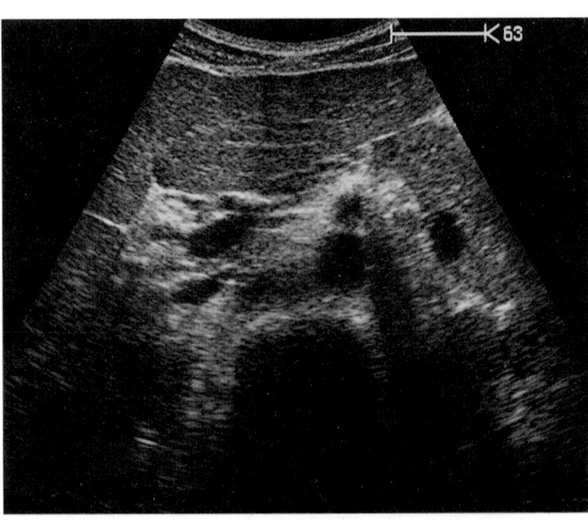

▶ **8** Superior mesenteric artery

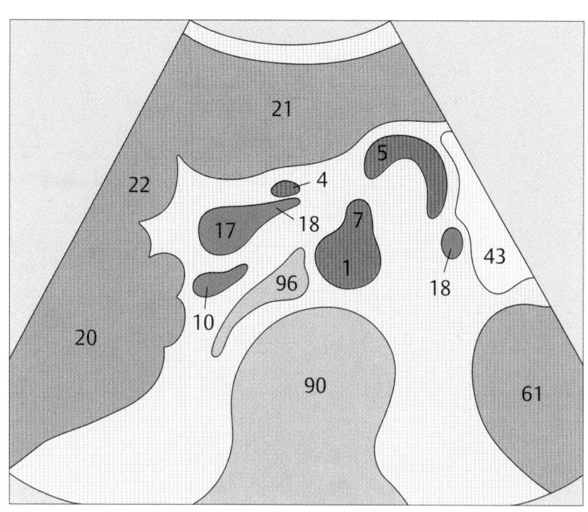

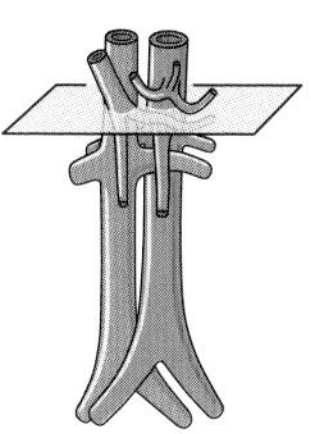

The superior mesenteric artery arises just below the celiac trunk and runs parallel to the aorta.

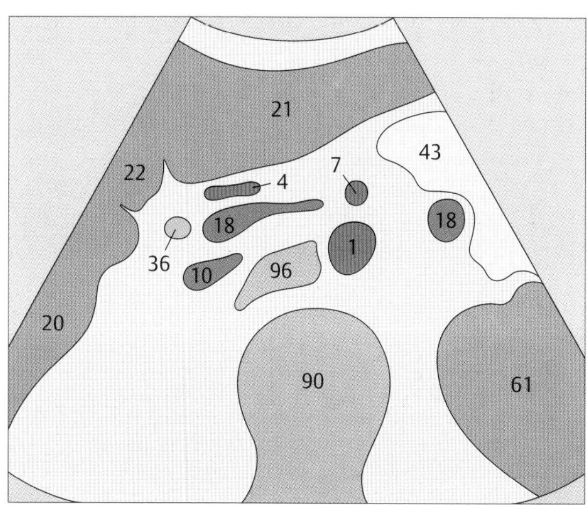

The root of the superior mesenteric artery is usually surrounded by an echodense fat pad.

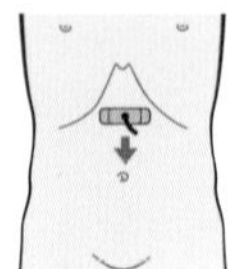

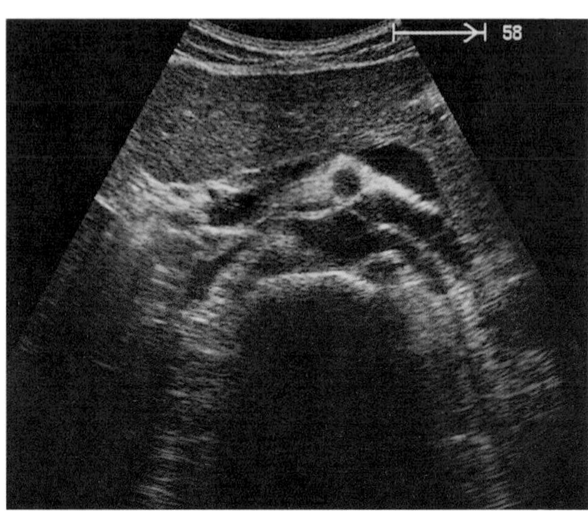

▶ **9** Superior mesenteric artery and splenic vein

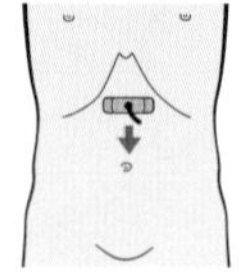

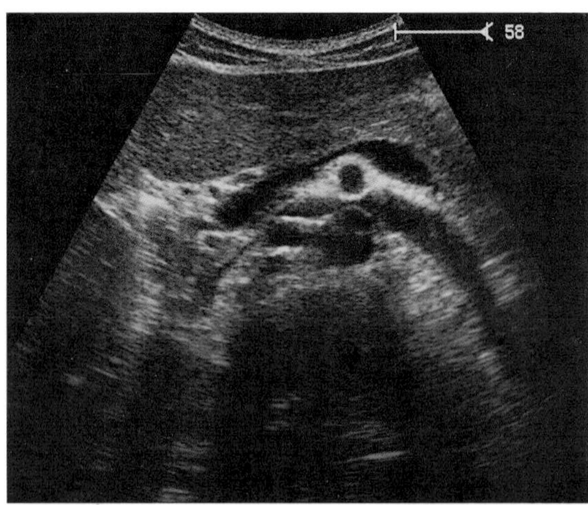

▶ **10** Left renal vein and right renal artery

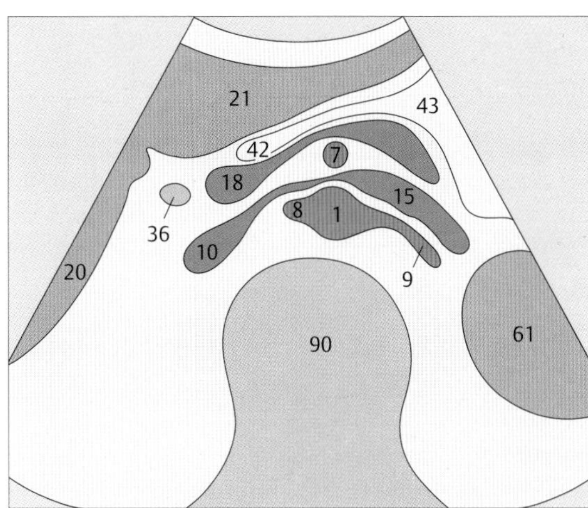

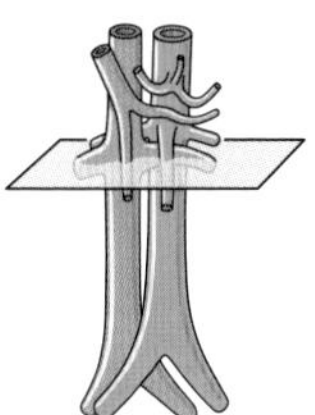

The aorta, the superior mesenteric artery, and the splenic vein crossing over the superior mesenteric artery provide landmarks for identifying the head of the pancreas.

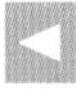

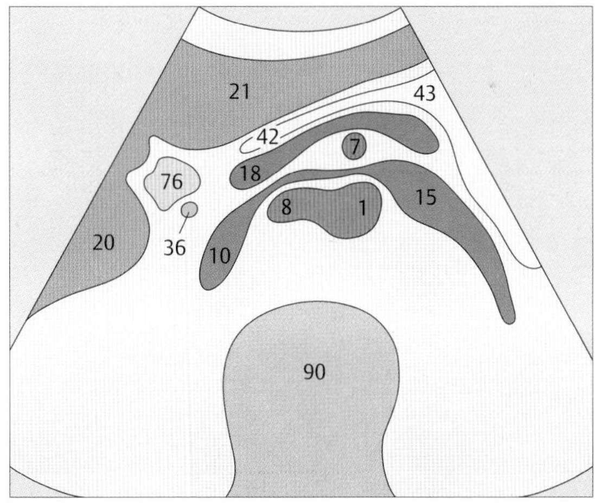

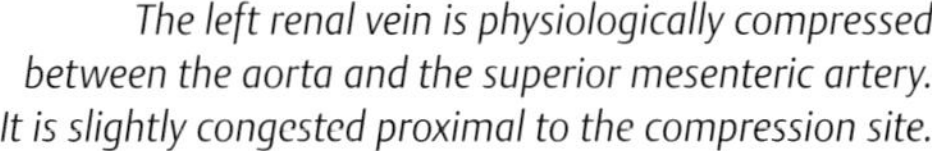

The left renal vein is physiologically compressed between the aorta and the superior mesenteric artery. It is slightly congested proximal to the compression site.

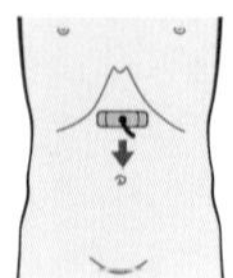

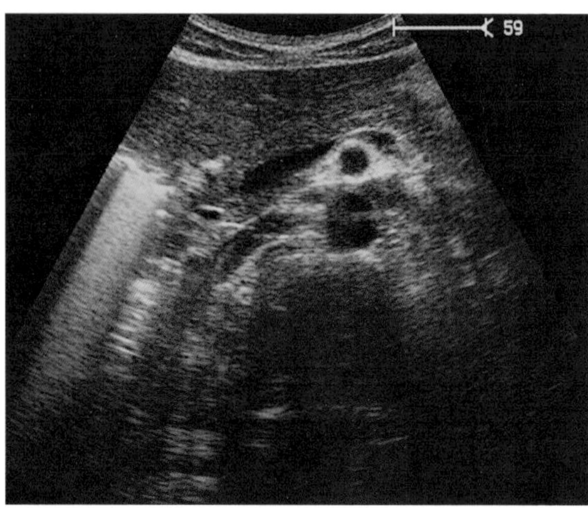

▶ **11** Infrarenal aorta and vena cava

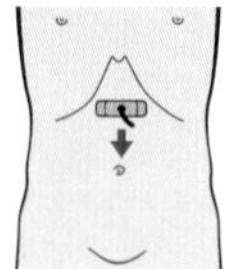

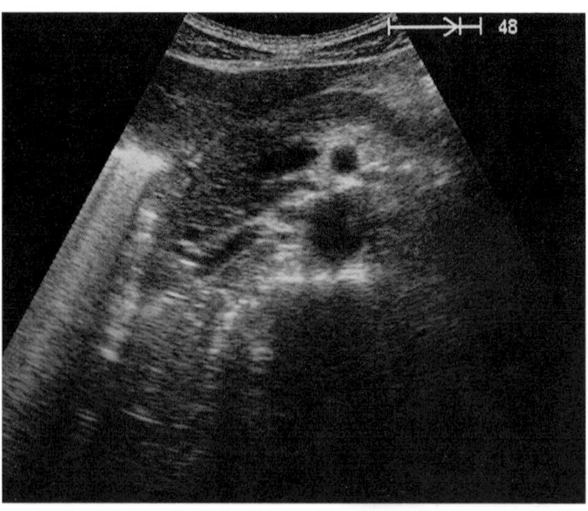

▶ **12** Infrarenal aorta and vena cava

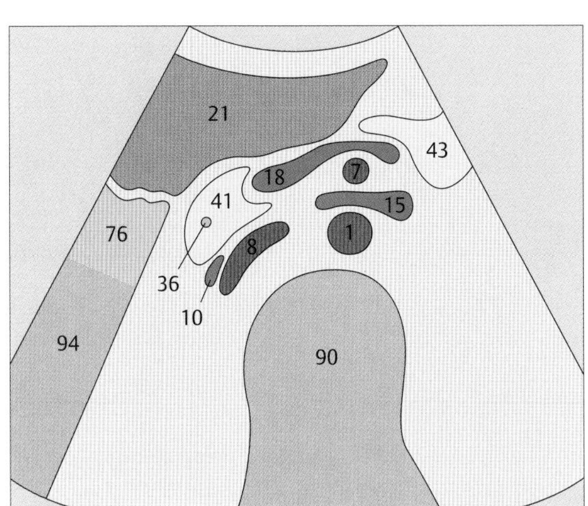

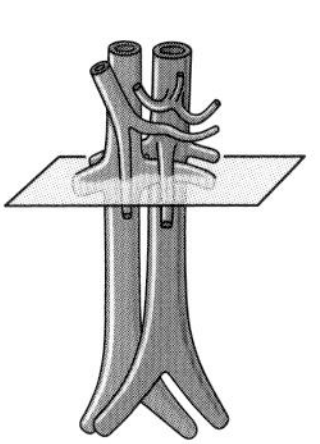

The vena cava is easily compressible with the transducer, and it bears impressions from adjacent organs.

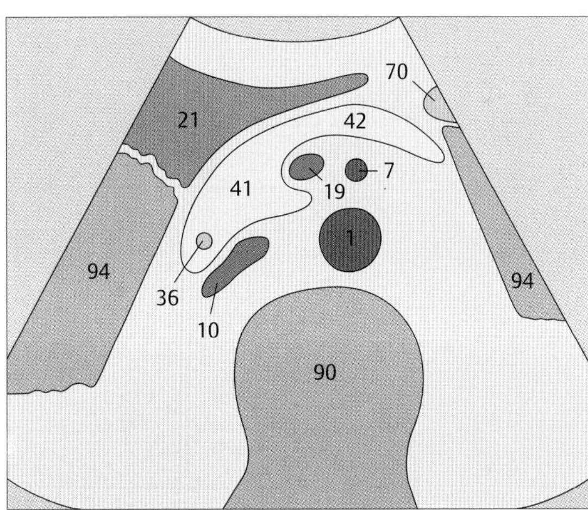

The aorta has a circular cross section, whereas the vena cava is somewhat flattened.

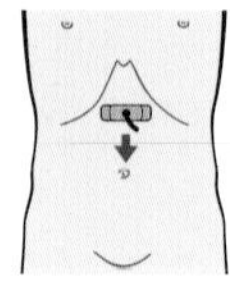

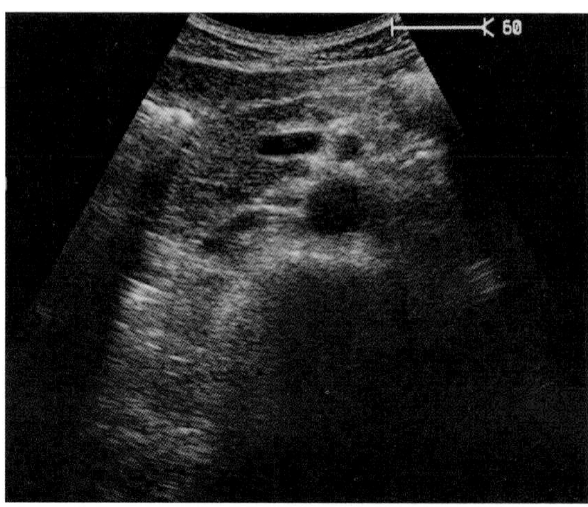

▶ **13** Infrarenal aorta and vena cava

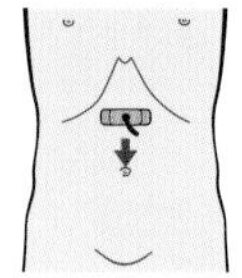

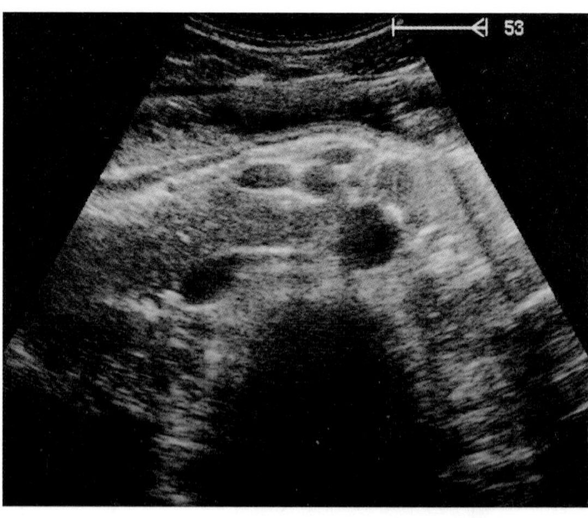

▶ **14** Infrarenal aorta, vena cava, and superior mesenteric artery and vein

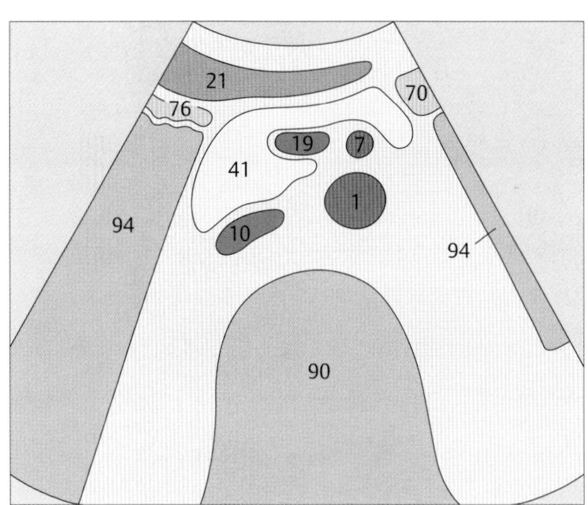

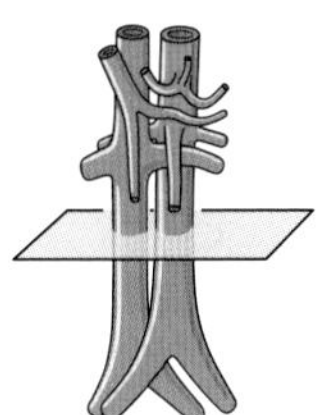

The caliber of the vena cava varies with the pulse and respirations. The diameter of the aorta measures 2.5 cm in its cranial portion, 2.0 cm in its caudal portion.

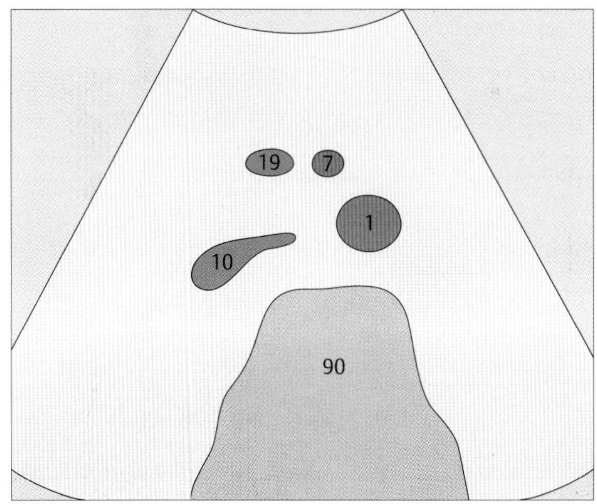

Together with the aorta and vena cava, the superior mesenteric artery and vein form a typical four-vessel pattern in a low transverse scan through the upper abdomen.

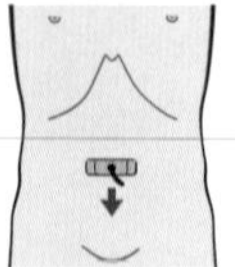

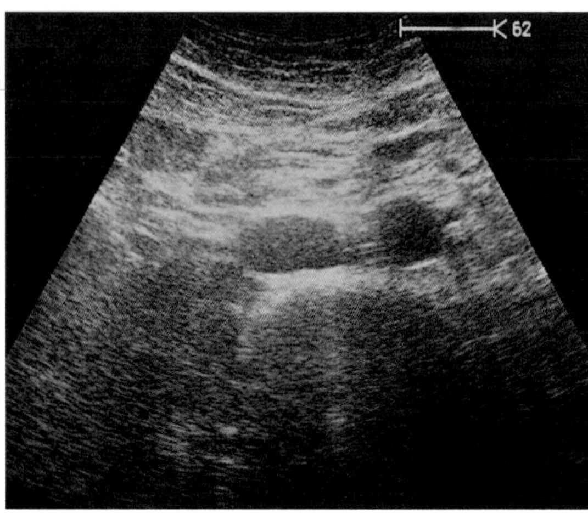

▶ **15** Infrarenal aorta and vena cava

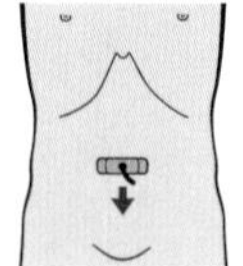

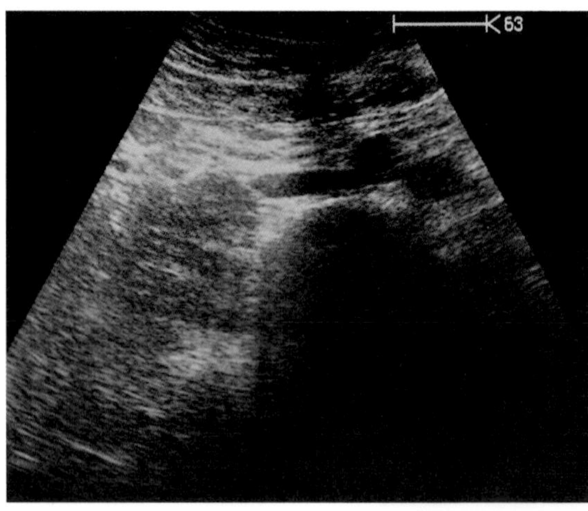

▶ **16** Aortic bifurcation

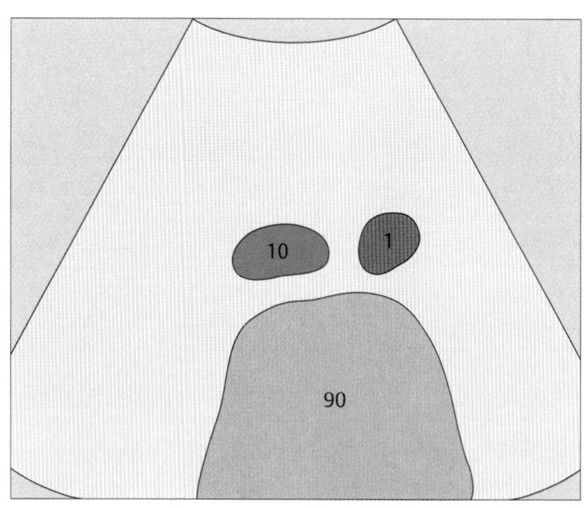

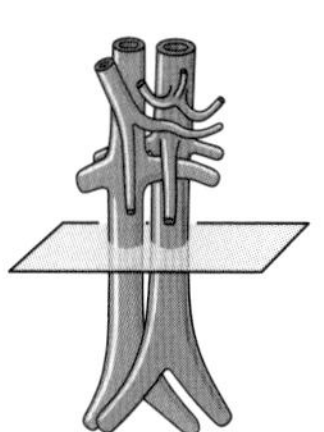

While the aorta and vena cava are relatively far apart in the upper abdomen, they converge at the level of the promontory, coming very close together.

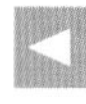

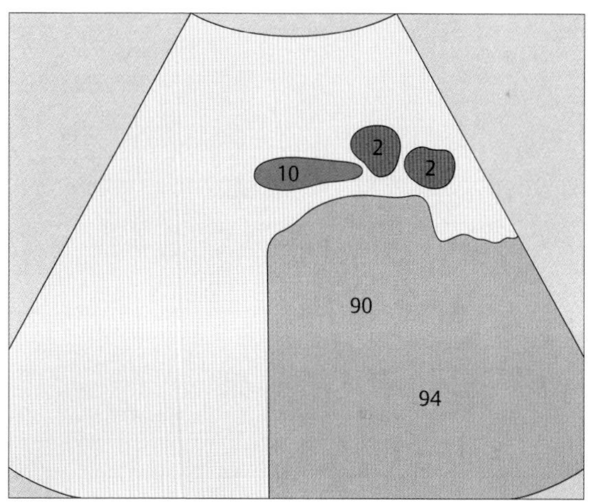

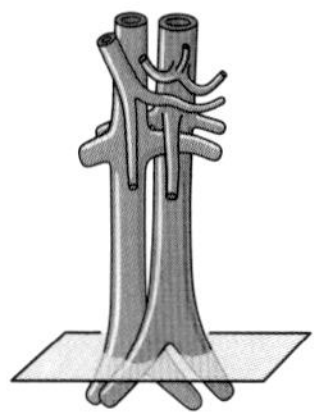

The aorta divides into the common iliac arteries at the level of the L4 vertebral body, above the promontory.

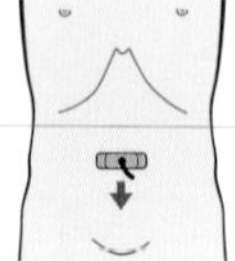

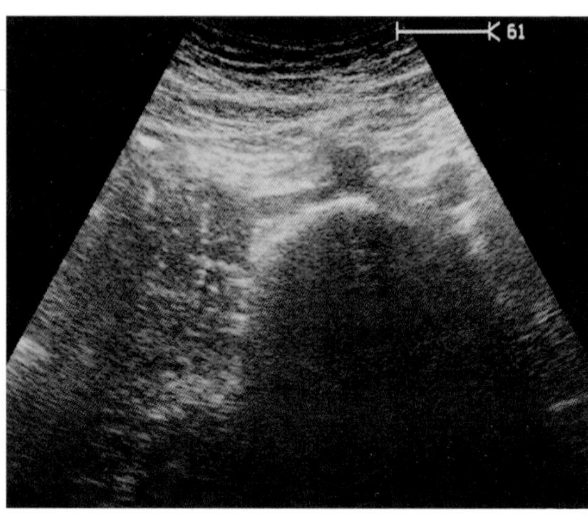

▶ **17** Iliac arteries

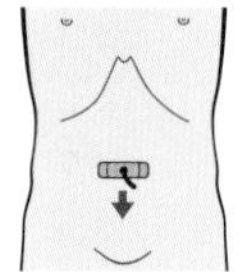

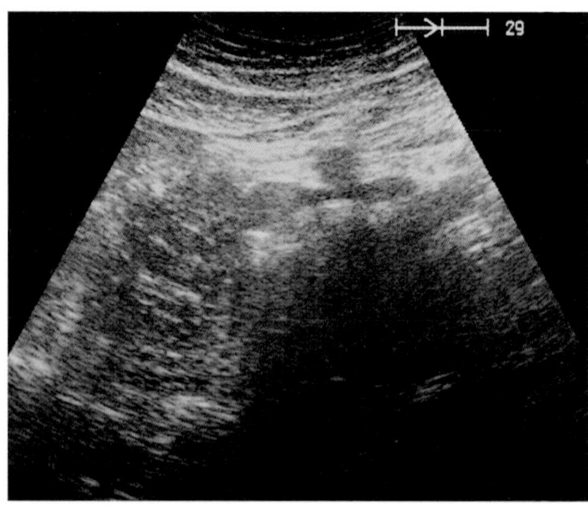

▶ **18** Confluence of iliac veins

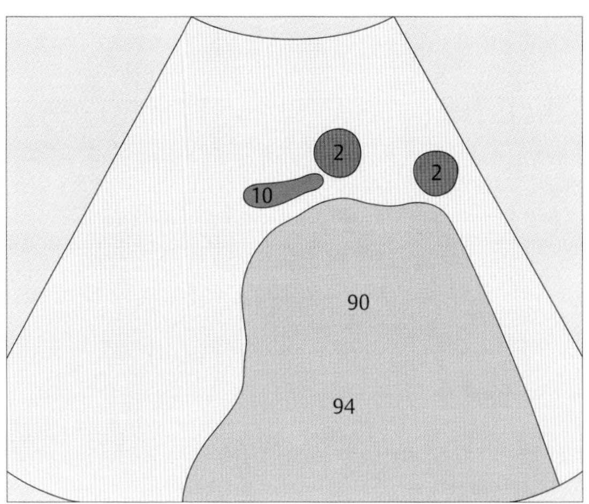

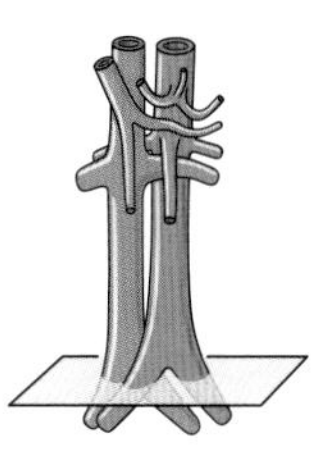

The aortic bifurcation is located slightly above the confluence of the iliac veins.

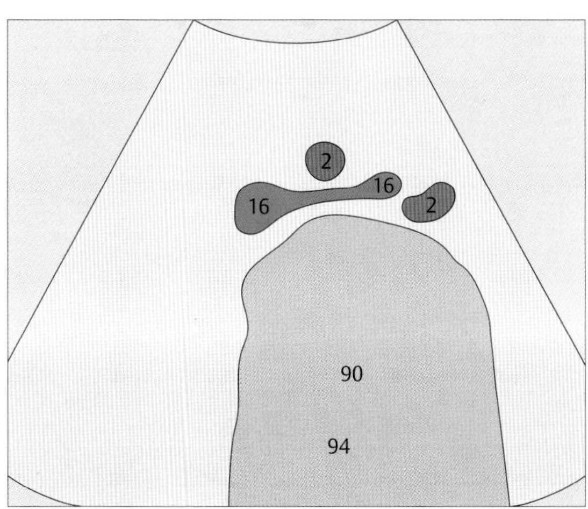

The confluence of the iliac veins lies approximately at the level of the umbilicus.

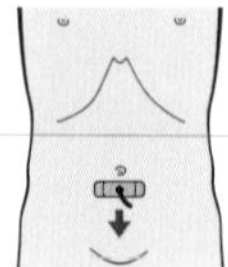

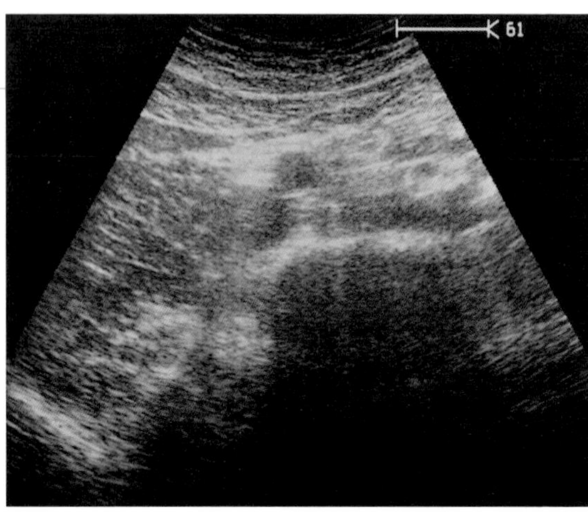

▶ **19** Iliac vessels

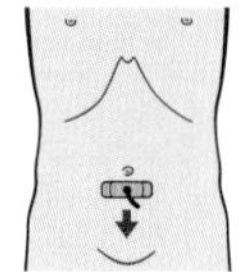

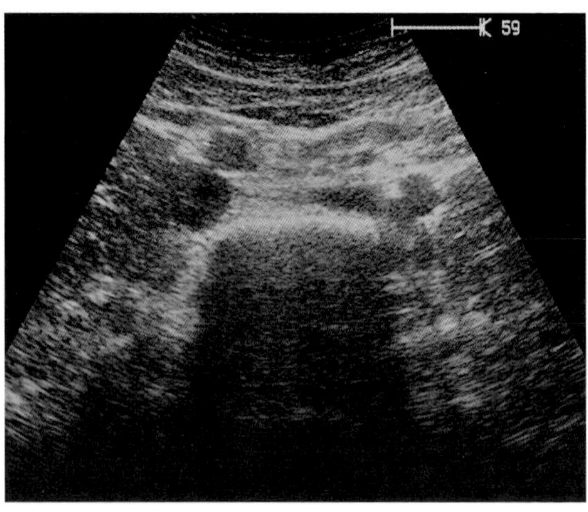

▶ **20** Iliac vessels

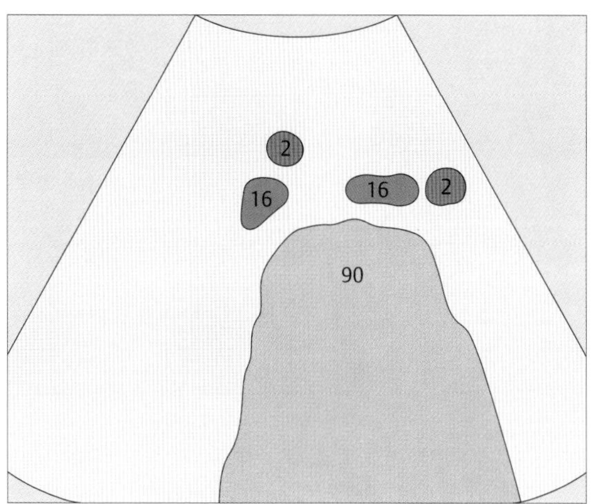

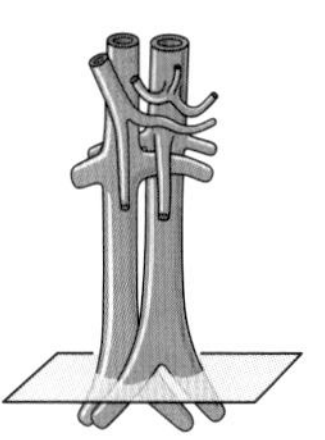

The iliac arteries are first anterior and then lateral to the iliac veins.

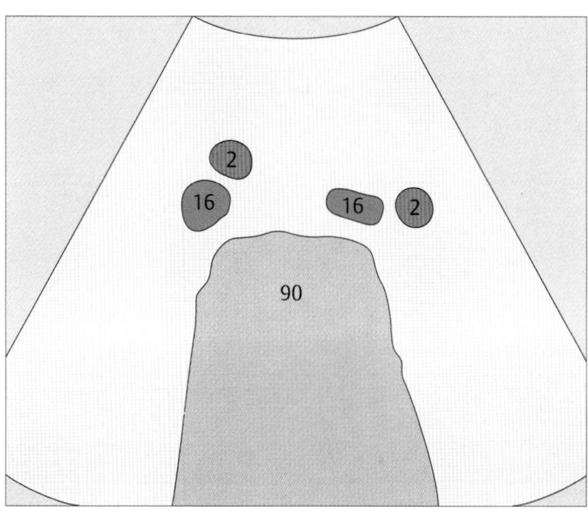

The iliac vessels follow the concavity of the lesser pelvis to the femoral arteries.

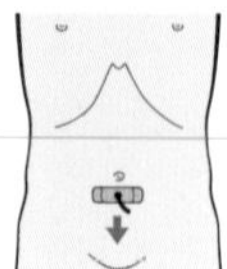

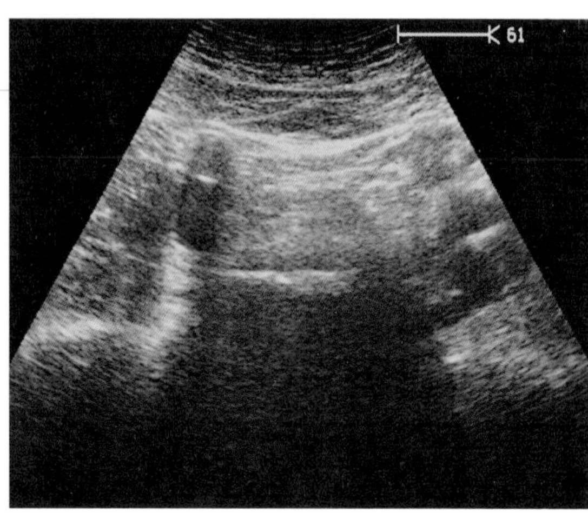

▶ **21** Iliac vessels

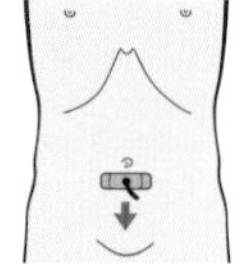

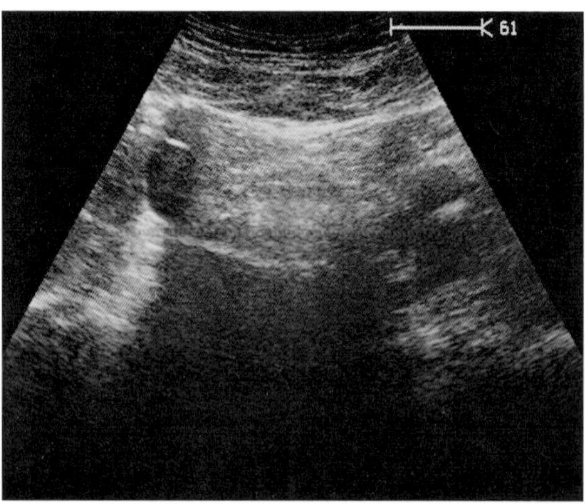

▶ **22** Iliac vessels

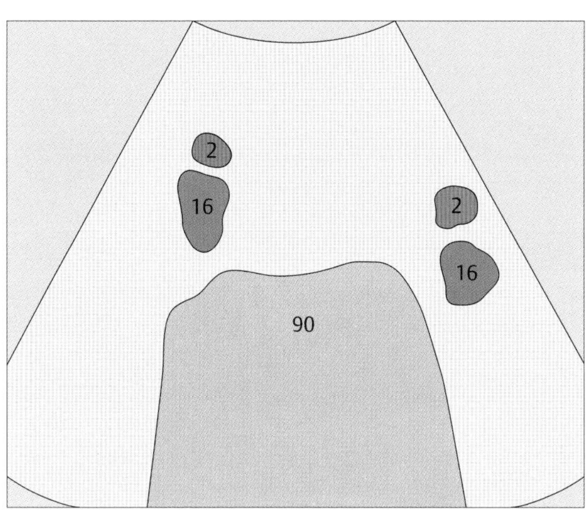

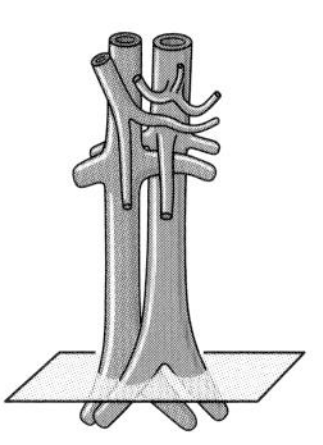

In serial transverse scans down the iliac vessels, the sections of the vessels are seen to move laterally and posteriorly.

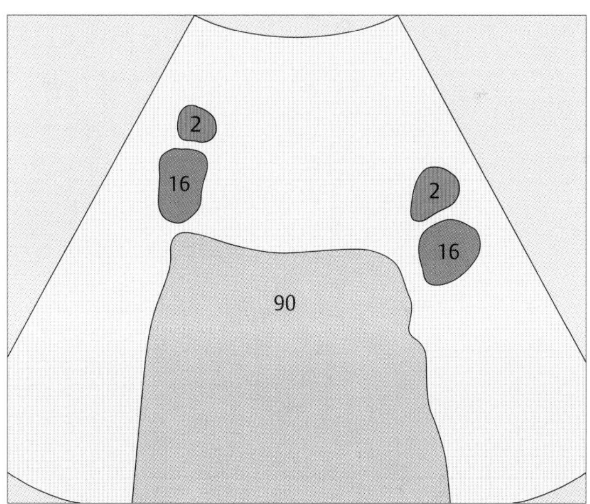

The iliac vessels are more difficult to scan at lower levels due to intervening bowel gas.

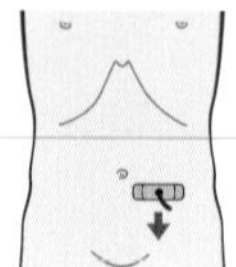

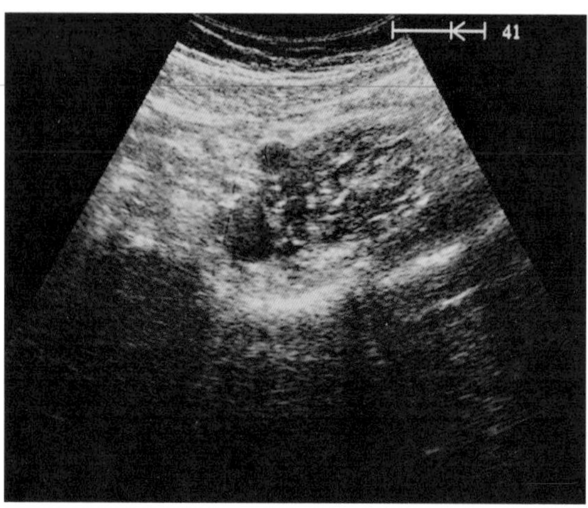

▶ **23** Left iliac vessels

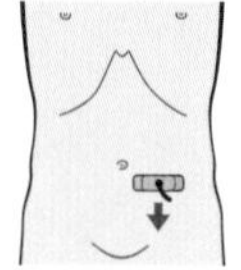

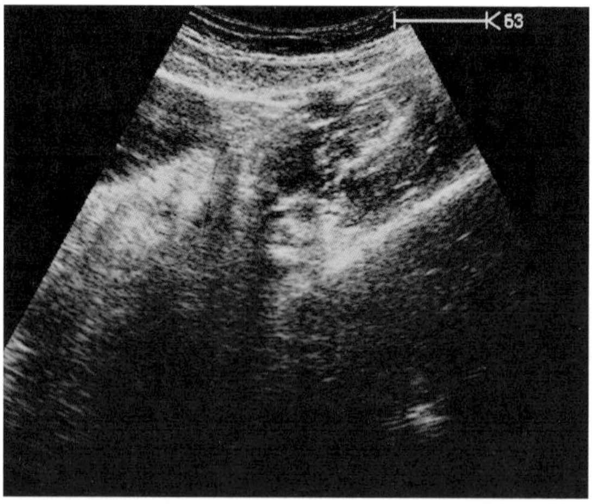

▶ **24** Left iliac vessels

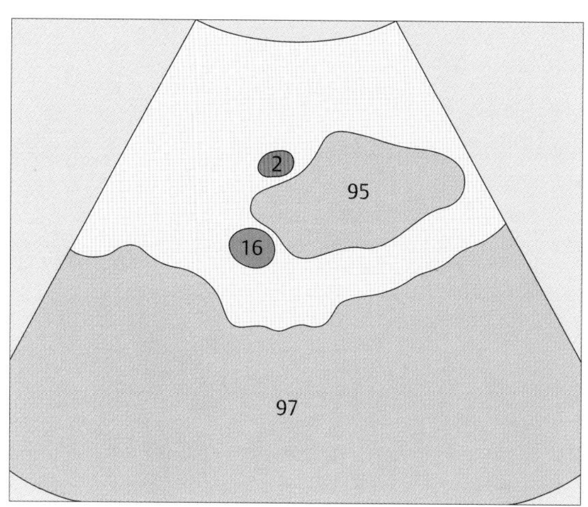

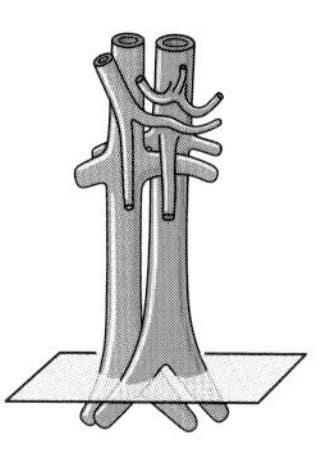

The iliac veins run dorsomedial to the iliac arteries in the lesser pelvis.

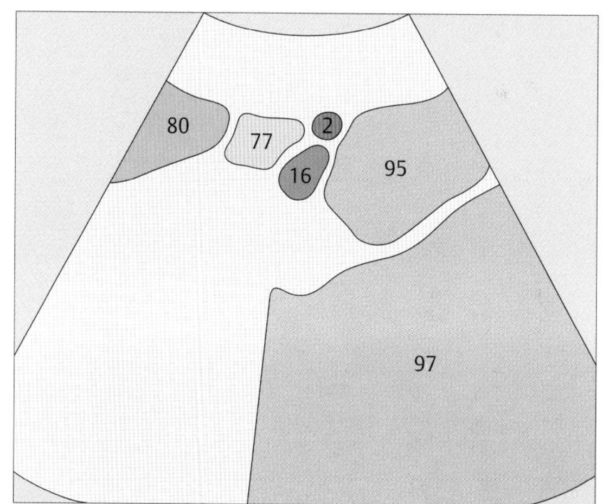

The iliac veins are always medial to the arteries at the level of the inguinal ligament.

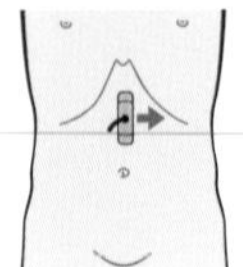

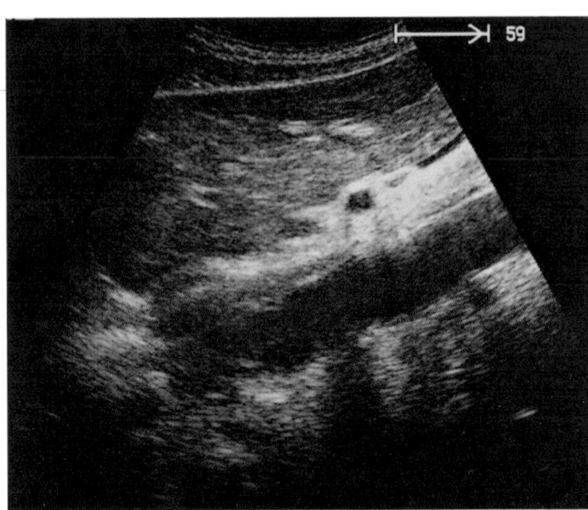

▶ **25** Aorta

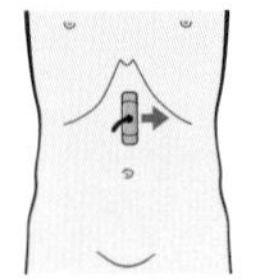

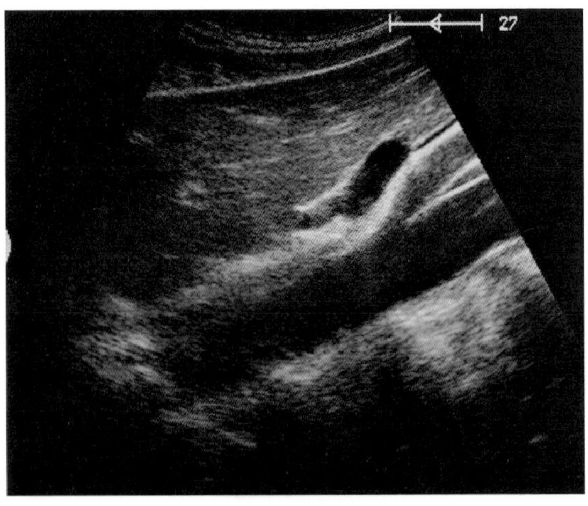

▶ **26** Splenic artery and left gastric artery

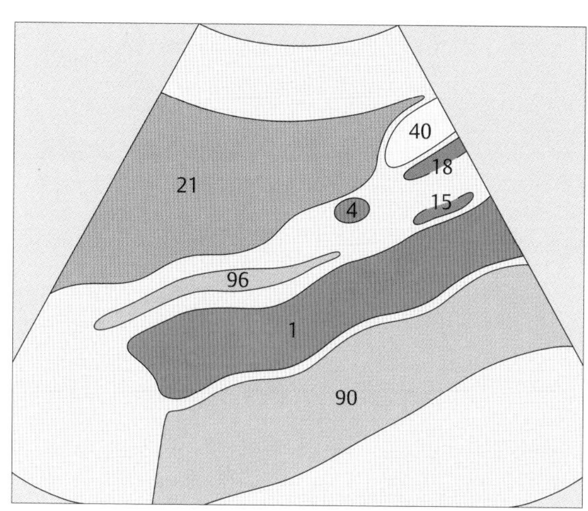

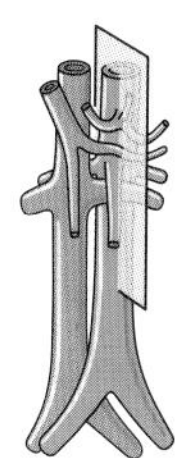

Because the celiac trunk runs slightly to the left initially, often it is not displayed in a longitudinal scan centered over the aorta.

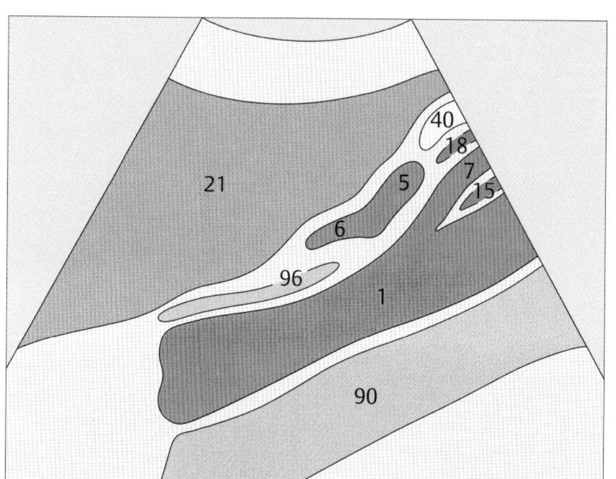

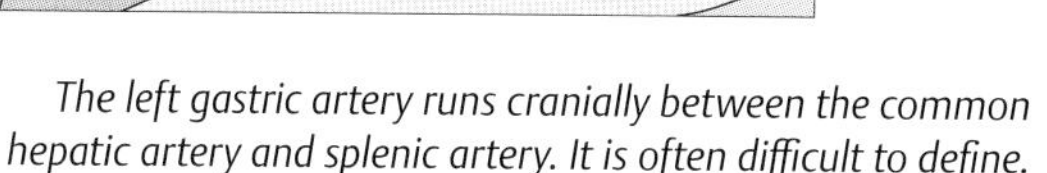

The left gastric artery runs cranially between the common hepatic artery and splenic artery. It is often difficult to define.

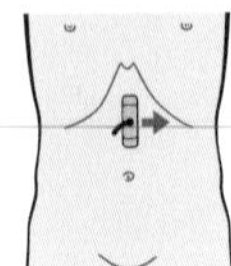

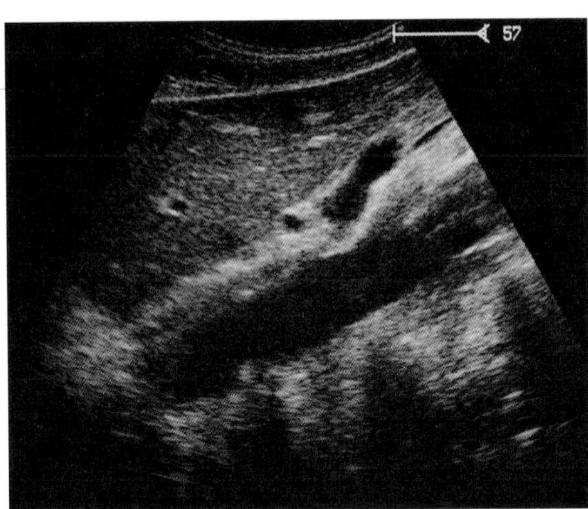

▶ **27** Splenic artery and vein, celiac trunk

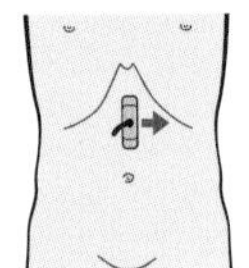

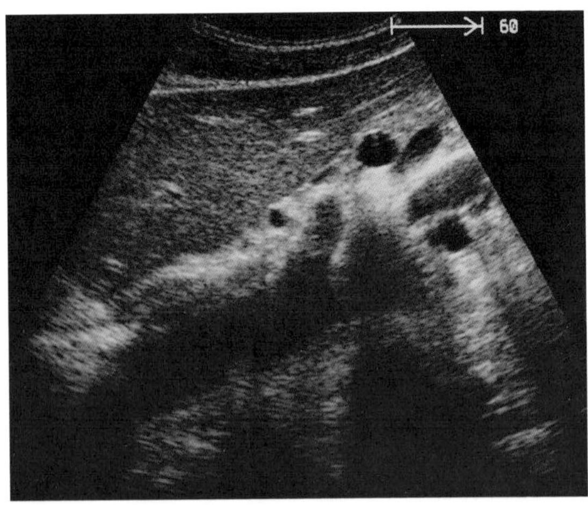

▶ **28** Splenic artery and vein, celiac trunk

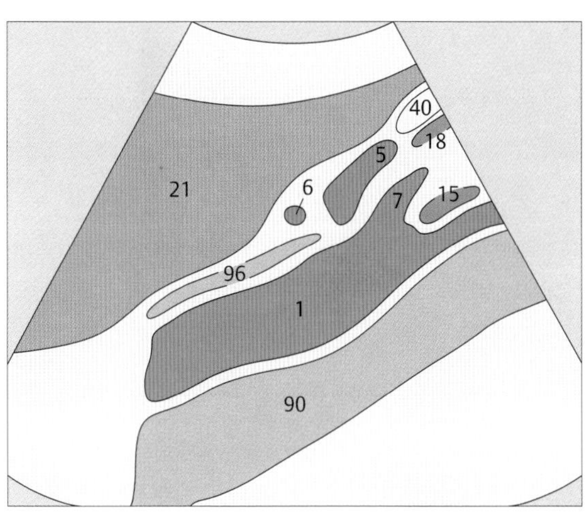

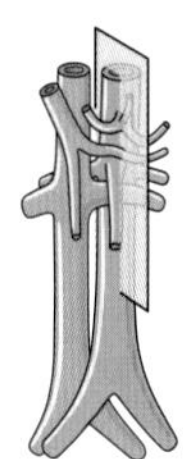

The celiac trunk divides into the left gastric artery, common hepatic artery, and splenic artery.

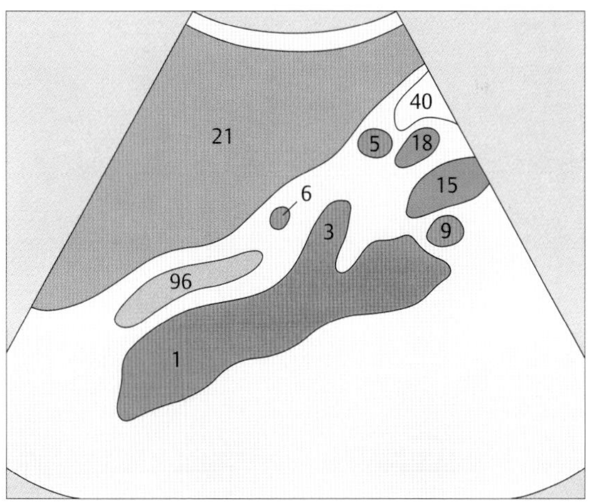

The curved course of the celiac trunk and splenic artery explains why both vessels appear in the same sagittal section.

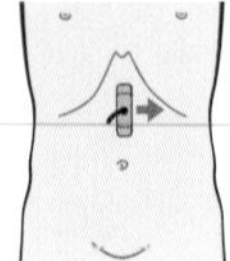

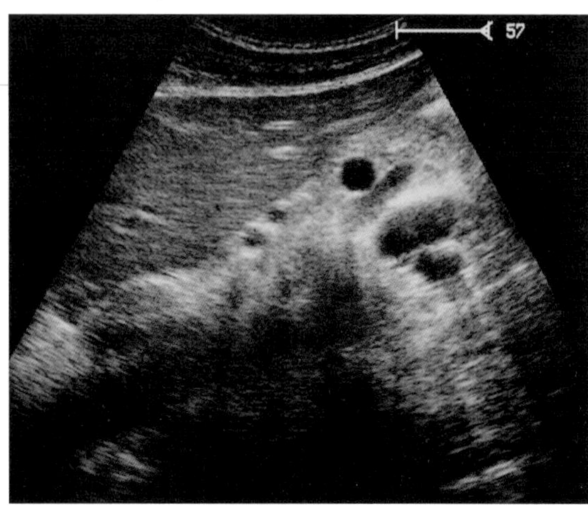

▶ **29** Splenic artery and vein, renal artery and vein

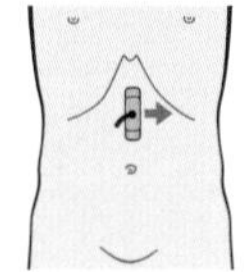

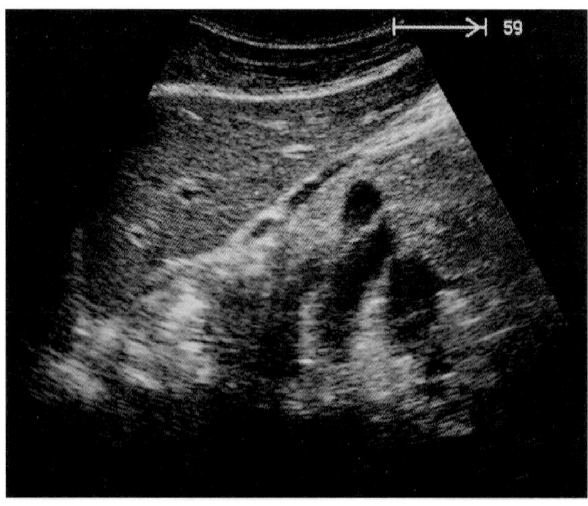

▶ **30** Splenic artery and vein, renal artery and vein

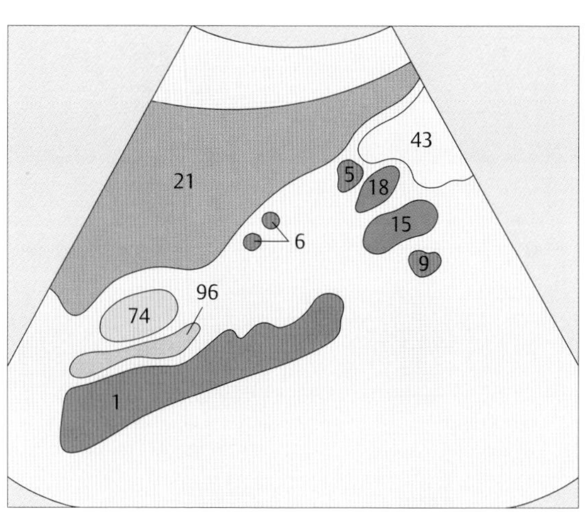

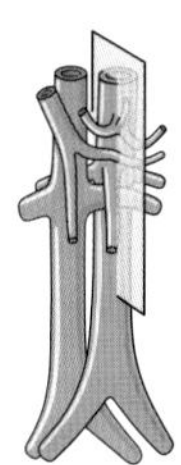

The splenic artery turns left and runs posteriorly with the splenic vein to the hilum of the spleen.

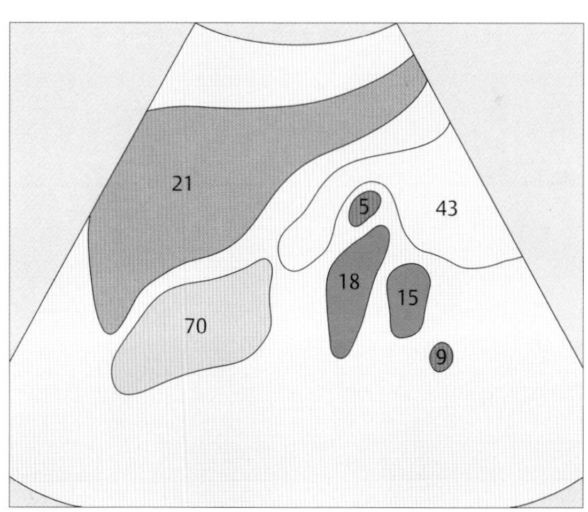

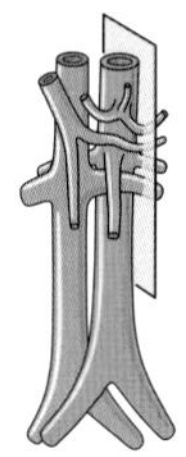

Longitudinal scan on the left side shows the typical appearance of the large splenic and renal veins and the smaller splenic and renal arteries.

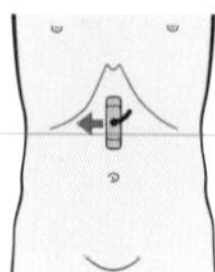

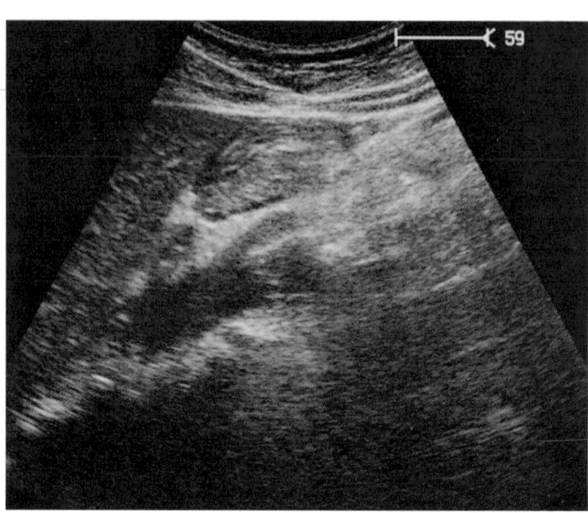

▶ **31** Celiac trunk

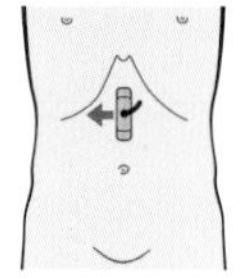

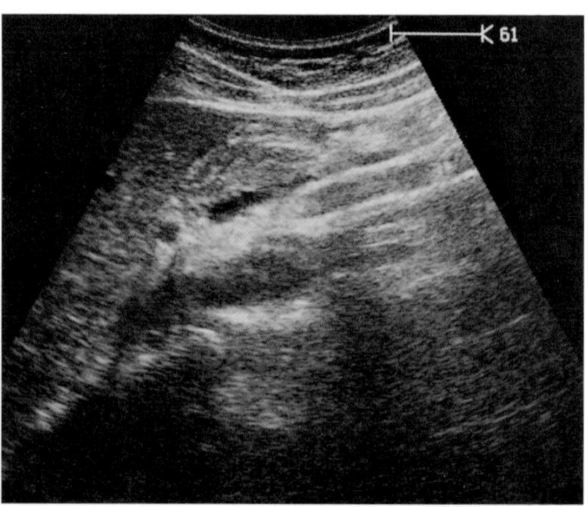

▶ **32** Hepatic artery and splenic vein

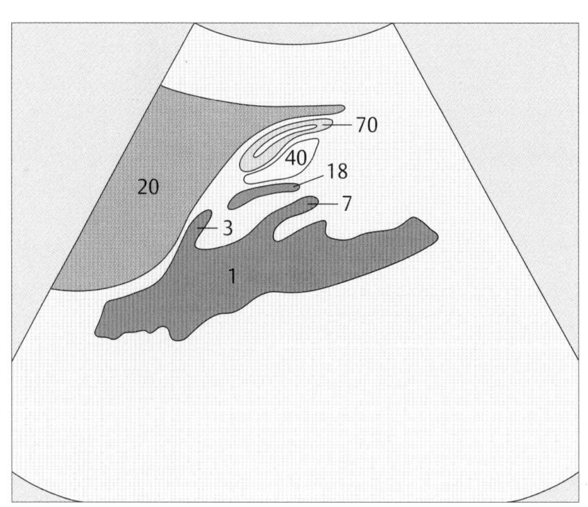

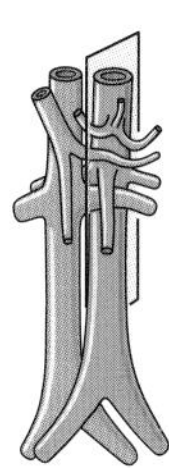

The origin of the celiac trunk and its division into branches are subject to numerous variations.

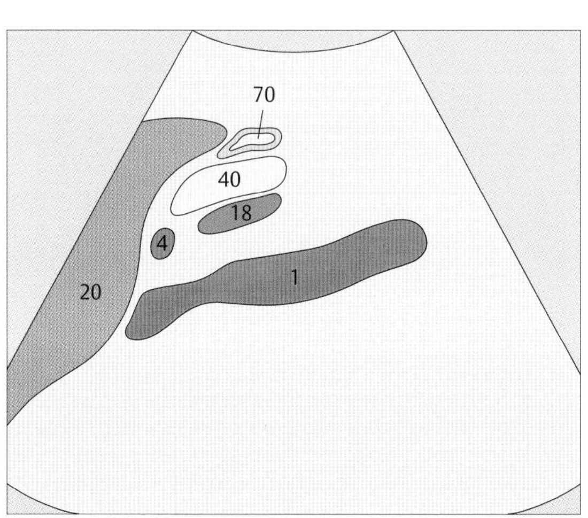

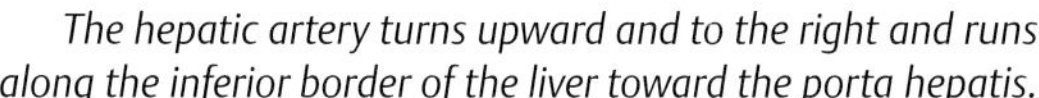

The hepatic artery turns upward and to the right and runs along the inferior border of the liver toward the porta hepatis.

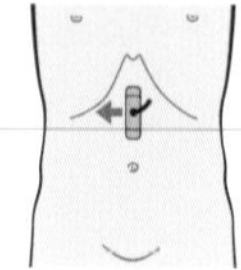

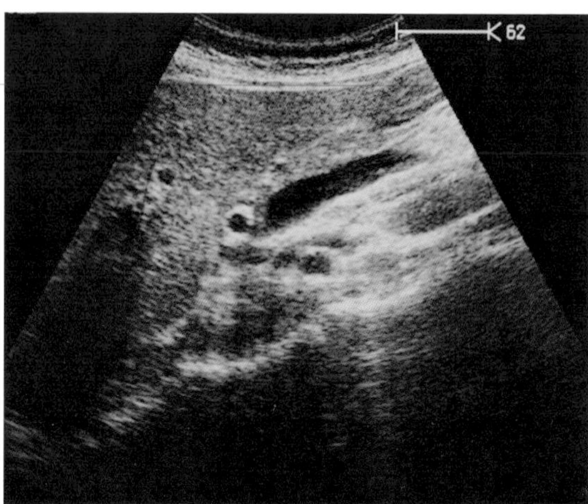

▶ **33** Hepatic artery and superior mesenteric vein

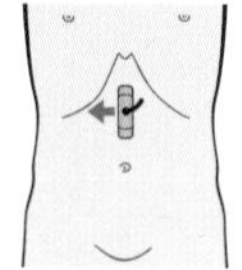

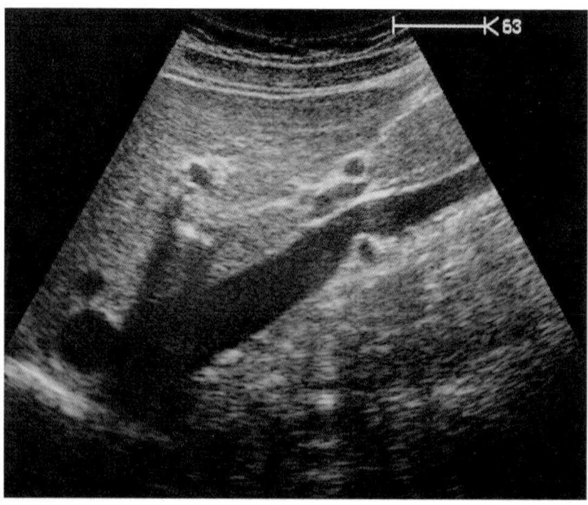

▶ **34** Hepatic artery and portal vein

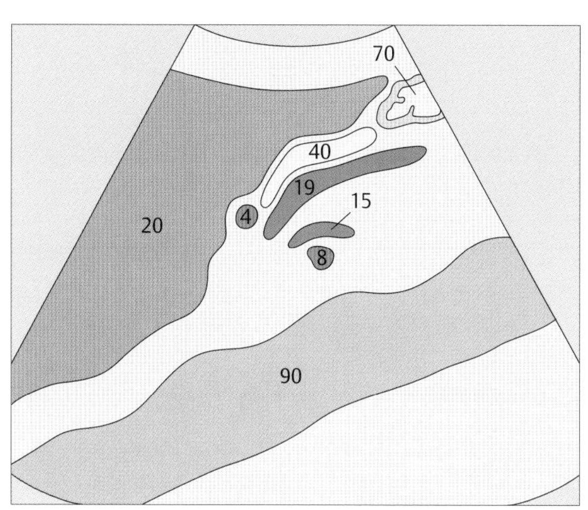

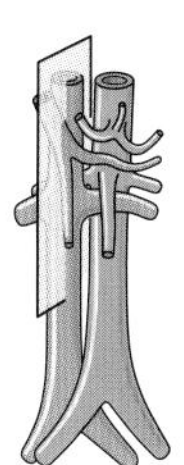

A longitudinal scan between the aorta and vena cava typically displays sections of four vessels: the hepatic artery, venous confluence, left renal vein, and right renal artery.

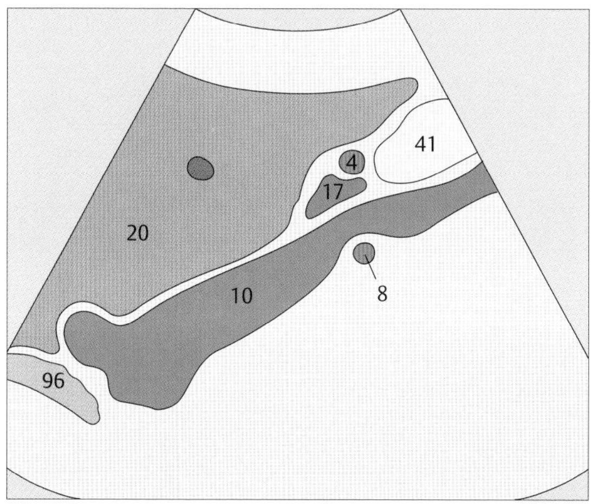

A longitudinal scan over the vena cava displays four typical vascular sections: the vena cava, portal vein, hepatic artery, and renal artery.

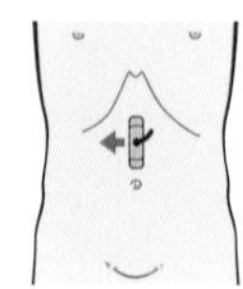

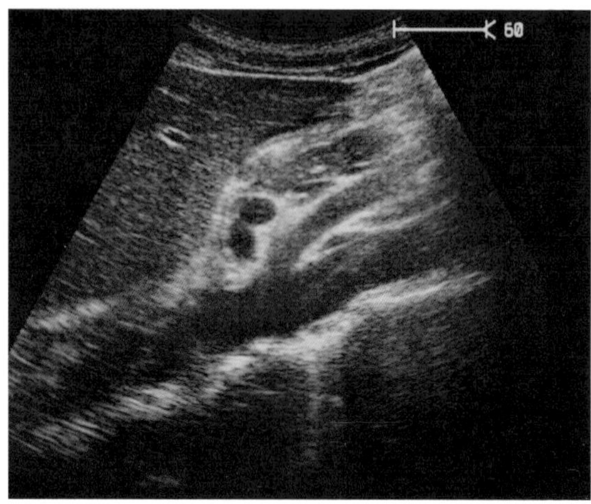

▶ **35** Aorta

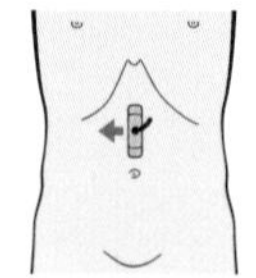

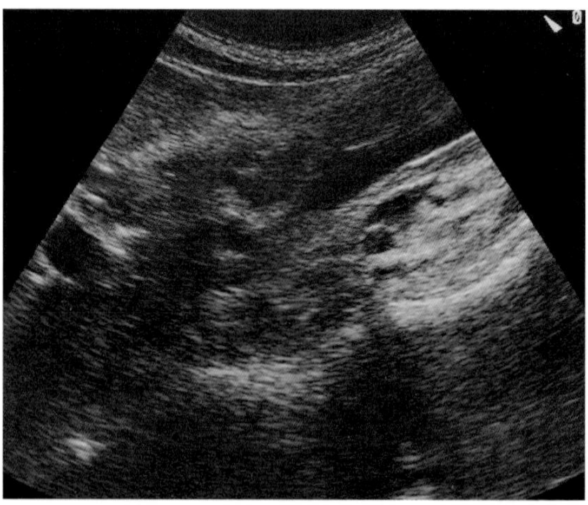

▶ **36** Right renal artery and left renal vein

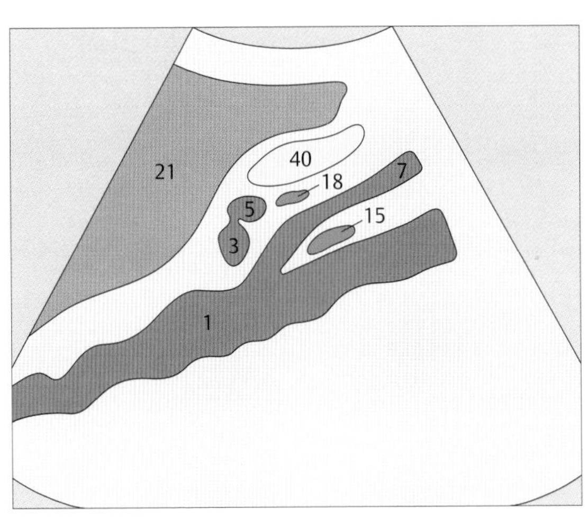

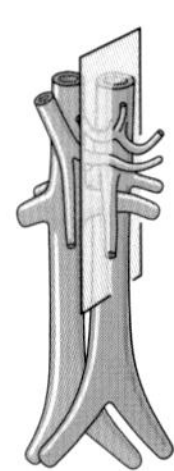

The left renal vein runs between the aorta and superior mesenteric artery, where it is subject to physiologic compression.

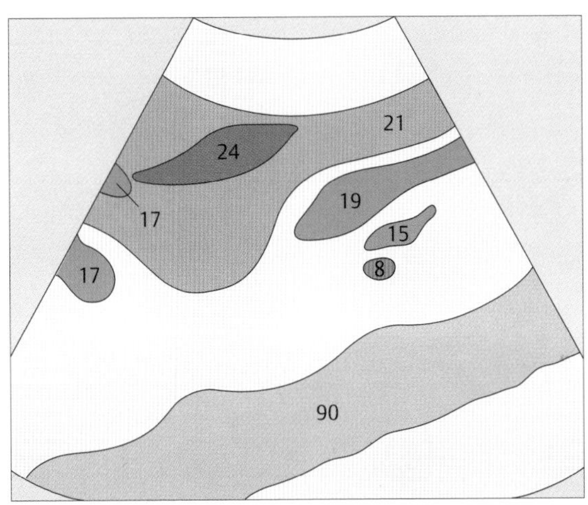

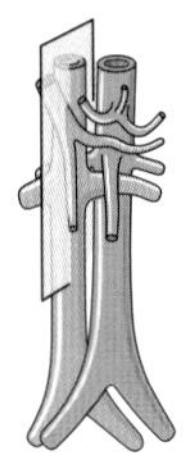

The section of the right renal artery can be identified between the aorta and vena cava. Just above the renal artery are the left renal vein and a longitudinal section of the superior mesenteric vein.

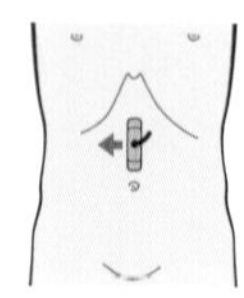

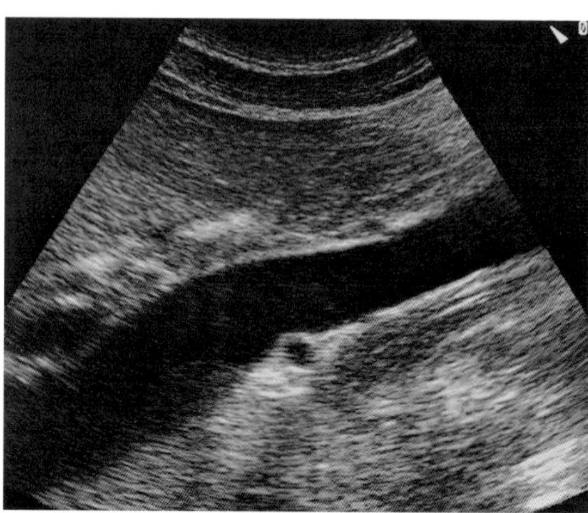

▶ **37** Vena cava and right renal artery

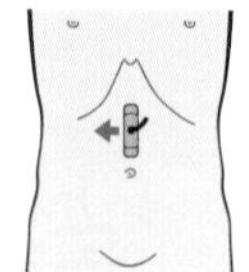

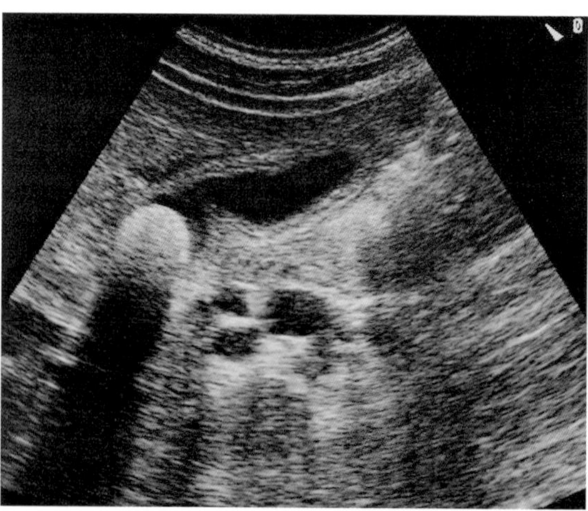

▶ **38** Right renal artery and right renal vein

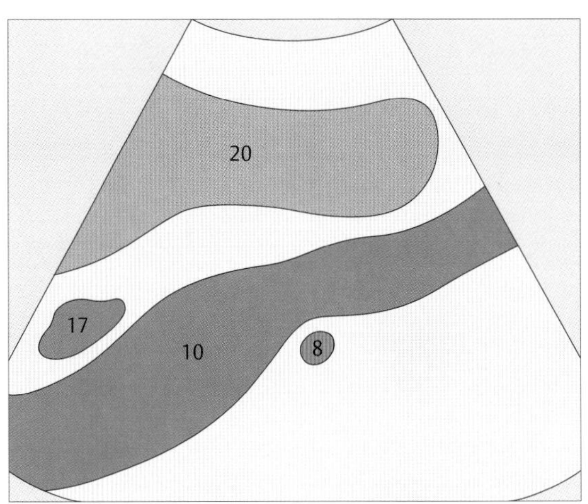

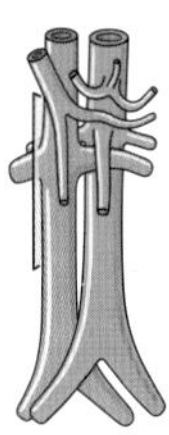

The right renal artery usually impresses the posterior surface of the vena cava, although variants may occur.

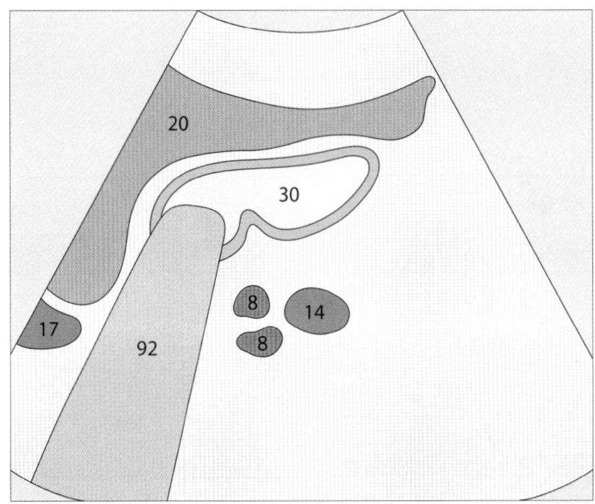

The renal veins are often more than twice the diameter of the renal arteries.

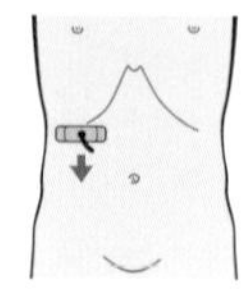

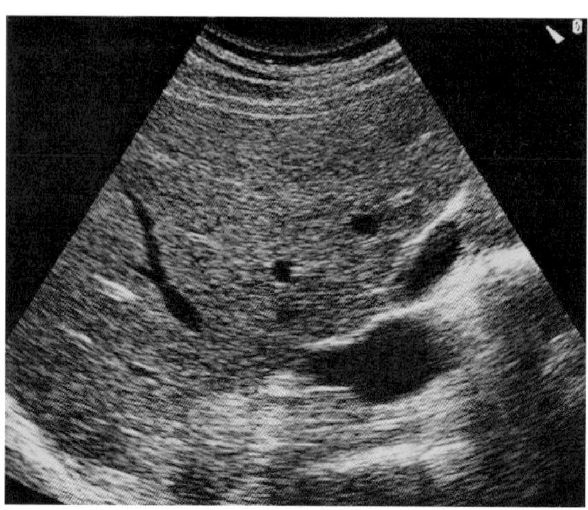

▶ **39** Opening of renal vein

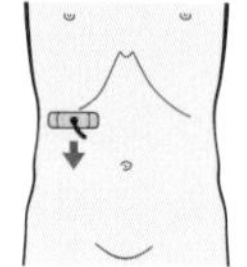

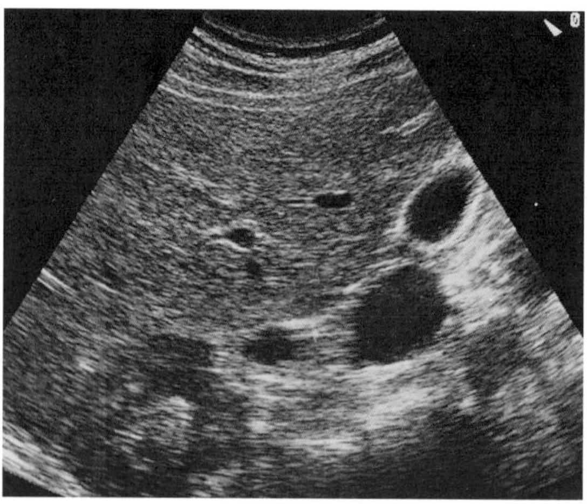

▶ **40** Renal vein

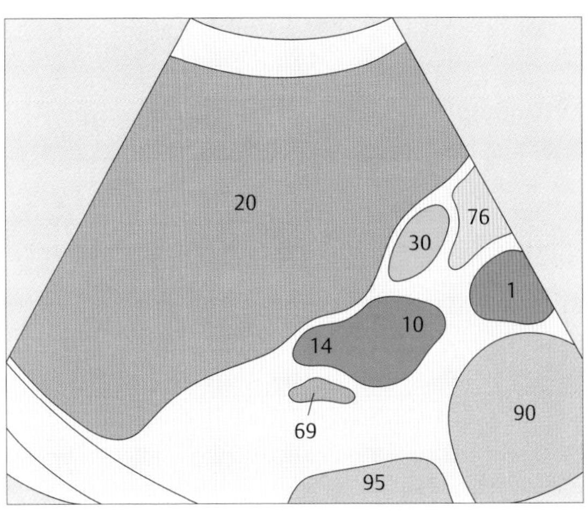

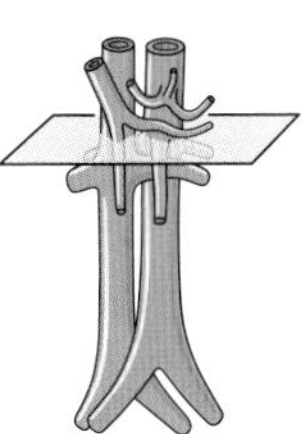

The opening of the right renal vein at the vena cava can be clearly defined above the kidney in most subjects.

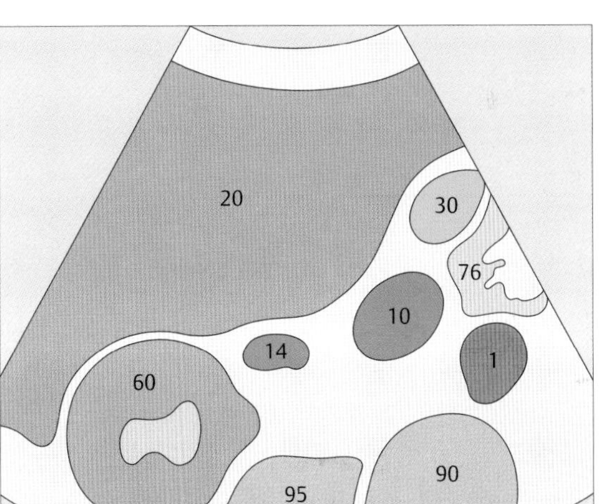

In serial transverse scans down the vena cava, the oval cross section of the renal vein separates from the vena cava and moves laterally toward the kidney.

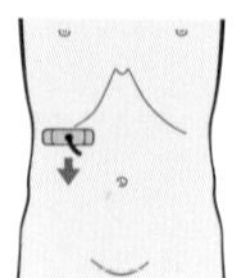

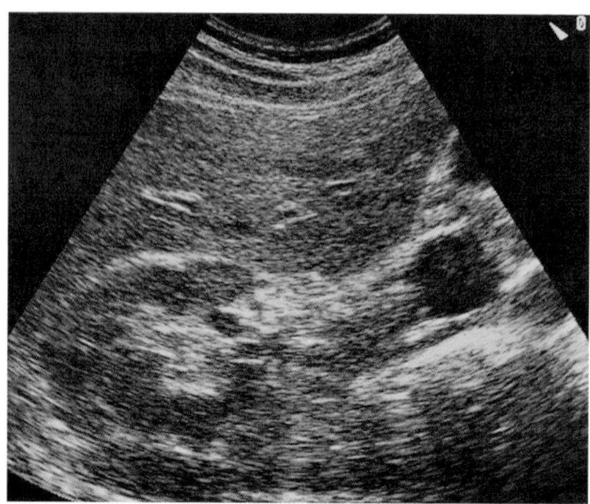

▶ **41** Renal vein at hilum, renal artery

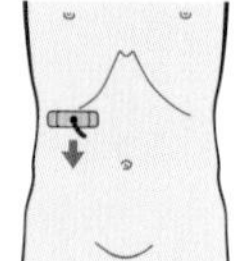

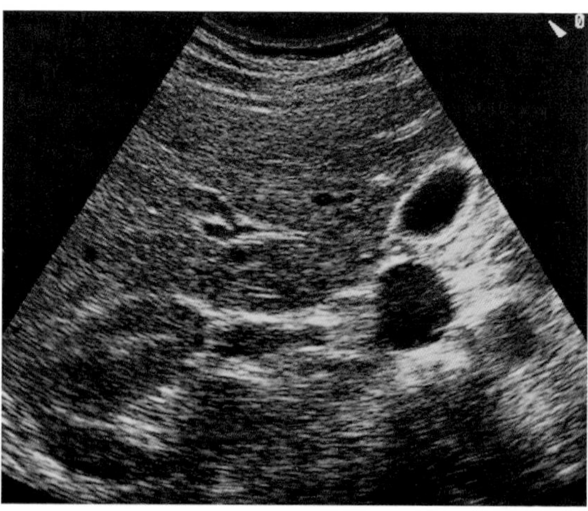

▶ **42** Renal artery

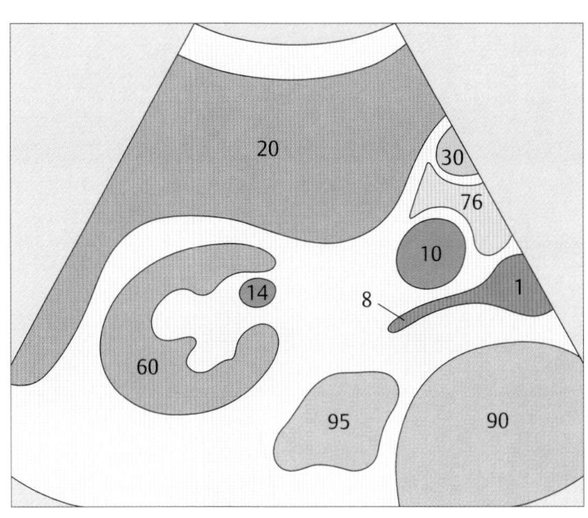

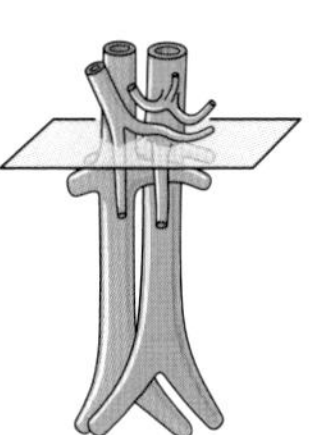

The renal artery follows the same course as the renal vein, but at a slightly more caudal level.

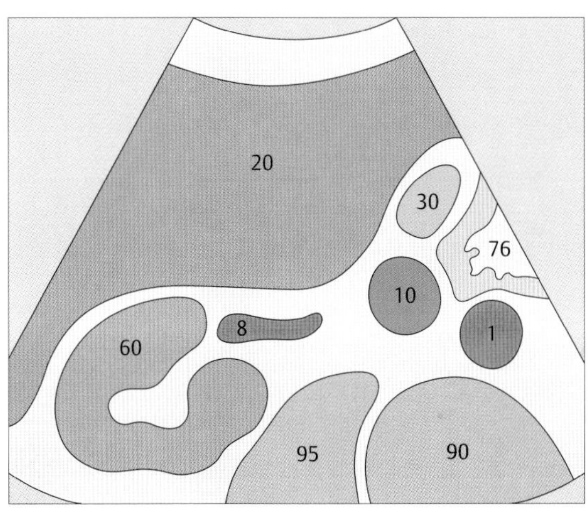

The renal arteries are located posterior and caudal to the renal veins.

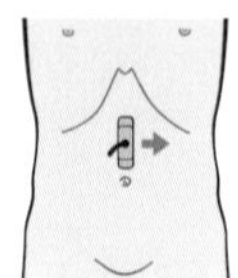

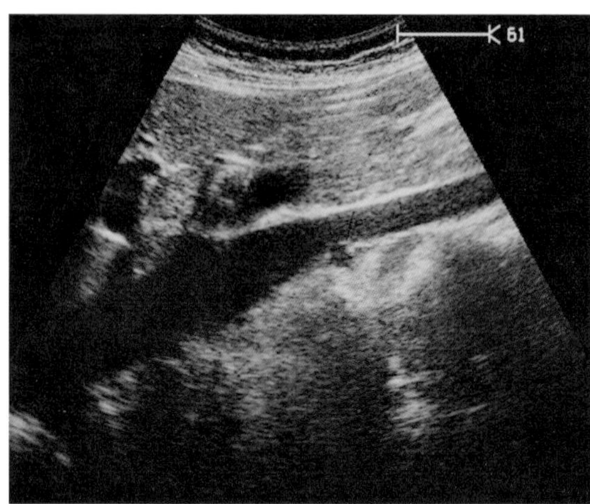

▶ **43** Vena cava

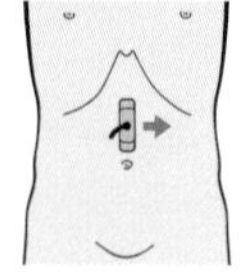

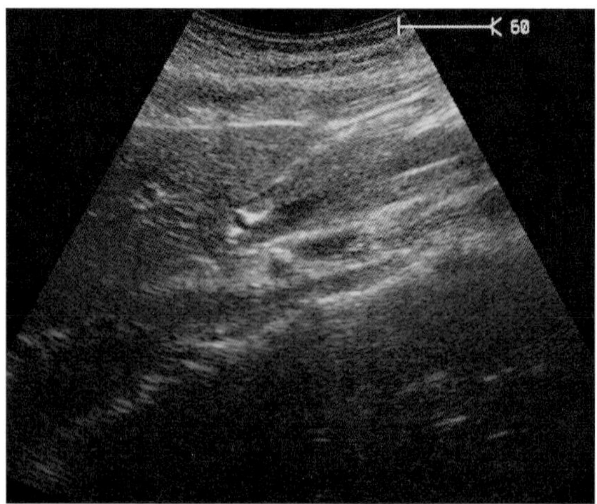

▶ **44** Right renal artery and left renal vein

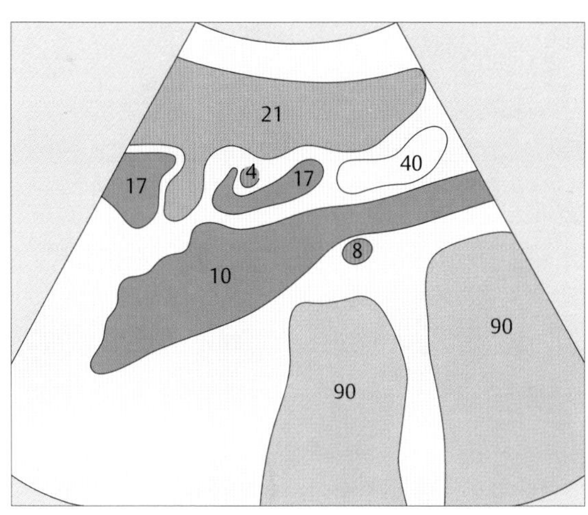

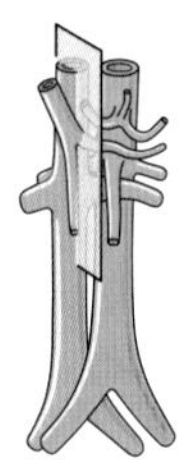

The right renal artery passes behind the vena cava, impressing its posterior surface.

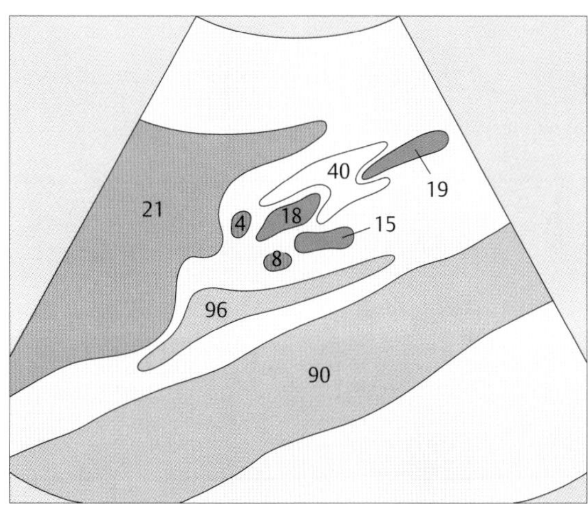

The scan plane cuts the left renal vein and right renal artery between the aorta and vena cava.

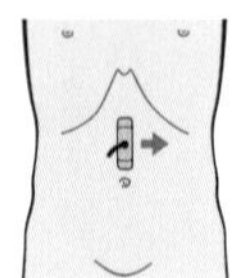

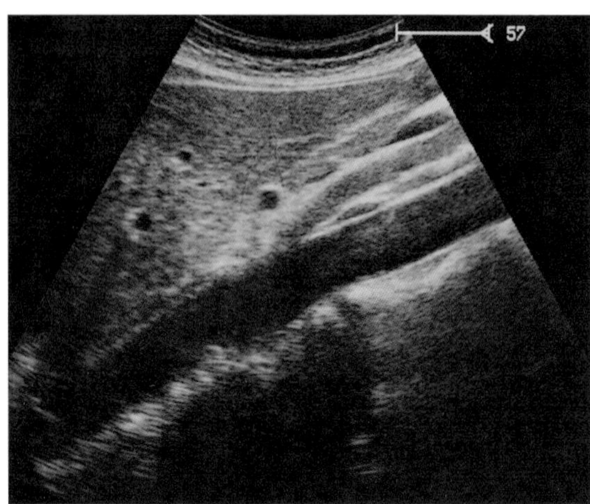

▶ **45** Aorta and left renal vein

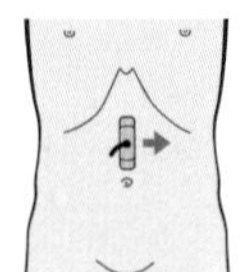

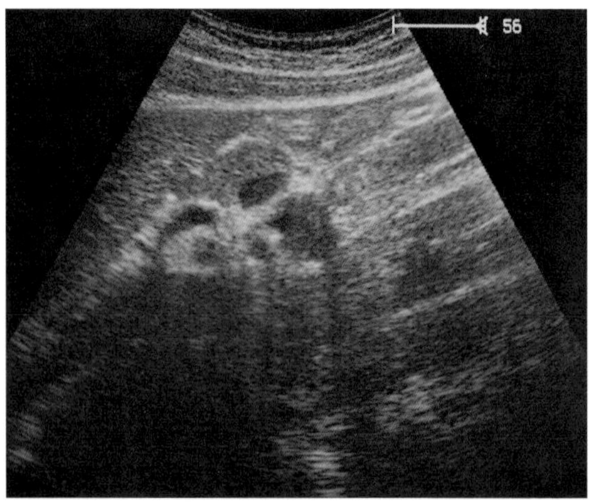

▶ **46** Left renal vessels, splenic artery and vein

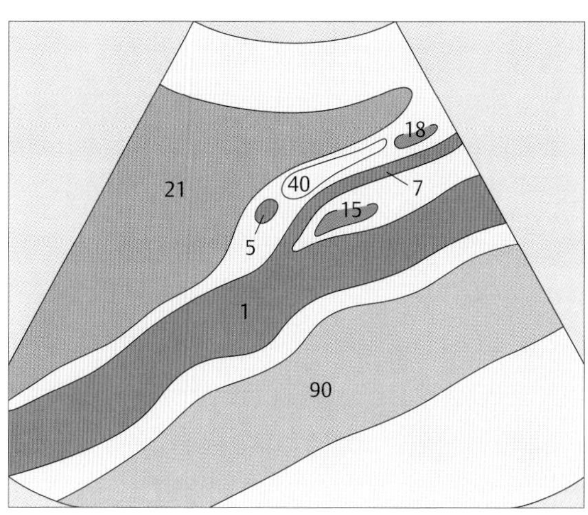

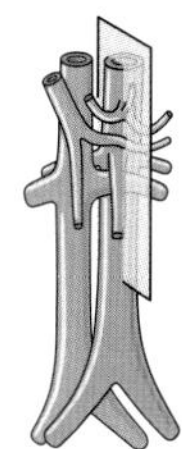

The left renal vein runs between the aorta and superior mesenteric artery.

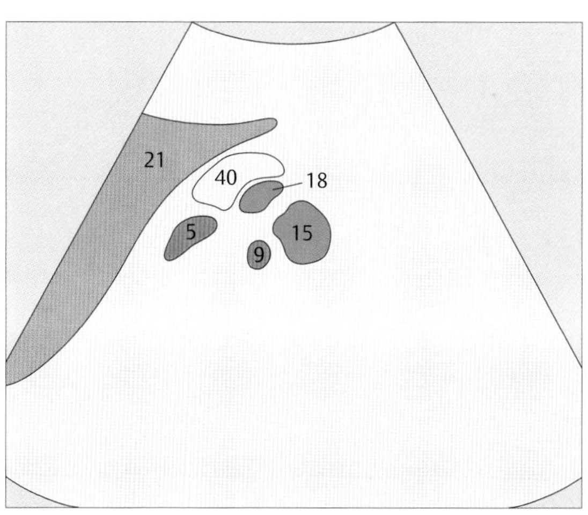

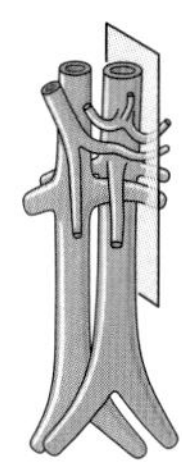

The left renal vessels are often difficult to scan because of overlying air.

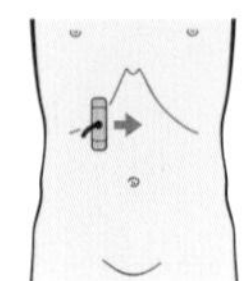

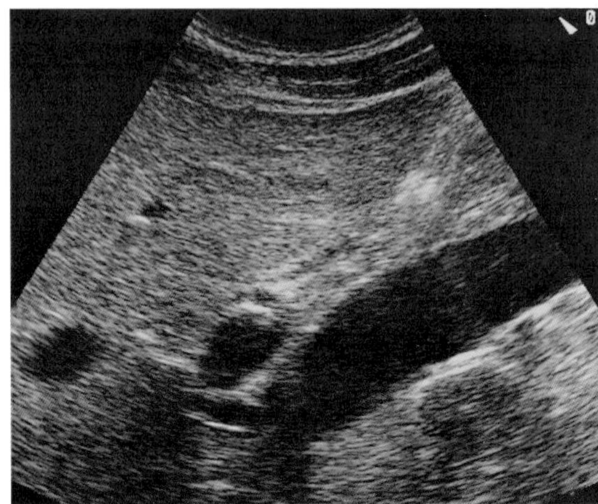

▶ **47** Portal vein, vena cava, right renal artery

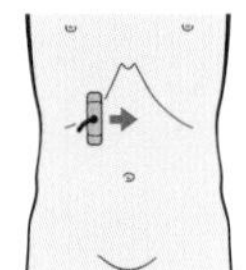

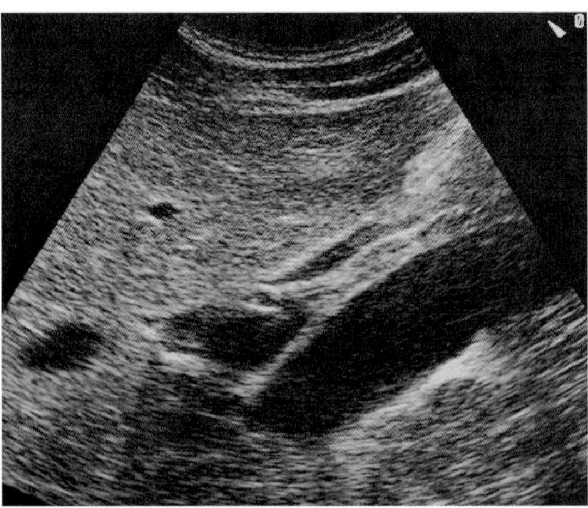

▶ **48** Portal vein, vena cava, right renal artery, and bile duct

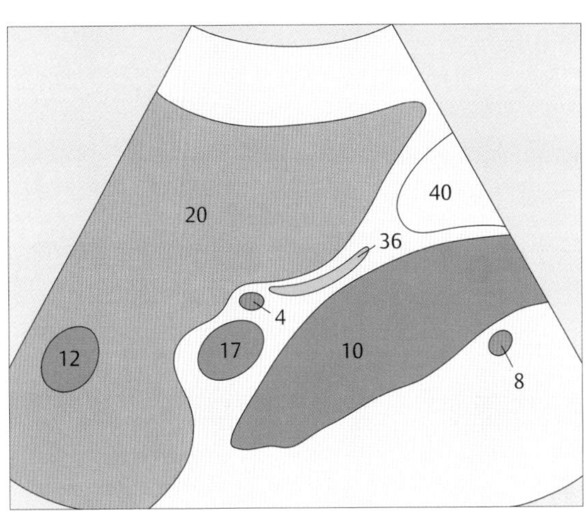

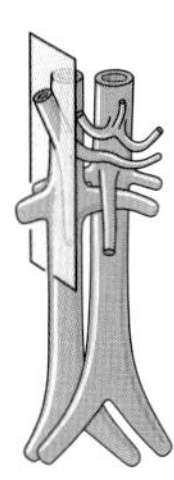

The triad of the portal vein, vena cava, and right renal artery provides a typical landmark in the upper abdominal longitudinal scan.

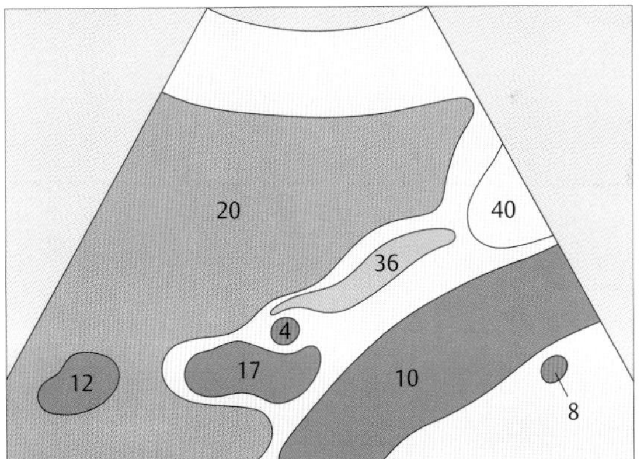

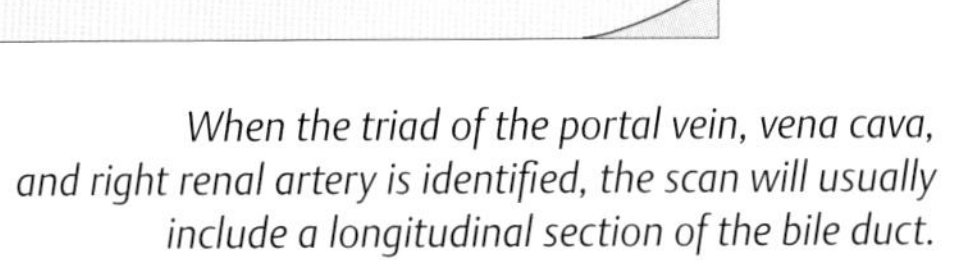

When the triad of the portal vein, vena cava, and right renal artery is identified, the scan will usually include a longitudinal section of the bile duct.

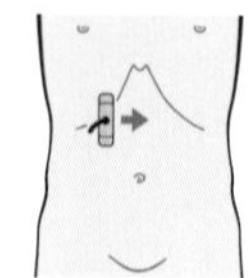

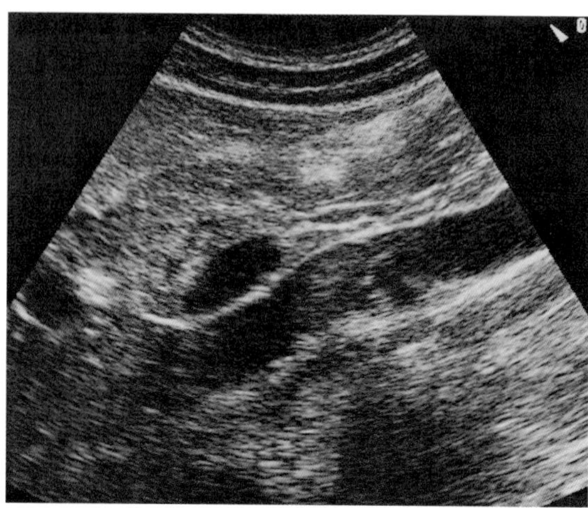

▶ **49** Portal vein, vena cava, and bile duct

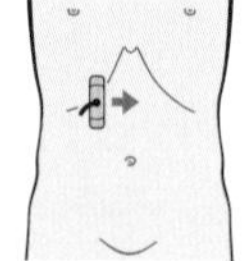

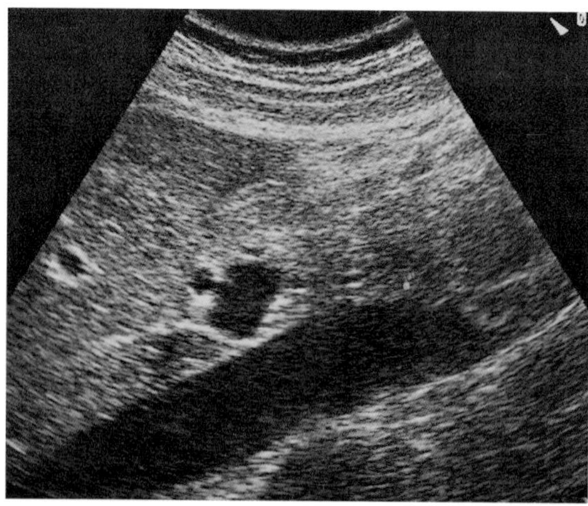

▶ **50** Portal vein and hepatic artery

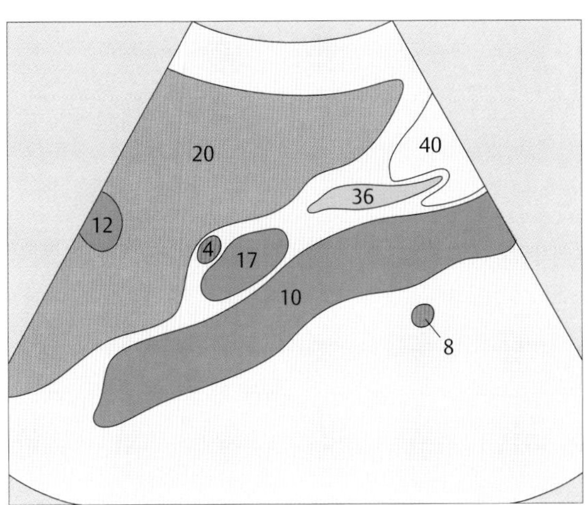

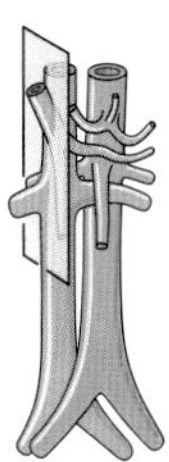

The bile duct enters the head of the pancreas anterior to the vena cava.

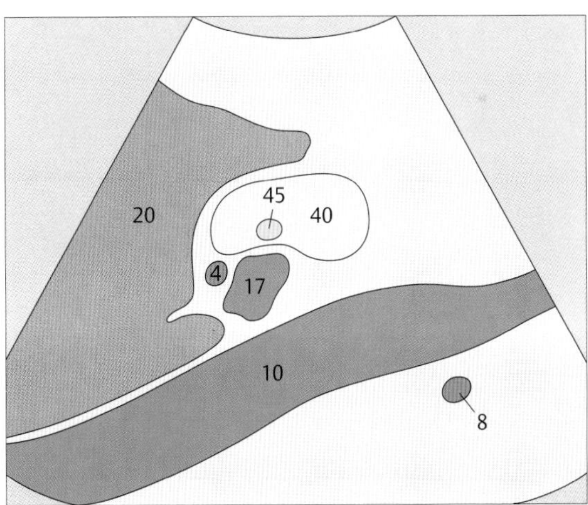

The portal vein and hepatic artery run side-by-side posterior to the head of the pancreas.

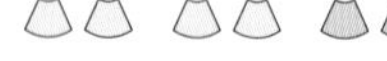

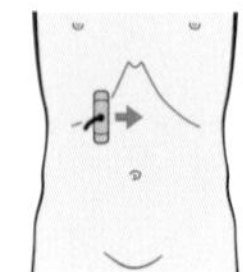

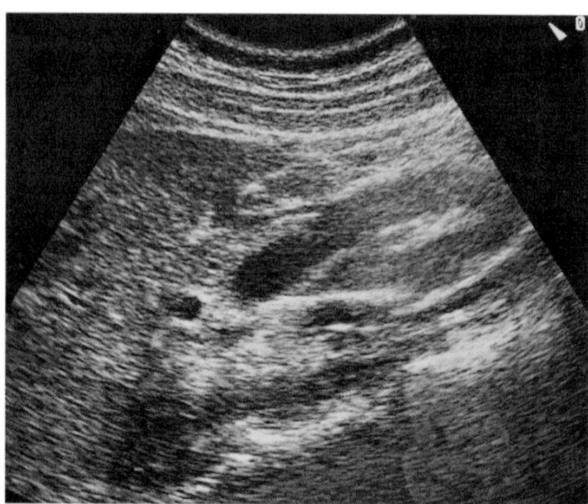

▶ **51** Hepatic artery, superior mesenteric vein

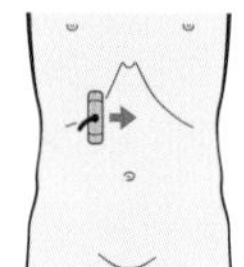

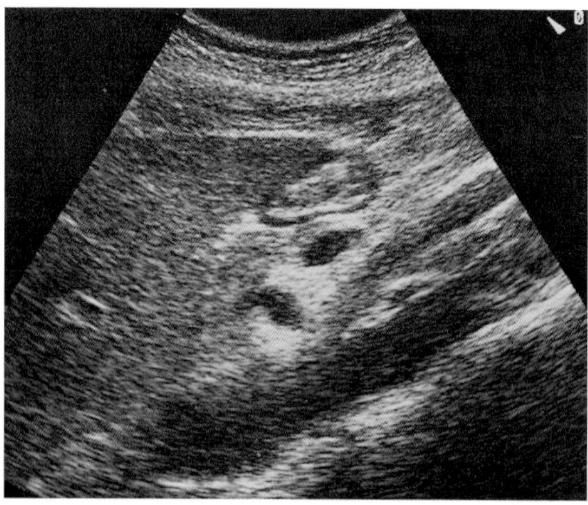

▶ **52** Hepatic artery, superior mesenteric artery, and splenic vein

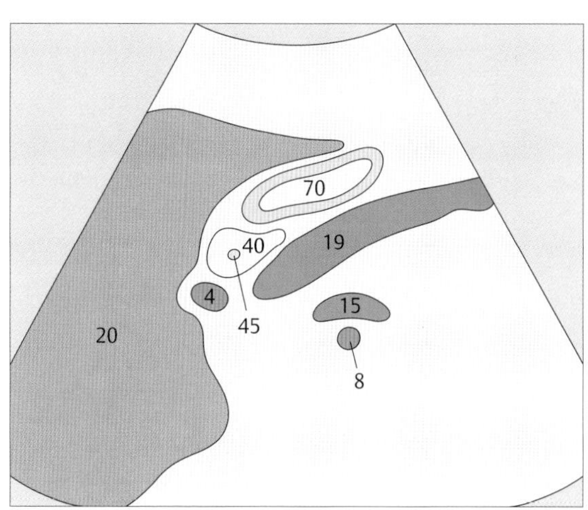

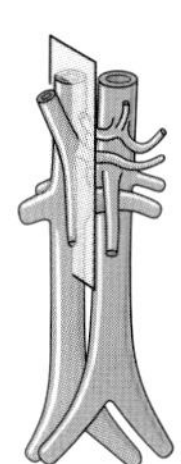

When the mesenteric vein is viewed in longitudinal section, typically the scan will also display the hepatic artery cranially and the right renal artery and left renal vein posteriorly.

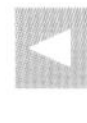

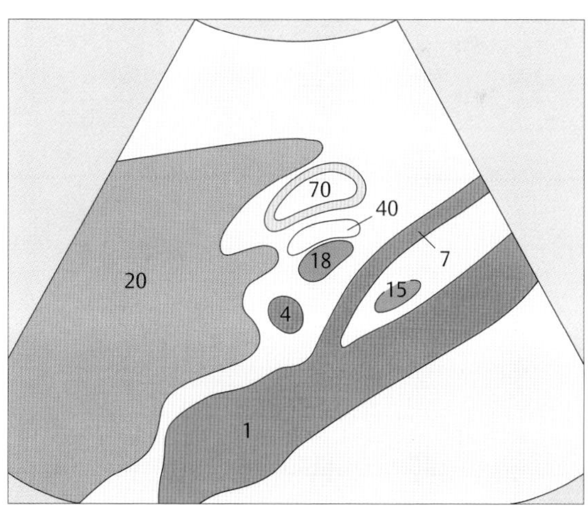

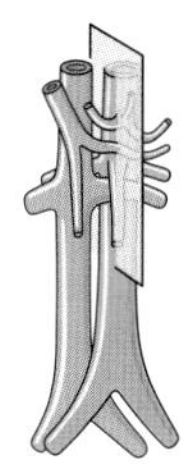

When the superior mesenteric artery is viewed in longitudinal section, typically the scan will also show the hepatic artery, splenic vein, and left renal vein.

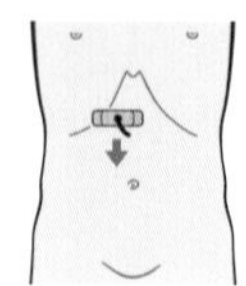

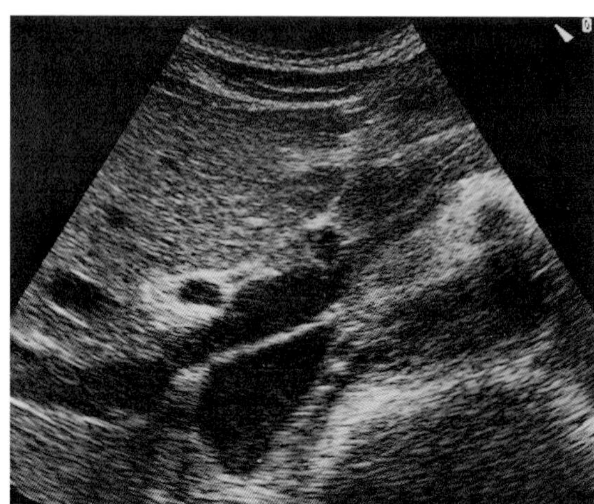

▶ **53** Hepatic artery, portal vein, vena cava

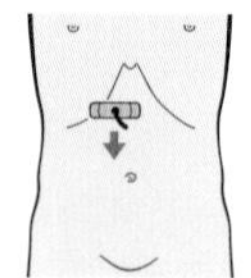

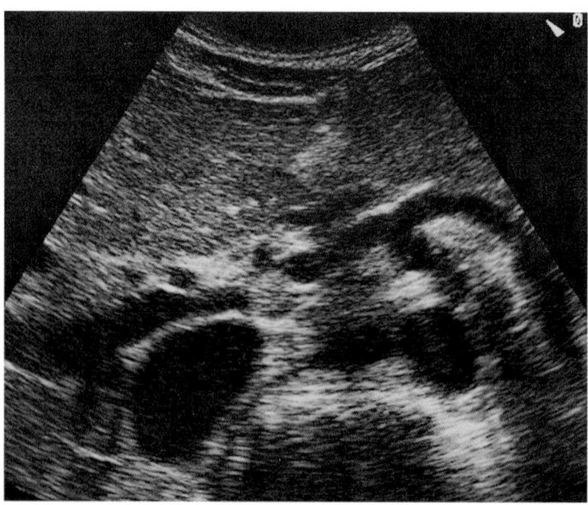

▶ **54** Hepatic artery, bile duct, portal vein

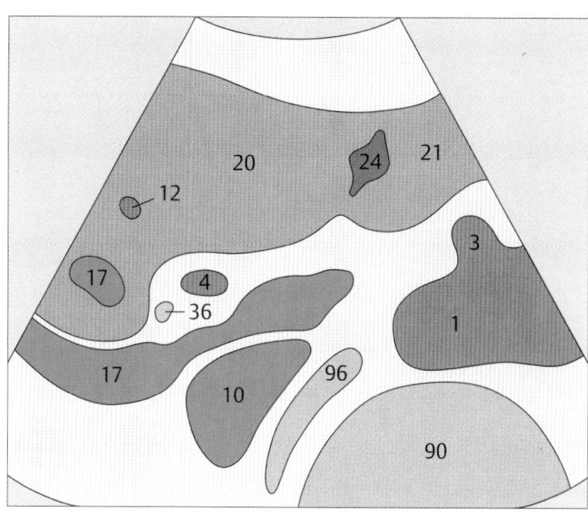

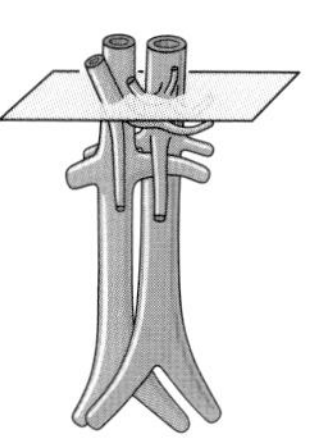

The portal vein runs between the vena cava and hepatic artery.

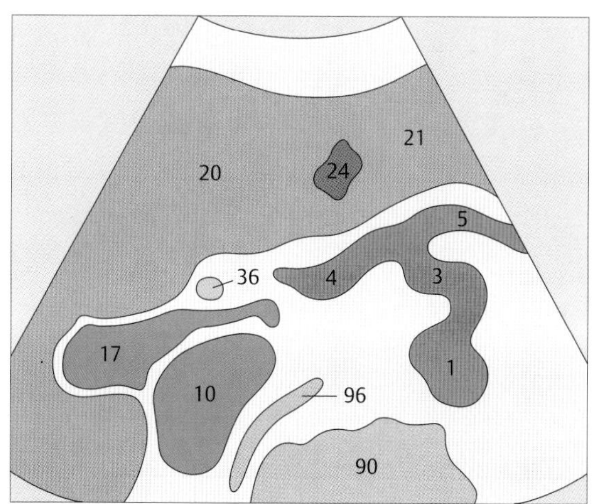

The hepatic artery runs cephalad into the porta hepatis.

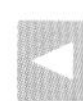

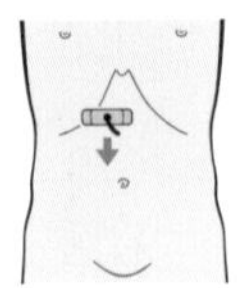

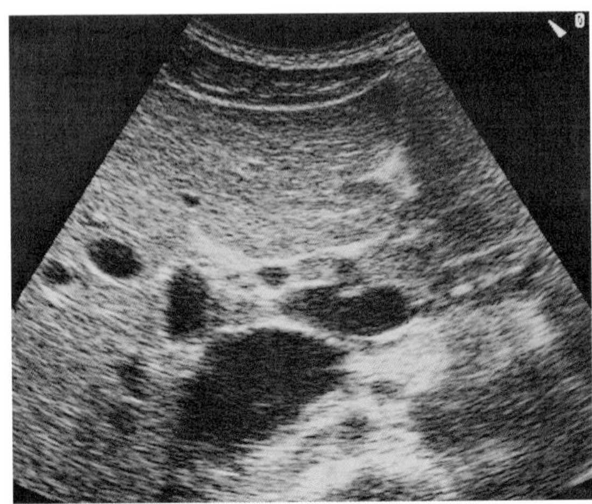

▶ **55** Bile duct, gallbladder, vena cava

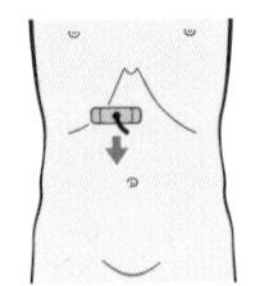

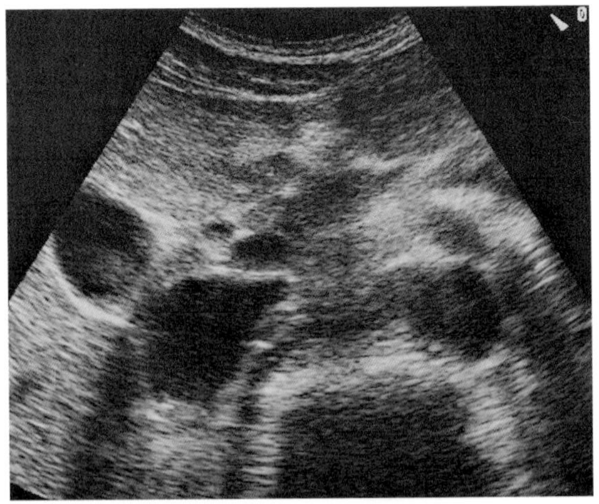

▶ **56** Bile duct, gallbladder, superior mesenteric vein

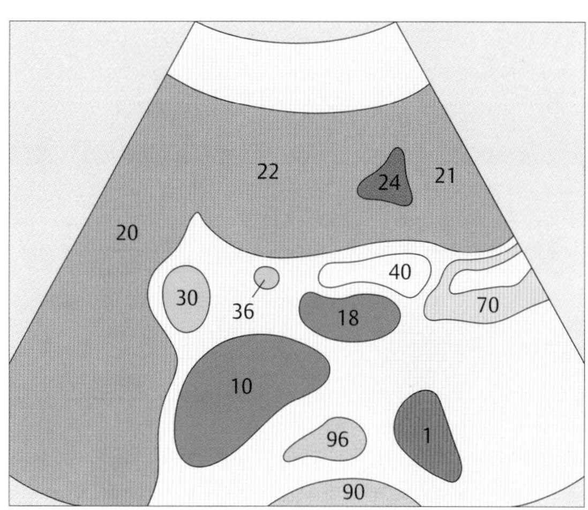

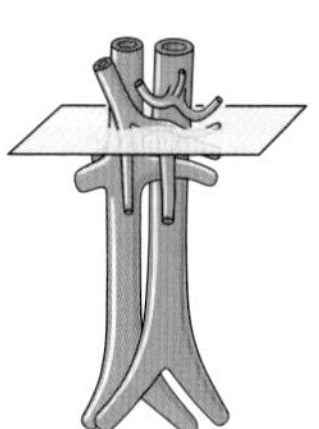

The bile duct is identified medial to the gallbladder and anterior to the vena cava.

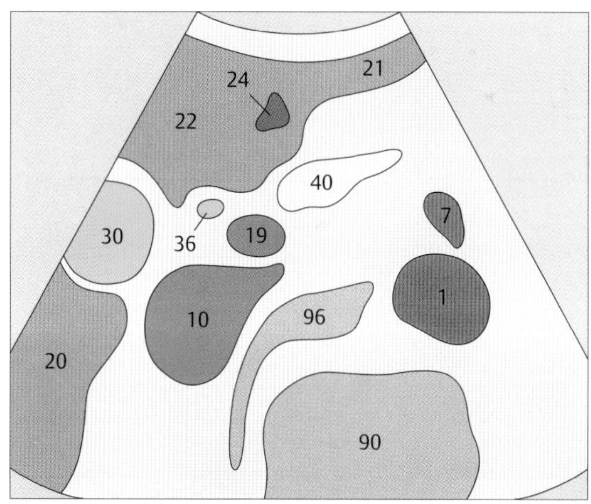

The bile duct runs parallel to the superior mesenteric vein for a short distance, then turns laterally to the right toward the papilla.

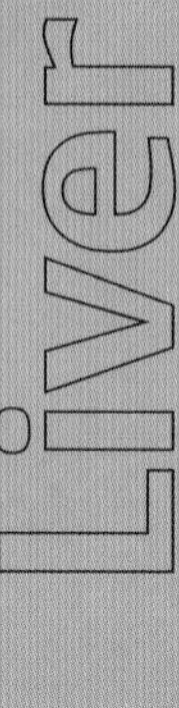

Liver in Longitudinal Sections ... p. 74

Left Portions of the Liver in Transverse Sections ... p. 88

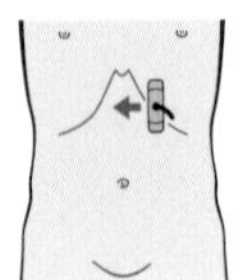

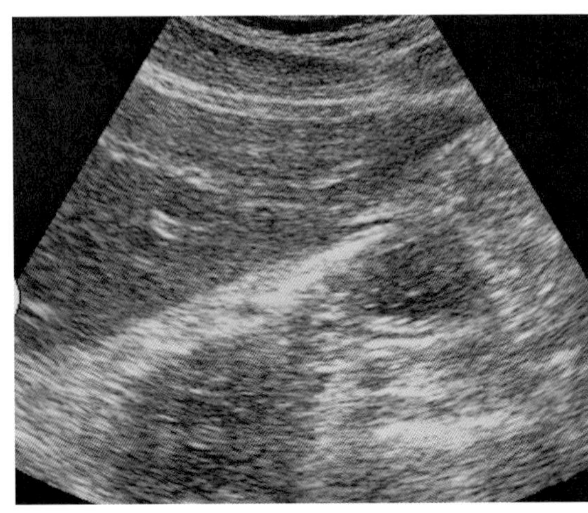

▶ **57** Left lobe of liver, lateral segment, subsegments II and III

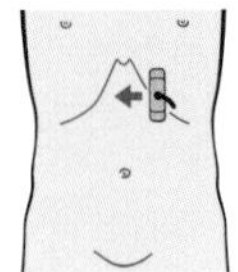

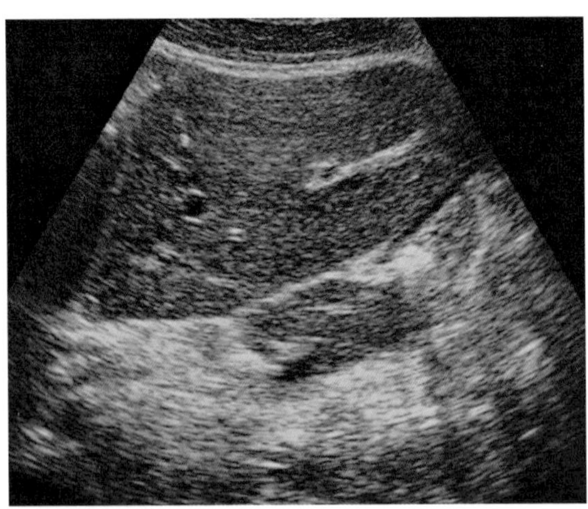

▶ **58** Left lobe of liver, ligamentum teres, boundary between lateral and medial segments

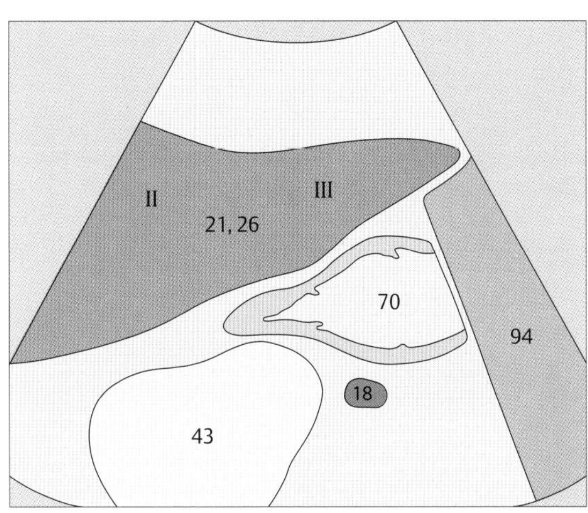

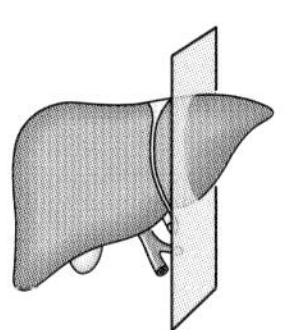

The liver is divided into a left and a right lobe on anatomical criteria. The left lobe corresponds to the lateral segment; the right lobe consists of the medial, anterior, and posterior segments.

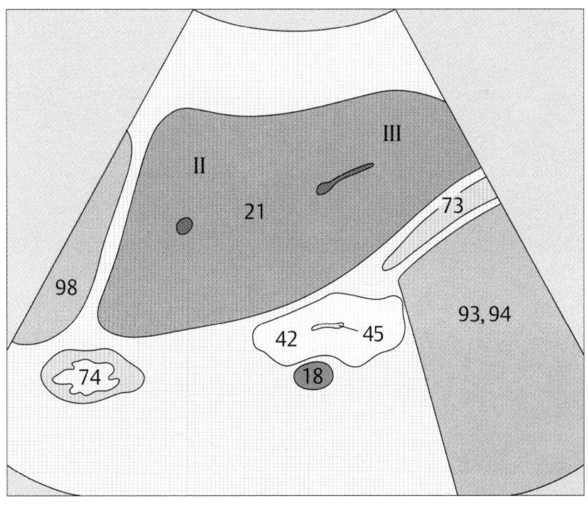

On functional criteria, the lateral and medial segments belong to the left lobe of the liver while the anterior and posterior segments belong to the right lobe.

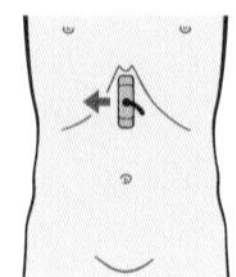

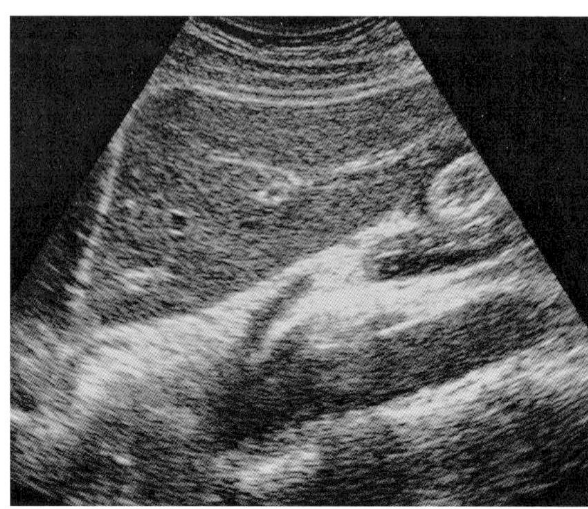

▶ **59** Left lobe of liver, ligamentum teres, boundary between lateral and medial segments

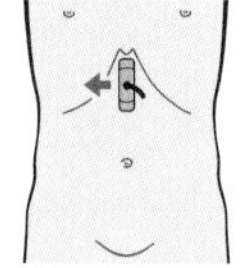

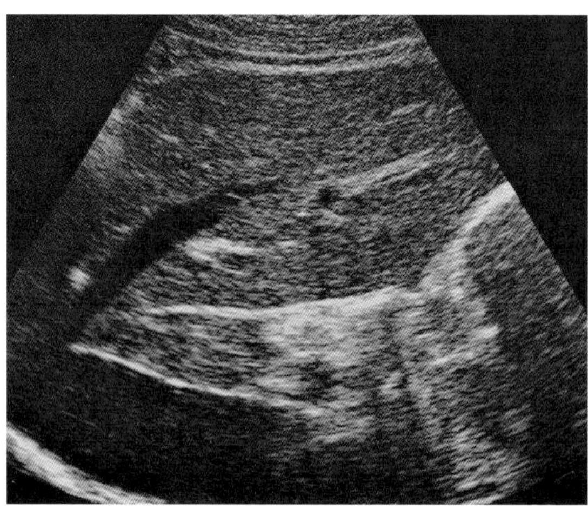

▶ **60** Left hepatic vein, ligamentum teres, boundary between lateral and medial segments, caudate lobe

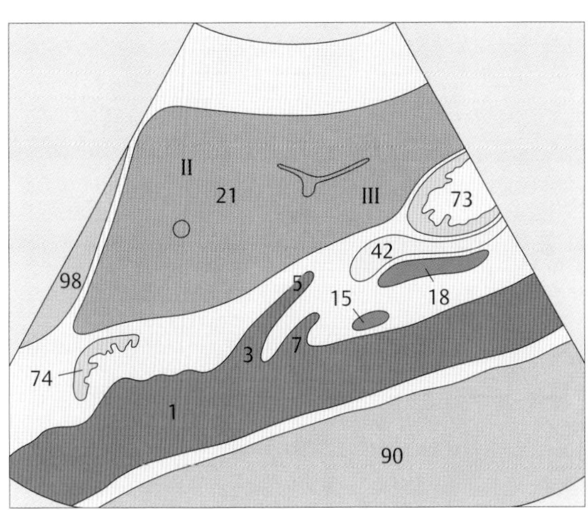

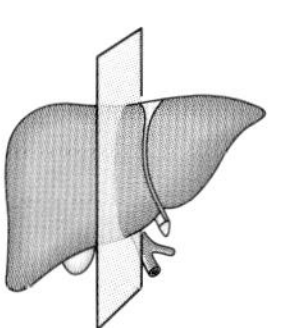

The lateral segment is composed of subsegment II cranially and subsegment III caudally.

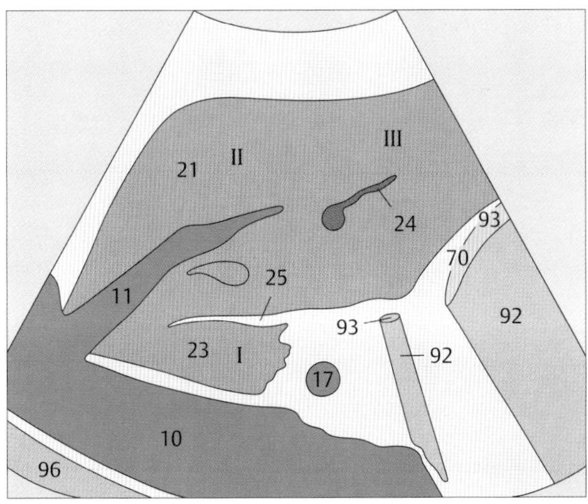

The boundary between the lateral and medial segments, i.e., between the anatomical left and right lobes of the liver, is the left hepatic vein.

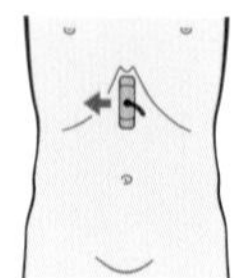

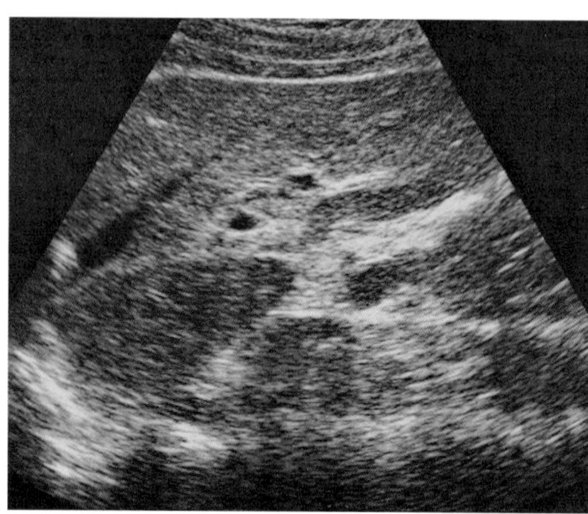

▶ **61** Left hepatic vein, ligamentum teres, boundary between lateral and medial segments, caudate lobe

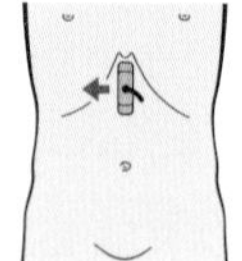

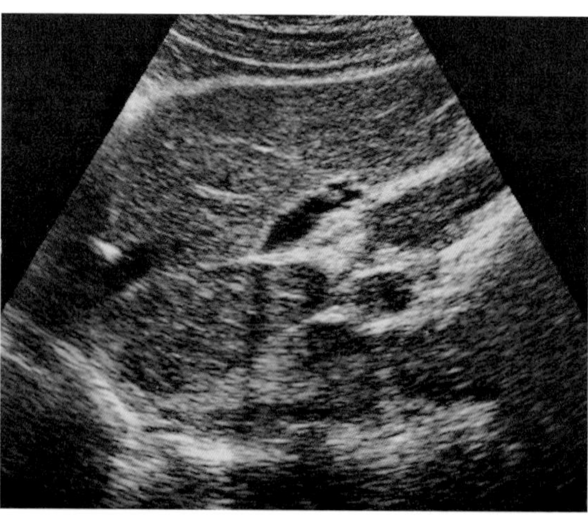

▶ **62** Left hepatic vein, ligamentum teres, boundary between lateral and medial segments, caudate lobe

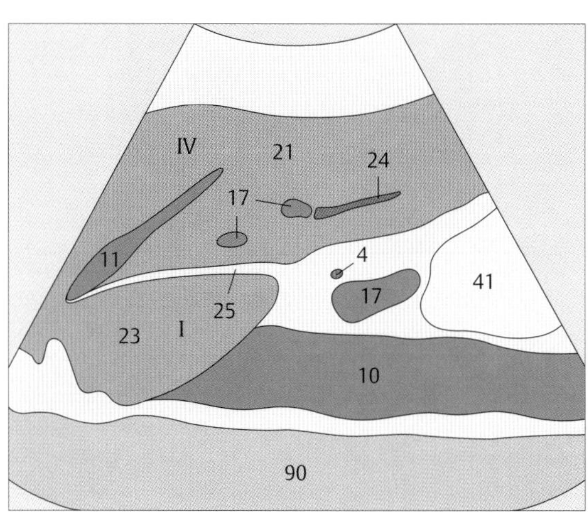

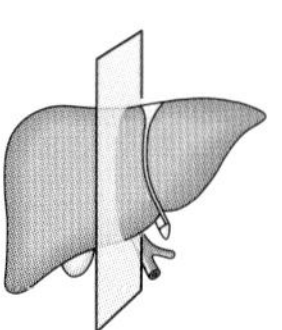

The caudate lobe corresponds to subsegment I of the medial segment and is located lateral and anterior to the vena cava. Most of the medial segment consists of subsegment IV.

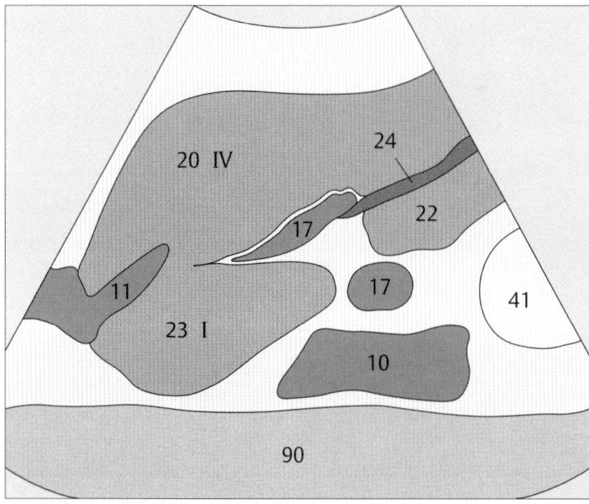

The boundary between the lateral and medial segments, i.e., between the anatomical left and right lobes of the liver, is the ligamentum teres.

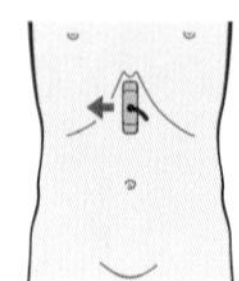

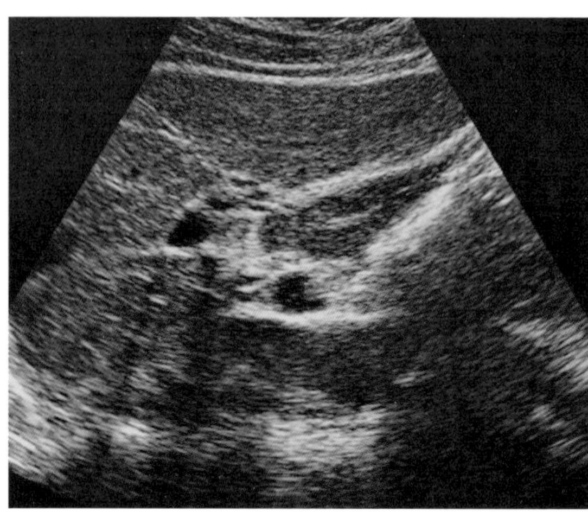

▶ **63** Left hepatic vein, ligamentum teres, boundary between lateral and medial segments, caudate lobe

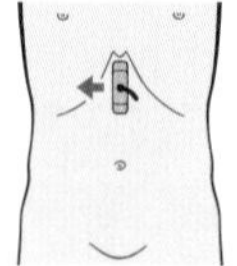

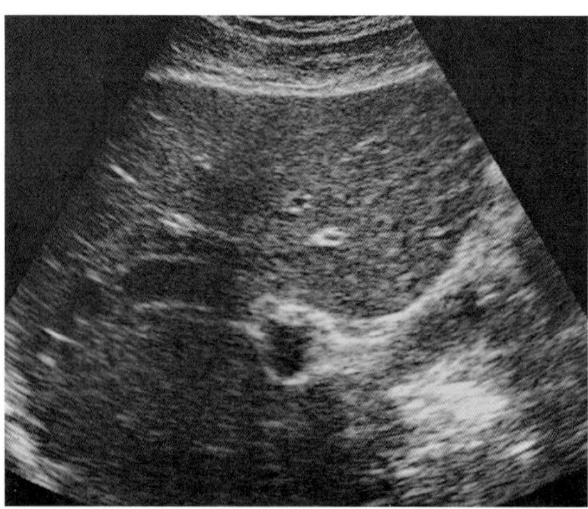

▶ **64** Medial segment, subsegment IV, quadrate lobe

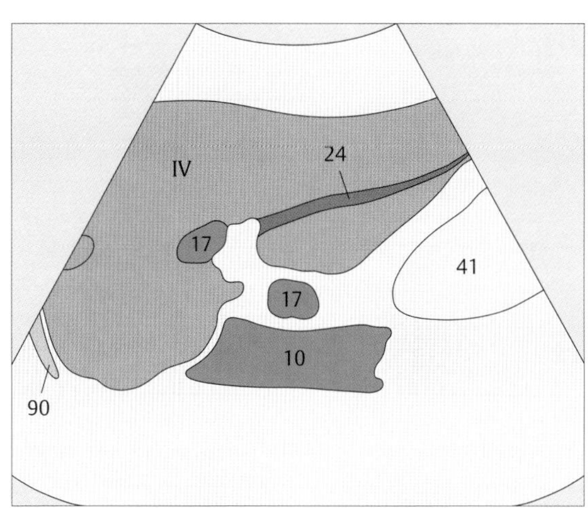

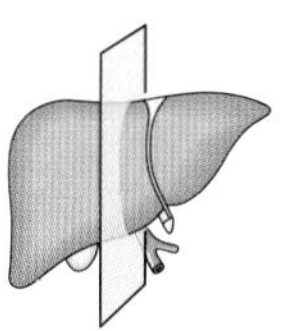

Ligamentum teres (the obliterated umbilical vein) extends from the left portal vein branch to the anterior inferior border of the liver.

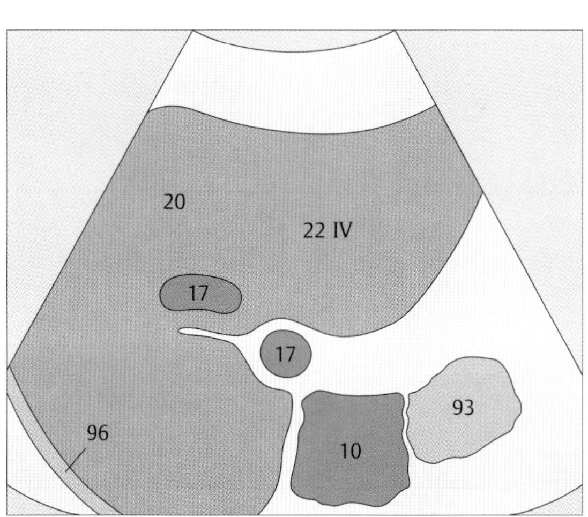

The caudal part of the medial segment, the quadrate lobe, is situated between ligamentum teres and the gallbladder. The quadrate lobe is part of subsegment IV.

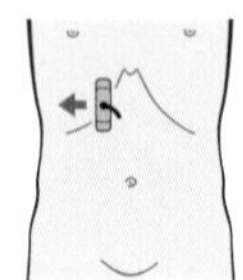

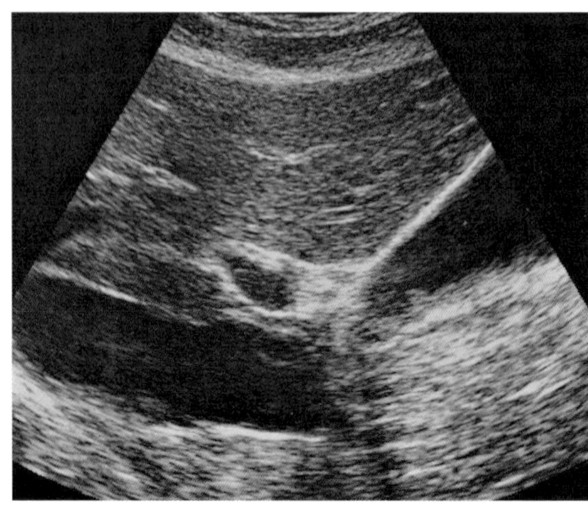

▶ **65** Gallbladder, portal vein, vena cava, boundary between medial and anterior segments

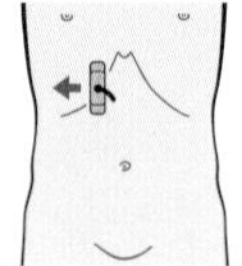

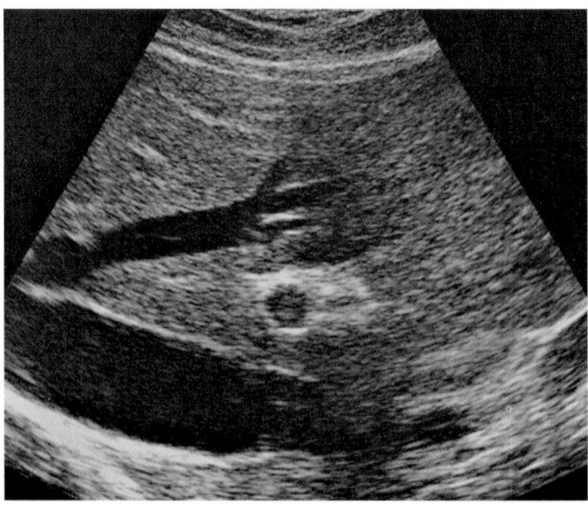

▶ **66** Middle hepatic vein, boundary between medial and anterior segments

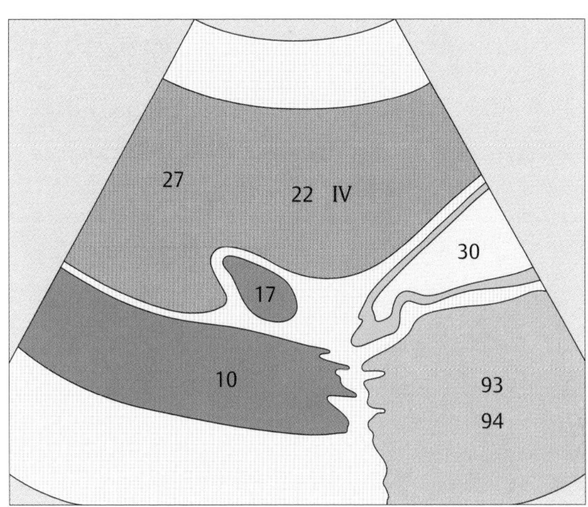

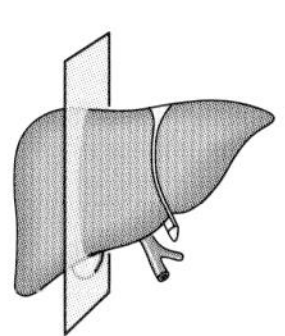

The plane of the gallbladder and vena cava forms the boundary plane between the medial and anterior segments of the liver.

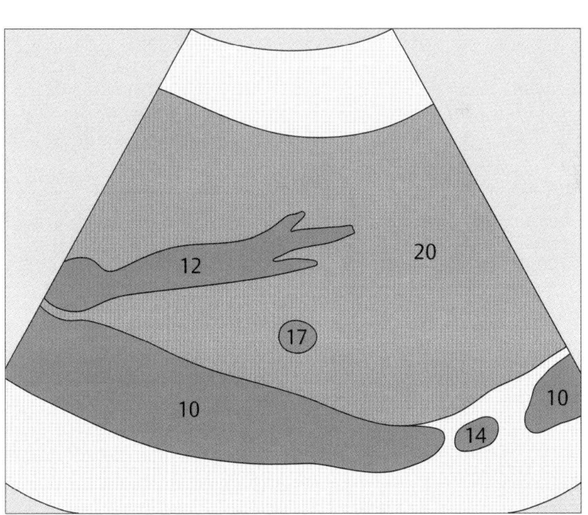

The middle hepatic vein marks the boundary between the medial and anterior segments in the cranial part of the liver.

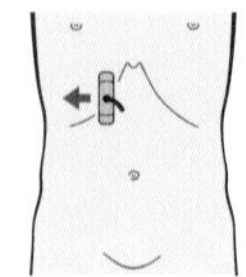

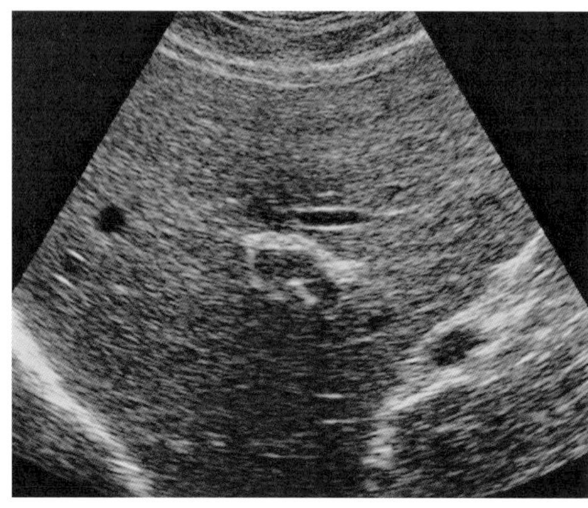

▶ **67** Anterior segment, subsegments VIII and V

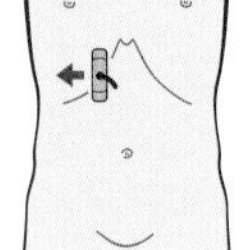

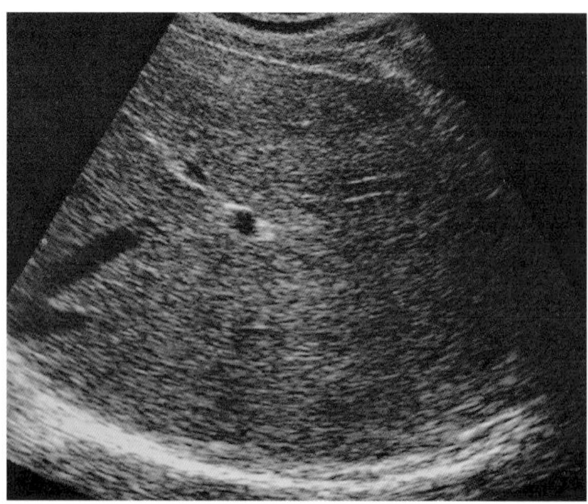

▶ **68** Right hepatic vein, boundary between anterior and posterior segments

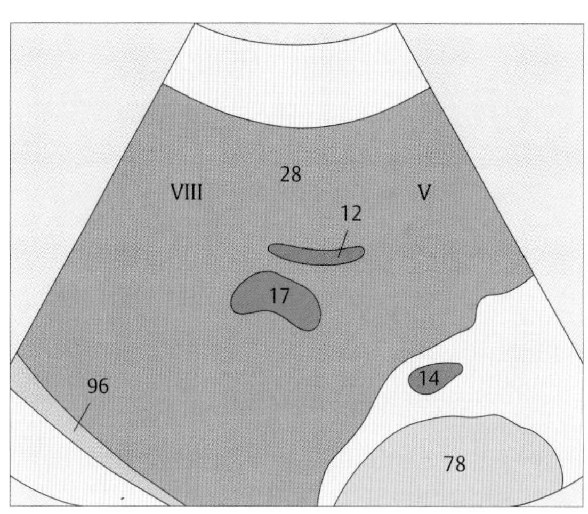

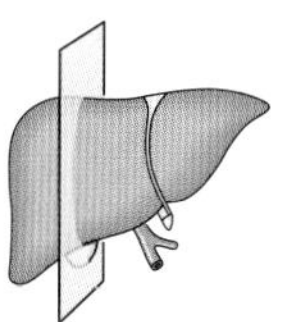

The anterior segment consists of subsegment VIII cranially and subsegment V caudally.

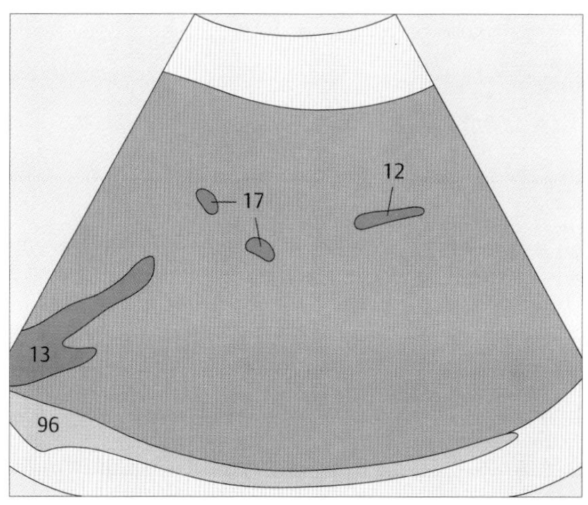

The right hepatic vein and the division of the right portal vein branch mark the boundary plane between the anterior and posterior segments.

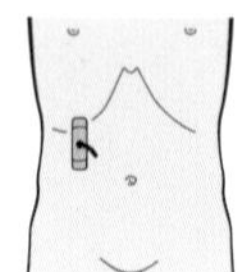

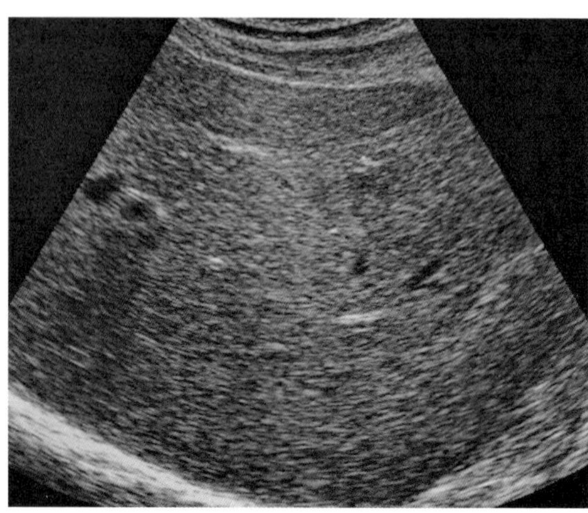

▶ **69** Posterior segment, subsegments VII and VI

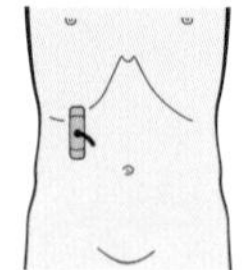

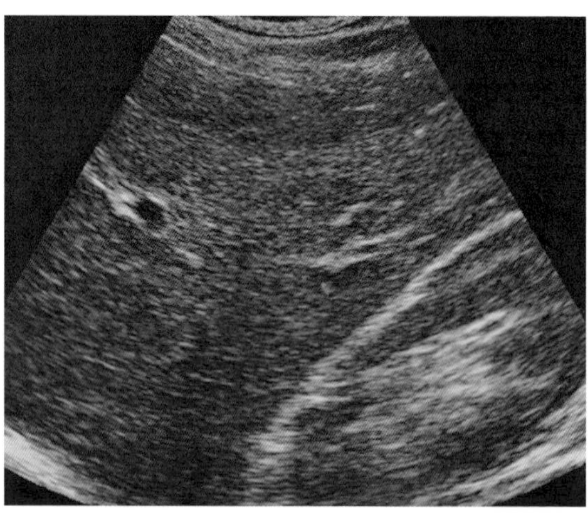

▶ **70** Posterior segment, lateral portions of liver, kidney

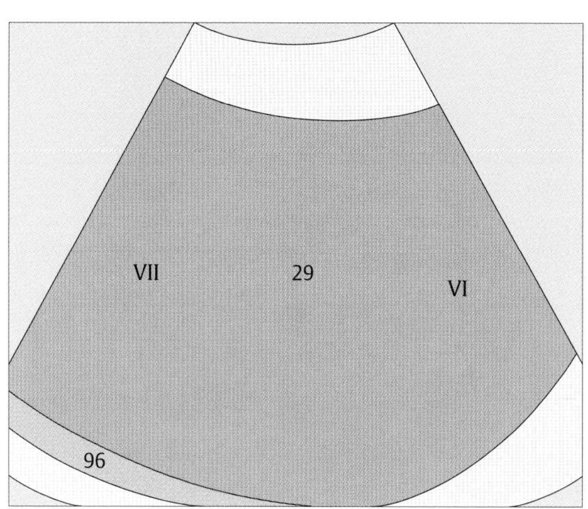

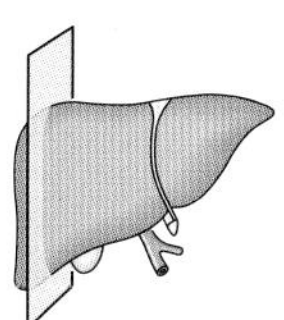

The posterior segment consists of subsegment VII cranially and subsegment VI caudally.

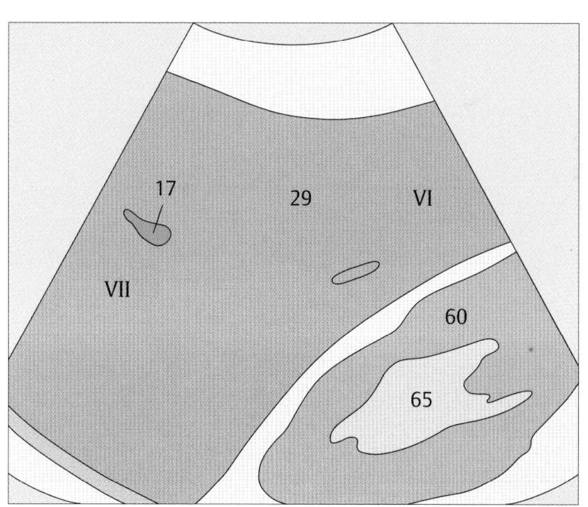

The right lobe of the liver is highly variable in its caudal extent.

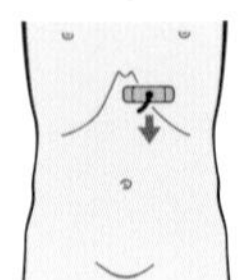

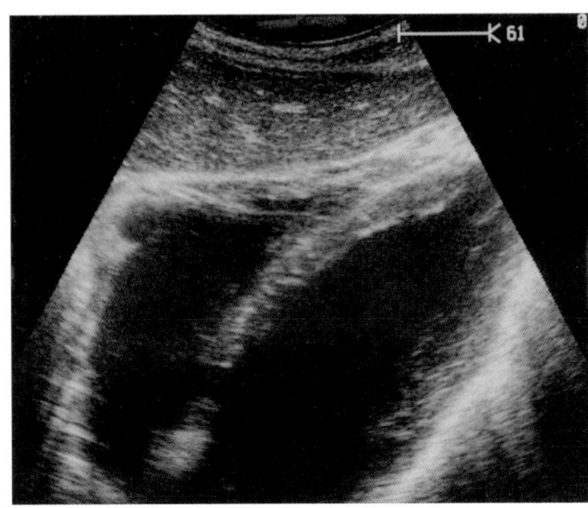

▶ **71** Left lobe of liver, lateral segment, heart

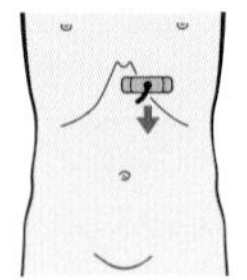

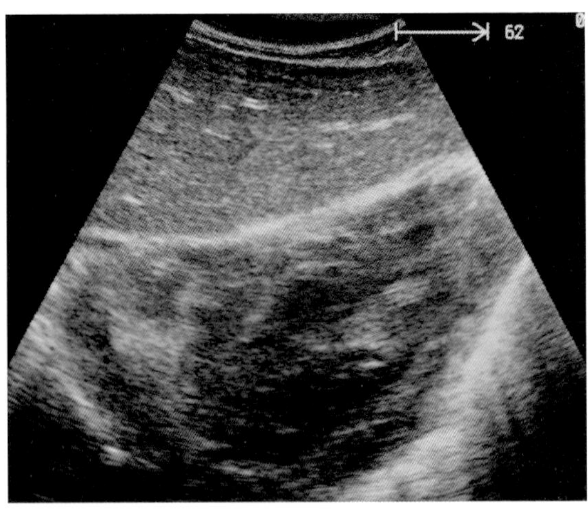

▶ **72** Left lobe of liver, lateral segment, heart

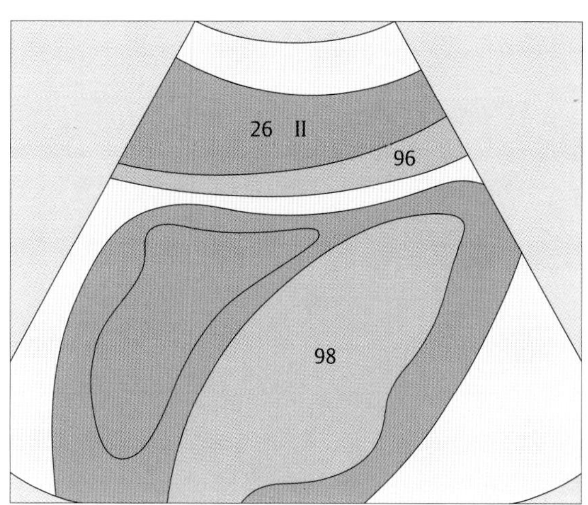

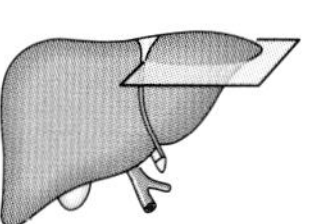

The left lobe of the liver is in close proximity to the heart, separated from it only by the diaphragm.

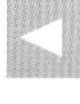

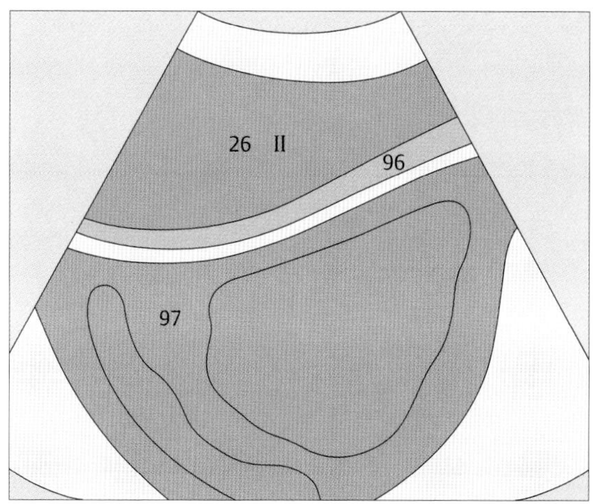

The anatomical left lobe of the liver corresponds to the lateral hepatic segment.

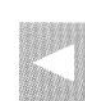

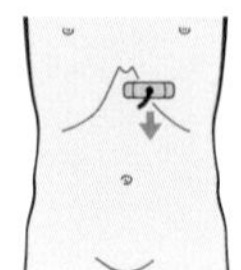

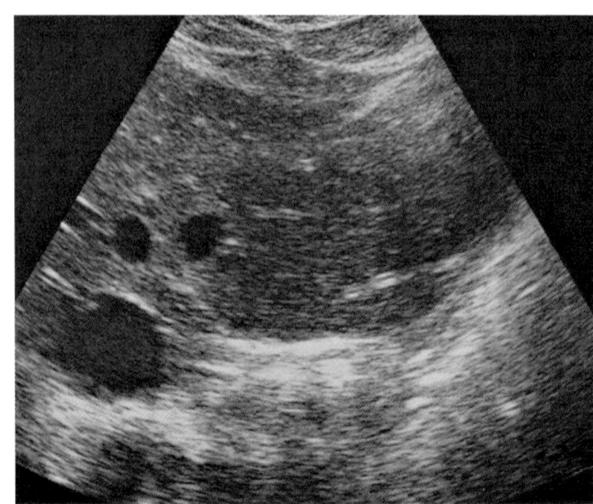

▶ **73** Left lobe of liver, lateral segment, hepatic veins

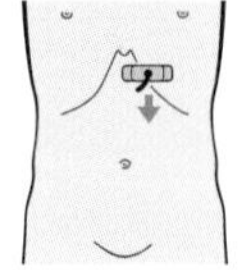

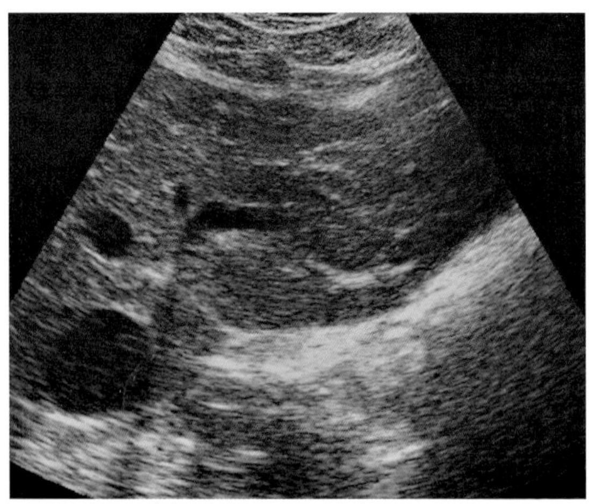

▶ **74** Left lobe of liver, lateral segment, caudate lobe

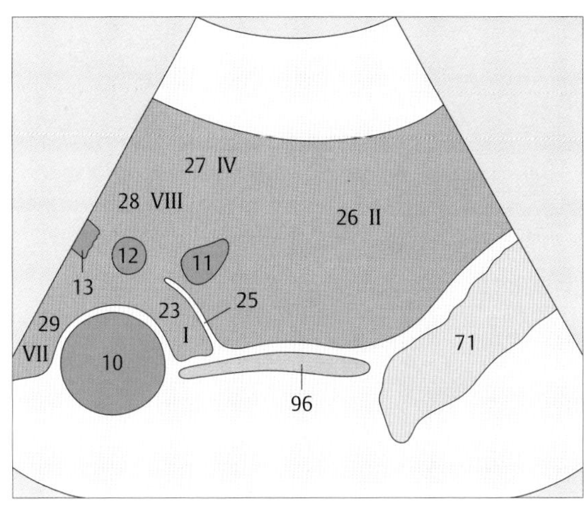

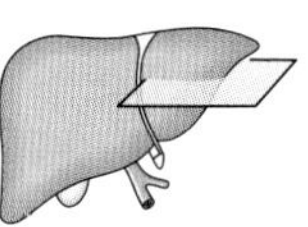

The left hepatic vein marks the boundary between the lateral and medial hepatic segments.

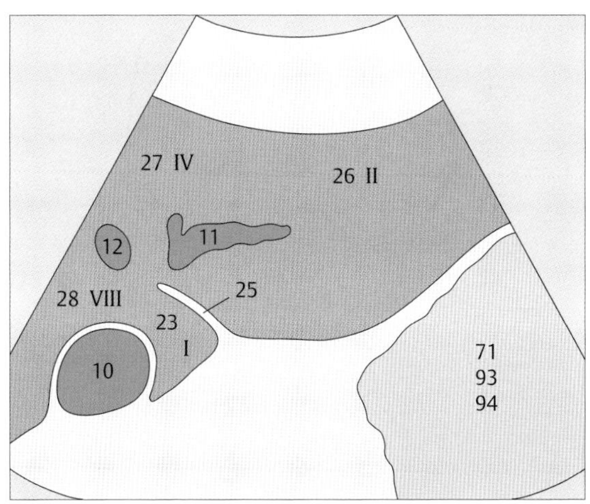

The cranial part of the lateral hepatic segment is designated as subsegment II.

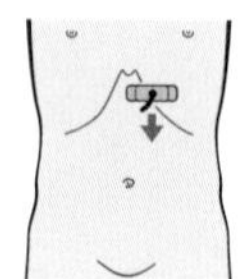

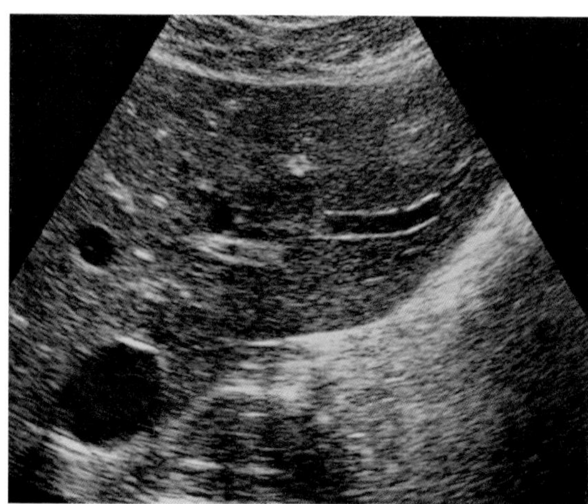

▶ **75** Left lobe of liver, lateral segment, caudate lobe

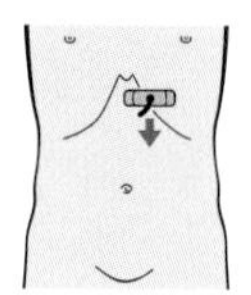

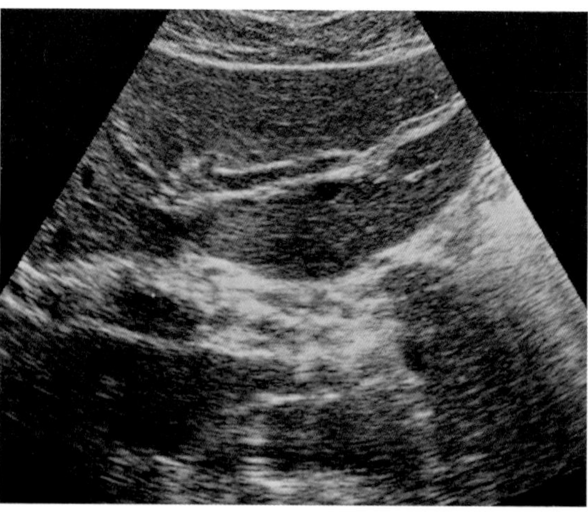

▶ **76** Left lobe of liver, lateral segment, left portal vein branch

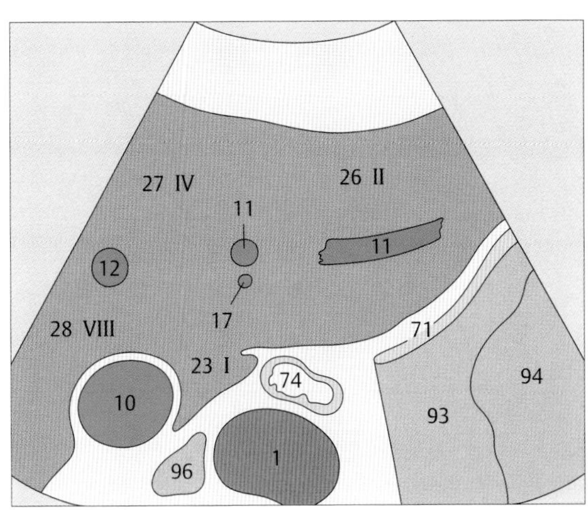

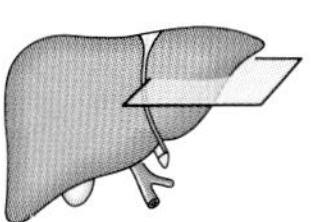

The caudate lobe is considered a separate entity, designated as subsegment I.

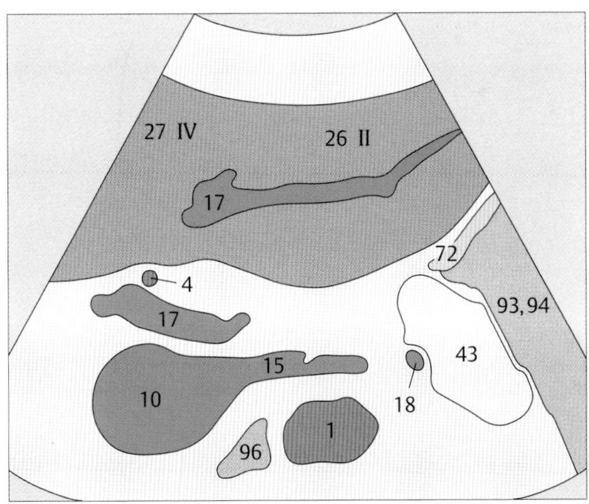

In scanning down the left lobe of the liver, the left branch of the portal vein marks the boundary between the cranial and caudal subsegments of the lobe.

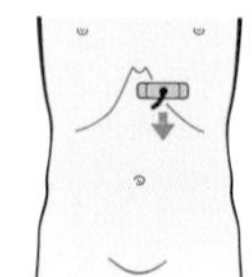

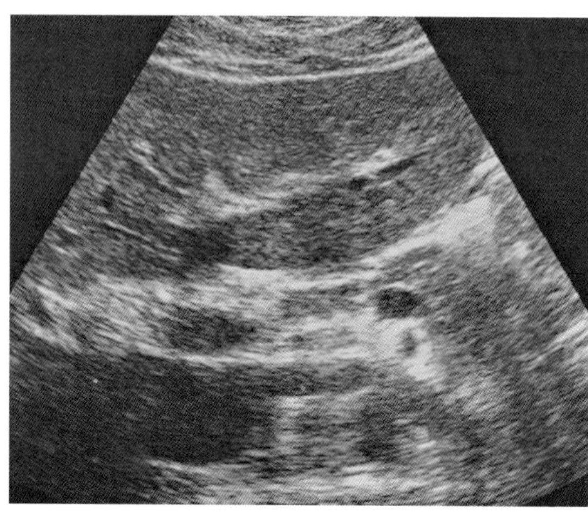

▶ **77** Left lobe of liver, lateral segment, ligamentum teres

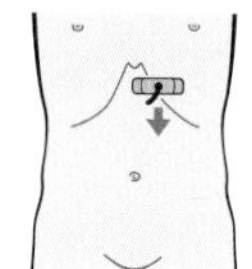

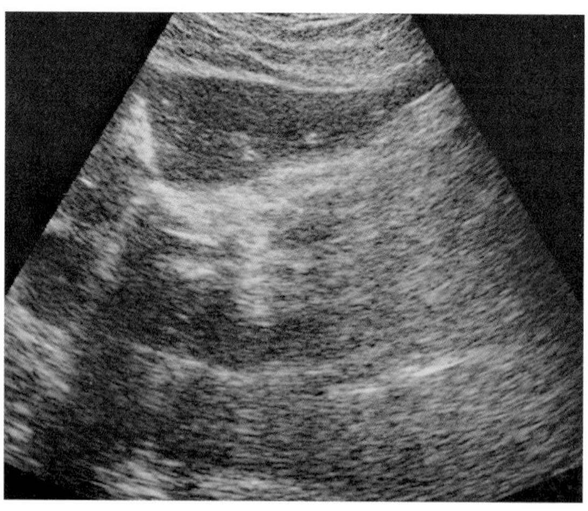

▶ **78** Left lobe of liver, subsegment III, ligamentum teres

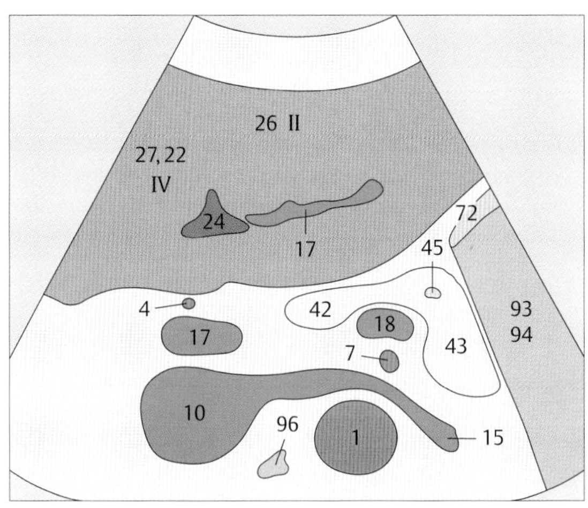

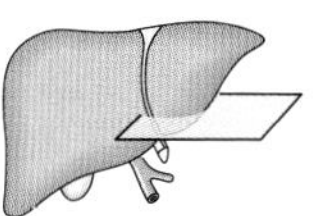

Ligamentum teres arises directly from the left portal vein branch and runs forward and downward.

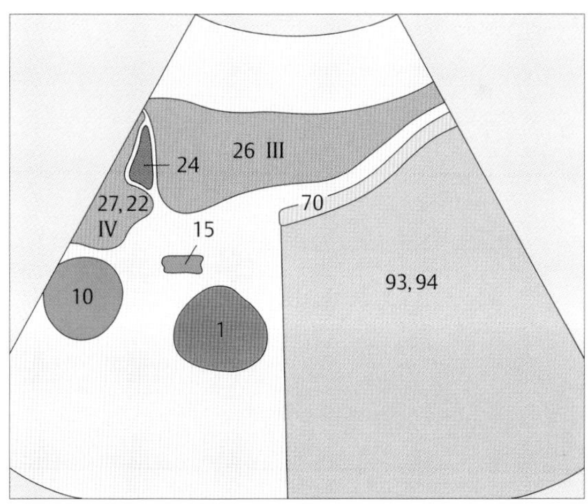

Ligamentum teres presents a triangular or polygonal shape in cross section. It marks the boundary between subsegment III and the quadrate lobe, which is designated as subsegment IVb.

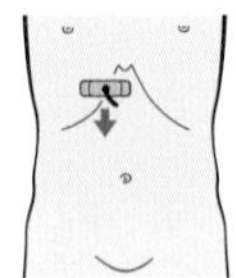

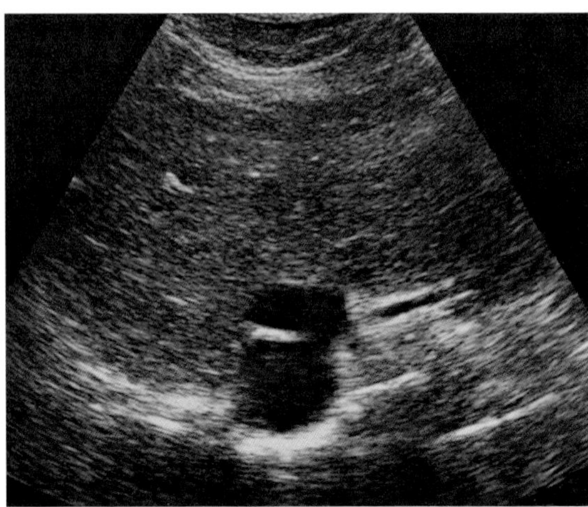

▶ **79** Medial and anterior hepatic segments, opening of hepatic veins

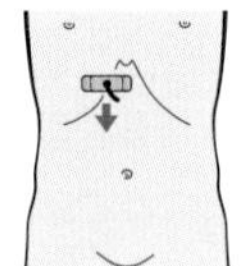

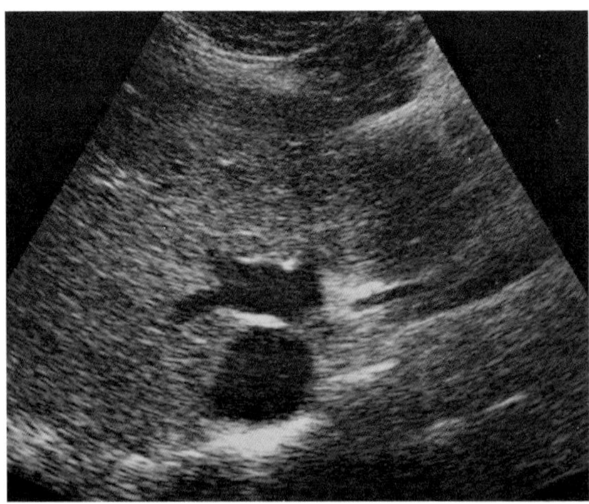

▶ **80** Medial and anterior hepatic segments, opening of hepatic veins

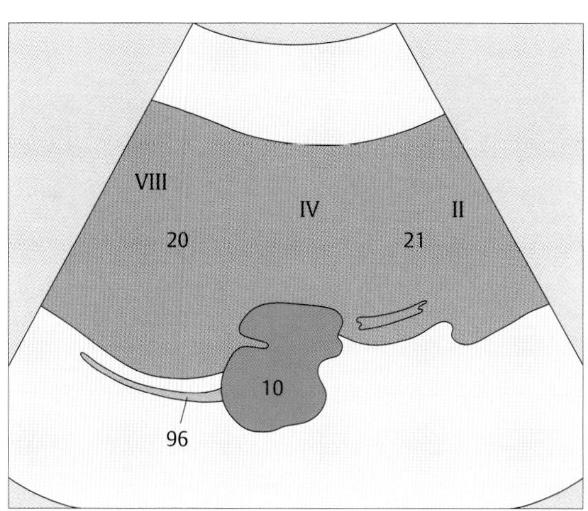

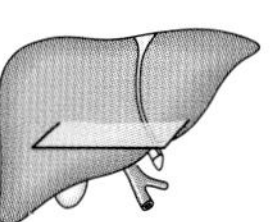

The hepatic veins converge and enter the vena cava just below the diaphragm.

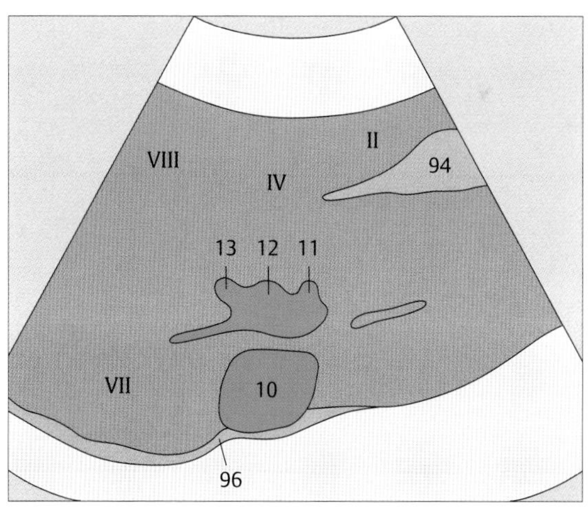

The opening of the hepatic veins at the vena cava forms a typical stellate pattern in transverse section.

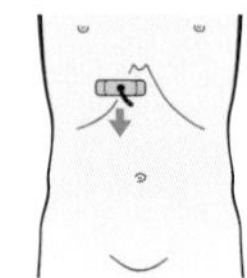

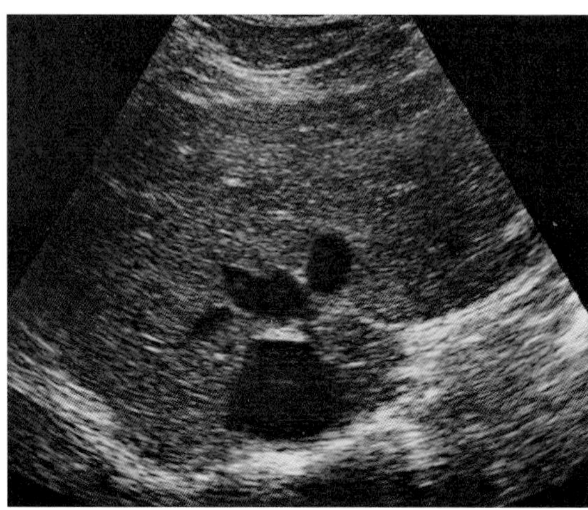

▶ **81** Medial and anterior hepatic segments, hepatic veins, caudate lobe

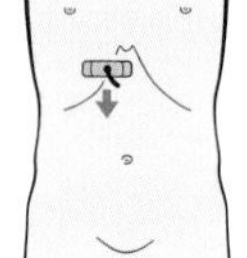

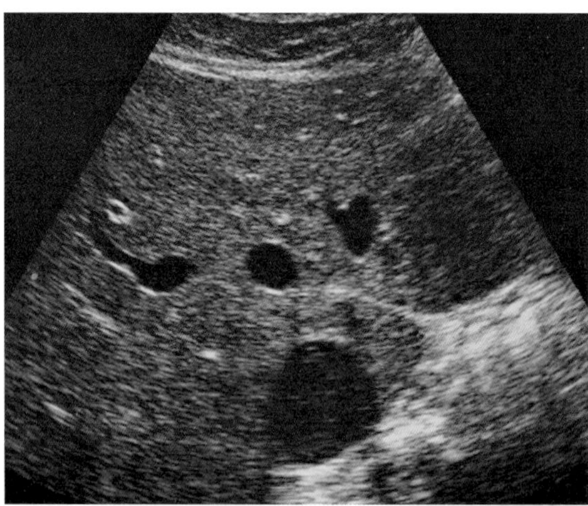

▶ **82** Medial and anterior hepatic segments, hepatic veins, caudate lobe

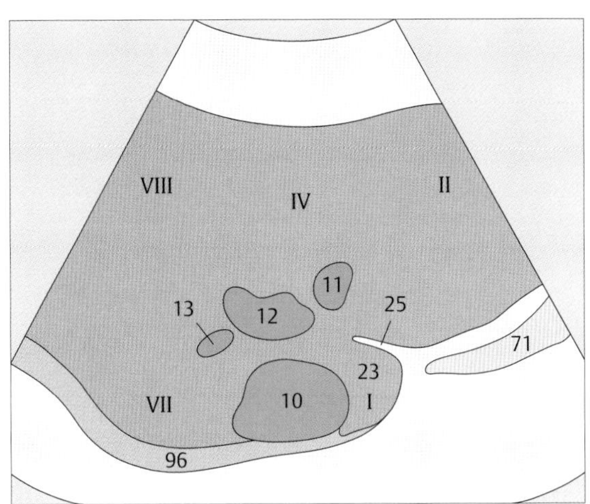

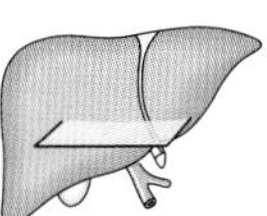

The upper pole of the caudate lobe extends to a point just below the opening of the hepatic veins into the vena cava.

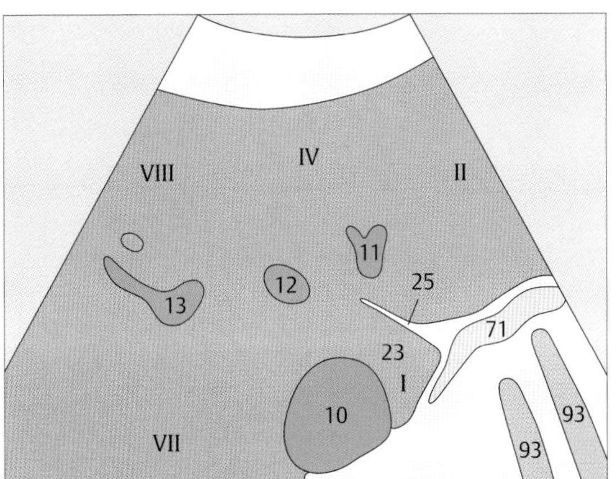

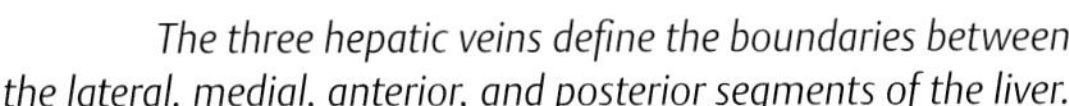

The three hepatic veins define the boundaries between the lateral, medial, anterior, and posterior segments of the liver.

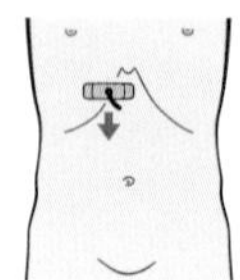

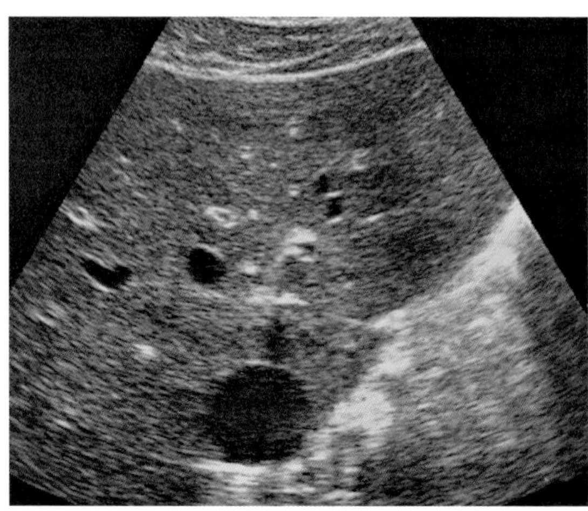

▶ **83** Medial and anterior hepatic segments, caudate lobe

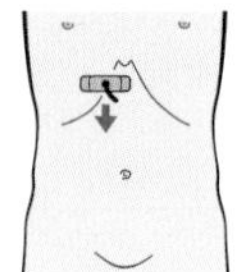

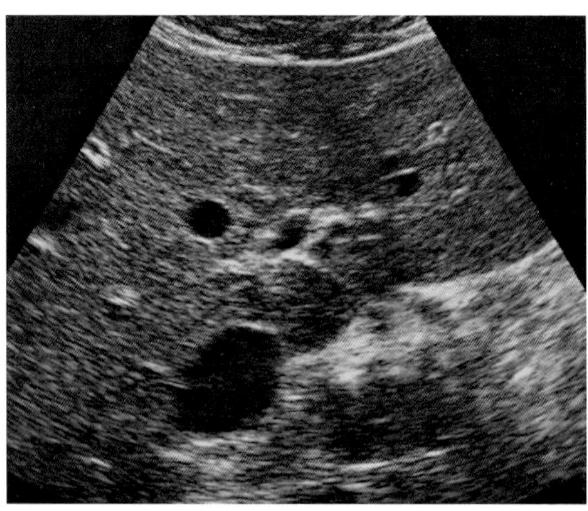

▶ **84** Medial and anterior hepatic segments, left portal vein branch, caudate lobe

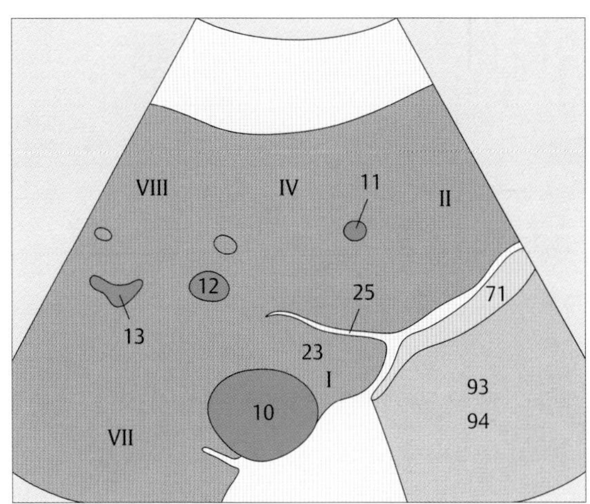

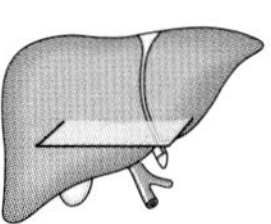

Ligamentum venosum separates the caudate lobe from subsegment II of the lateral hepatic segment.

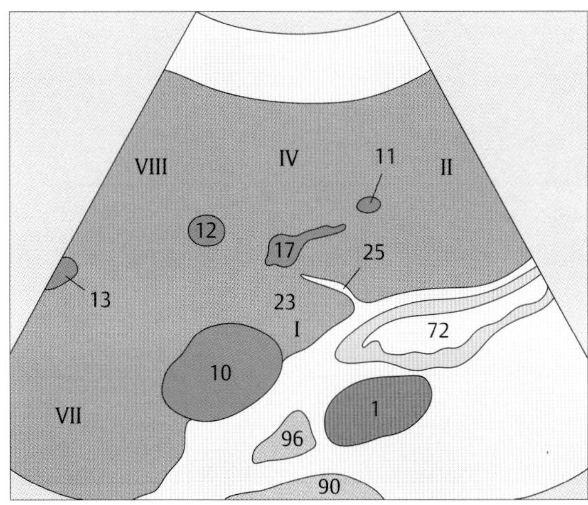

The caudate lobe of the liver is designated as subsegment I.

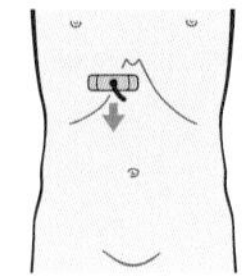

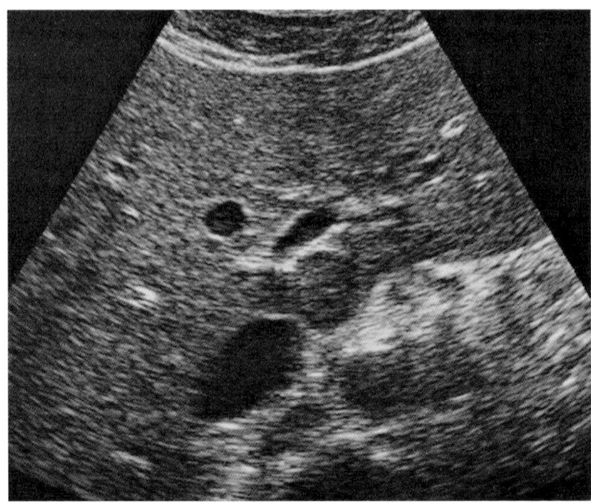

▶ **85** Medial and anterior hepatic segments, left portal vein branch, caudate lobe

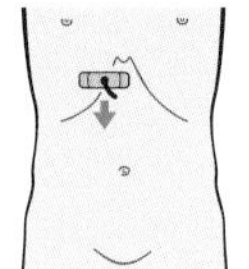

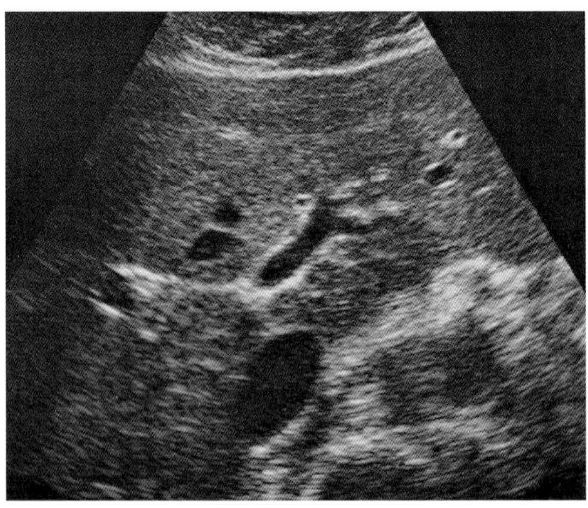

▶ **86** Medial and anterior hepatic segments, left portal vein branch, caudate lobe

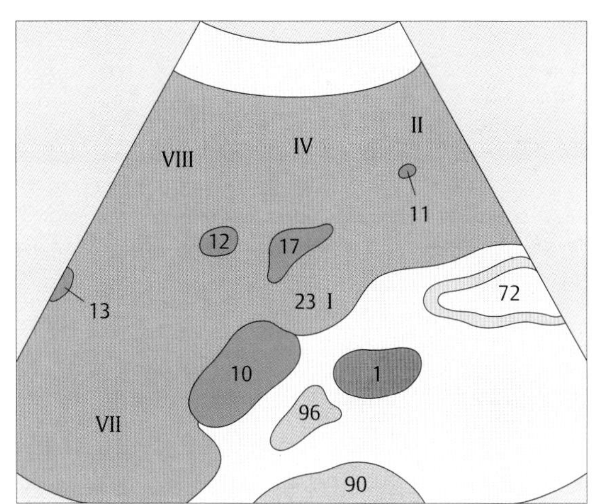

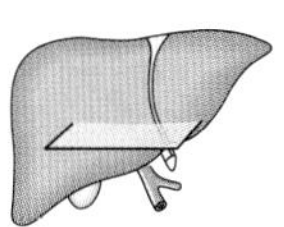

The caudate lobe is interposed between the vena cava and left portal vein branch.

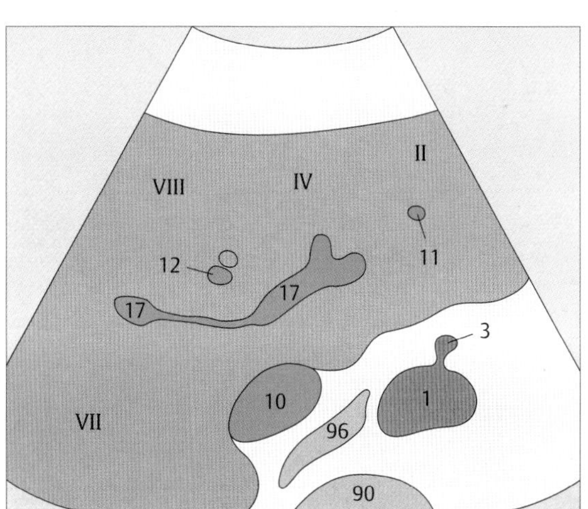

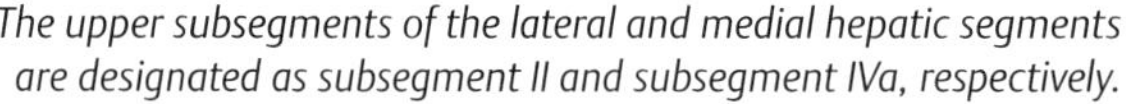

The upper subsegments of the lateral and medial hepatic segments are designated as subsegment II and subsegment IVa, respectively.

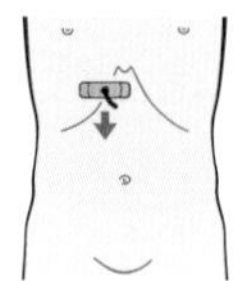

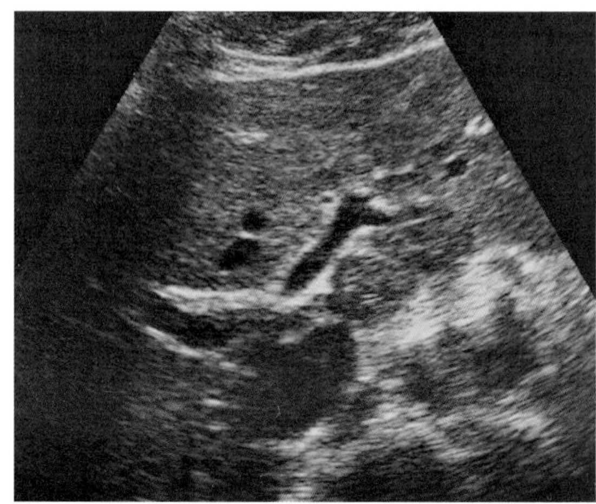

▶ **87** Medial and anterior hepatic segments, bifurcation of portal vein

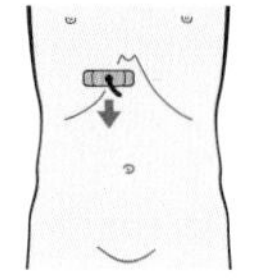

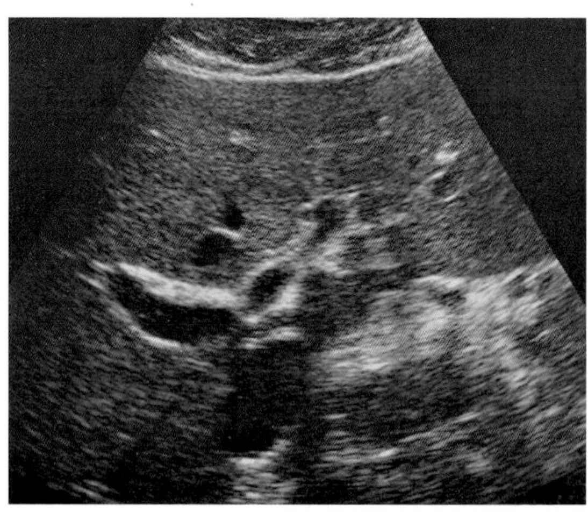

▶ **88** Medial and anterior hepatic segments, bifurcation of portal vein

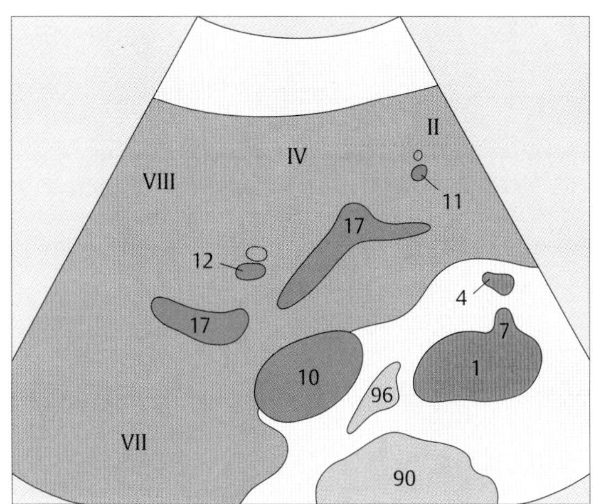

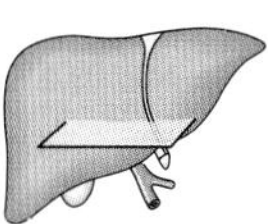

The upper subsegments of the anterior and posterior hepatic segments are designated as subsegments VIII and VII.

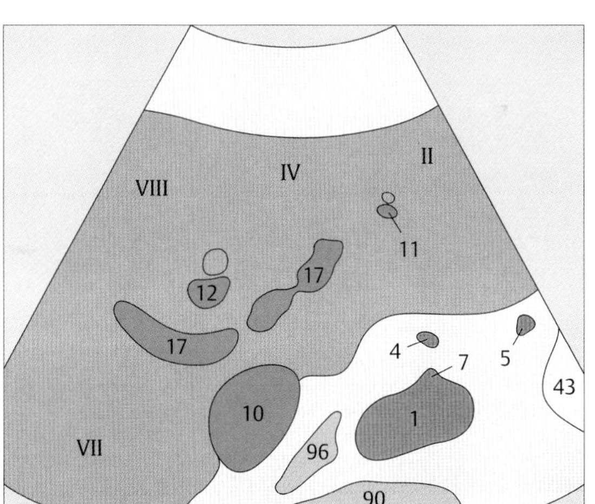

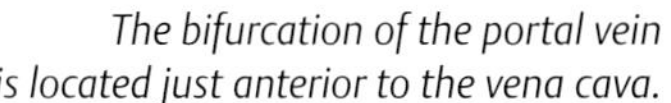

The bifurcation of the portal vein is located just anterior to the vena cava.

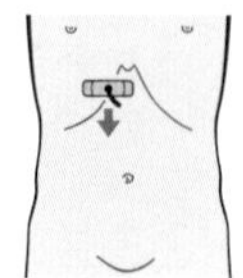

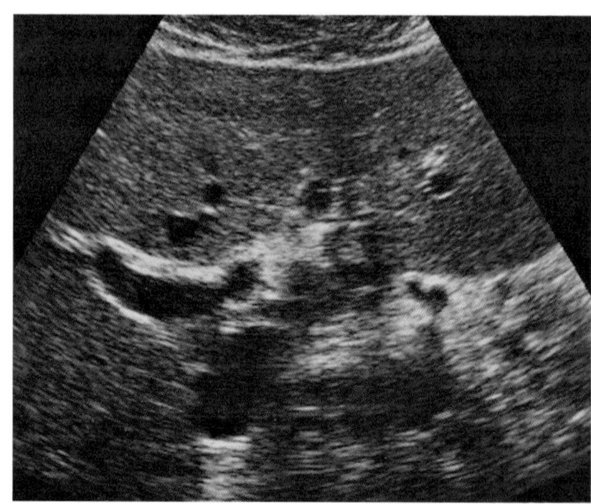

89 Medial and anterior hepatic segments, right portal vein branch

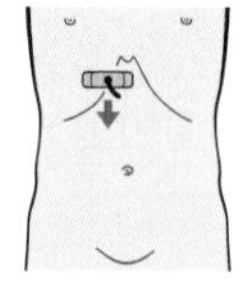

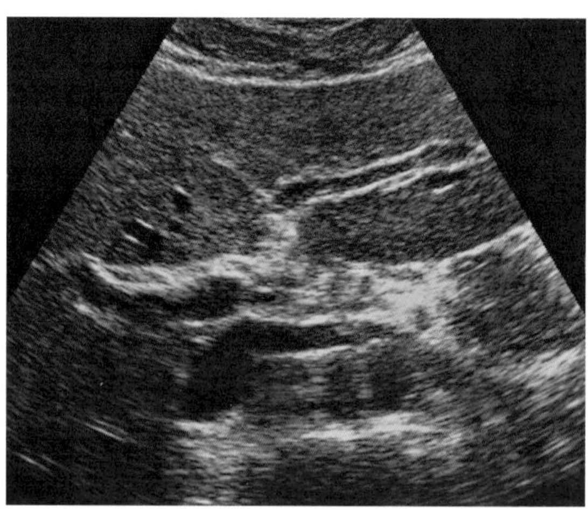

90 Medial and anterior hepatic segments, right and left portal vein branches

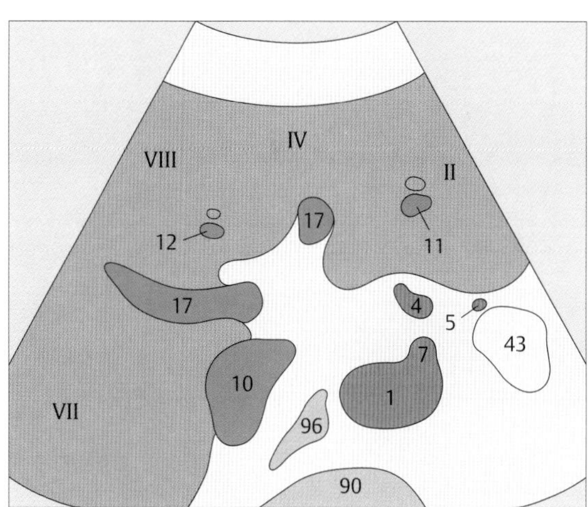

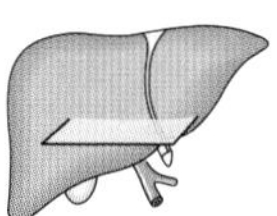

The division of the portal vein into right and left branches marks the approximate boundary between the upper and lower subsegments.

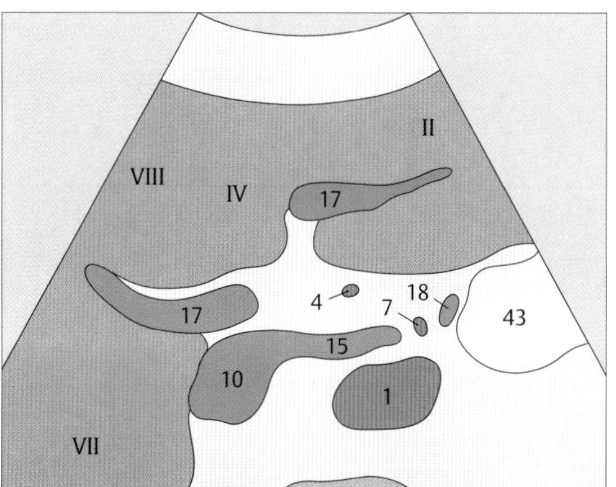

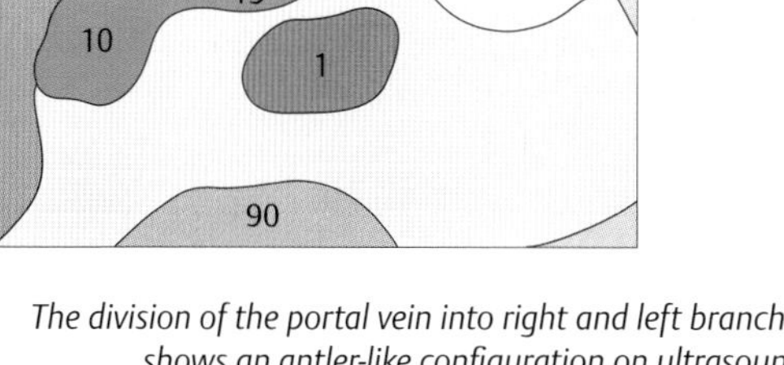

The division of the portal vein into right and left branches shows an antler-like configuration on ultrasound.

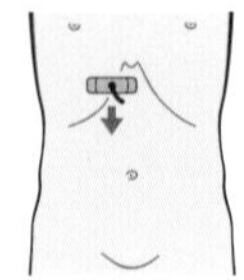

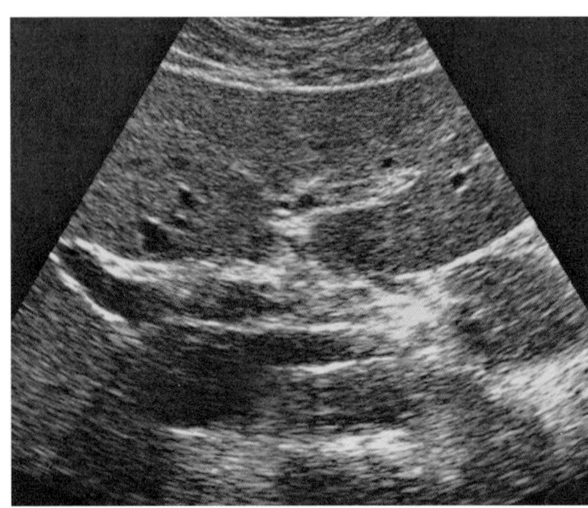

▶ **91** Medial and anterior hepatic segments, right and left portal vein branches

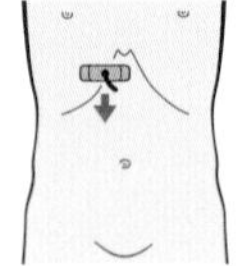

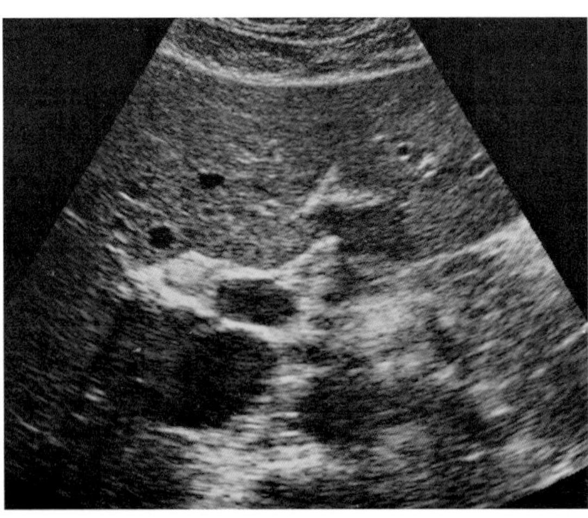

▶ **92** Medial and anterior hepatic segments, quadrate lobe, ligamentum teres, portal vein

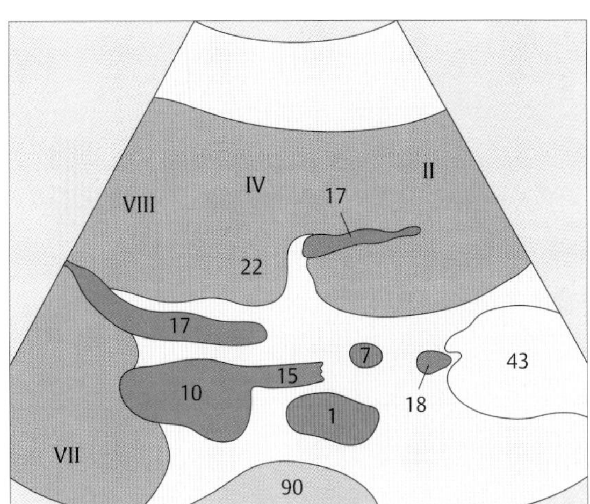

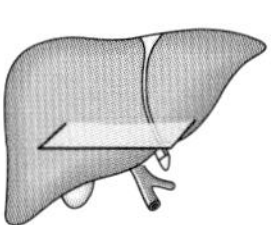

The right portal vein branch initially runs slightly caudally from the bifurcation.

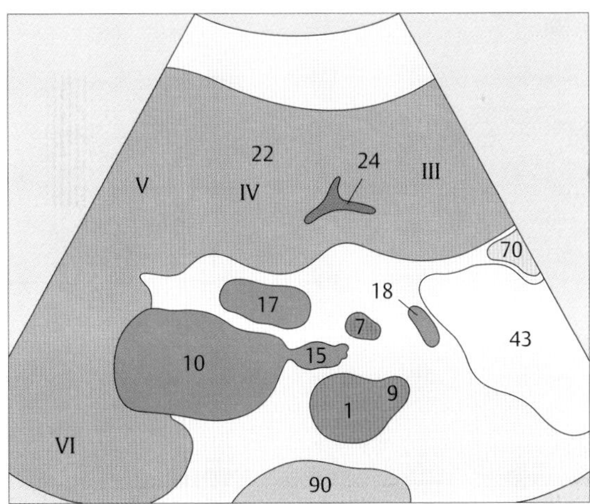

Ligamentum teres marks the boundary plane between the right and left lobes of the liver.

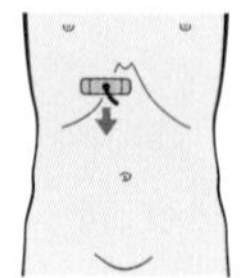

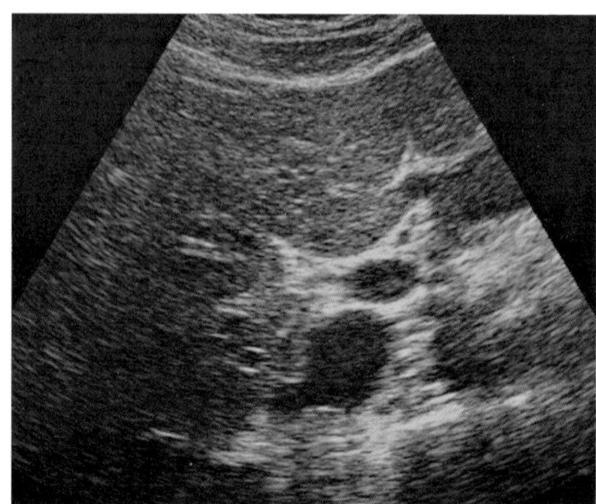

▶ **93** Medial and anterior hepatic segments, quadrate lobe, ligamentum teres, portal vein

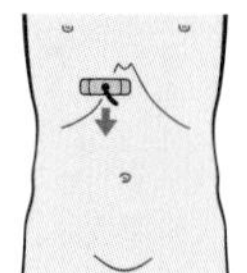

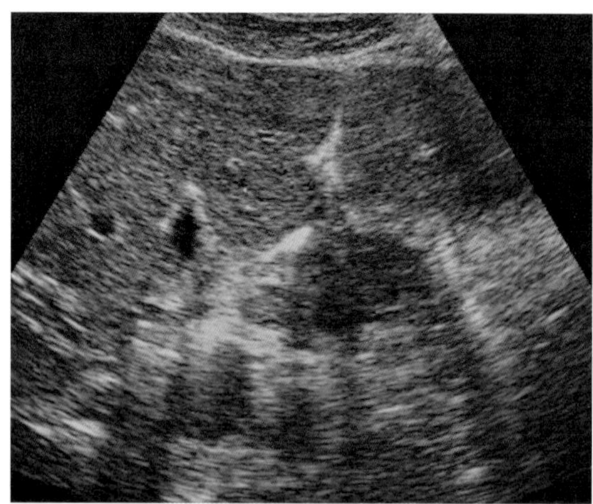

▶ **94** Medial and anterior hepatic segments, quadrate lobe, ligamentum teres, gallbladder

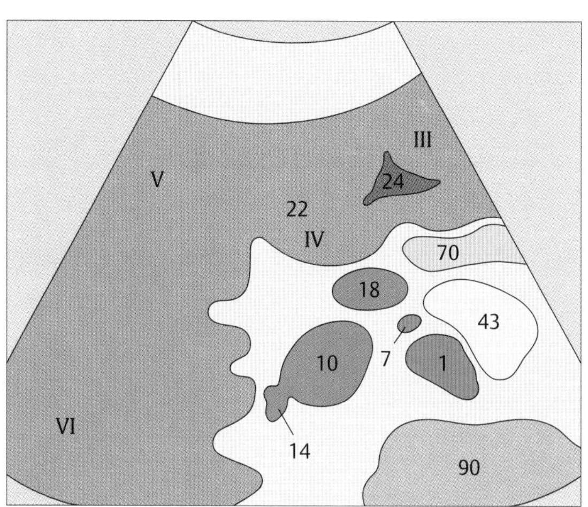

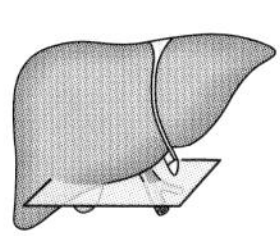

The lower subsegments of the lateral, medial, anterior, and posterior hepatic segments are designated, respectively, subsegments III, IVb, V, and VI.

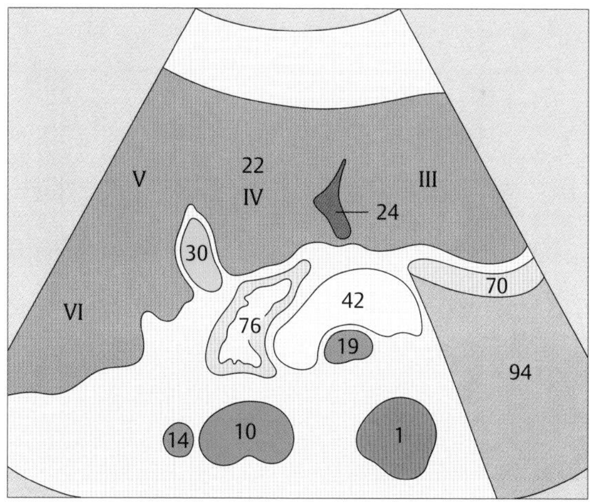

The gallbladder and ligamentum teres form the boundary structures of the quadrate lobe in transverse section.

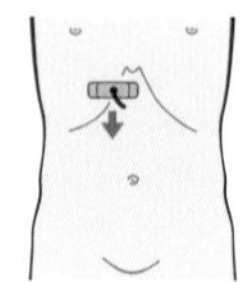

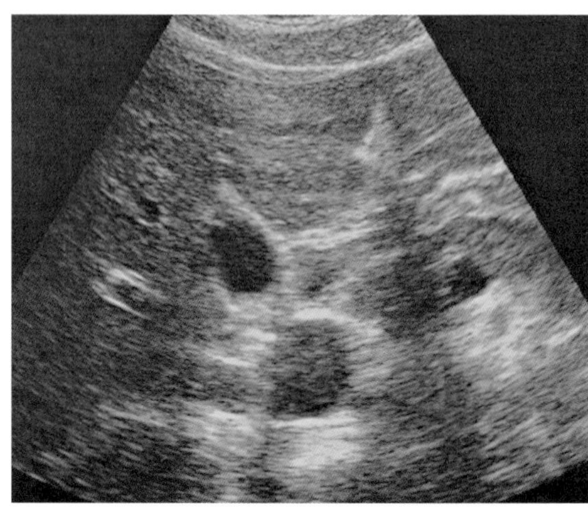

▶ **95** Medial and anterior hepatic segments, quadrate lobe, ligamentum teres, gallbladder

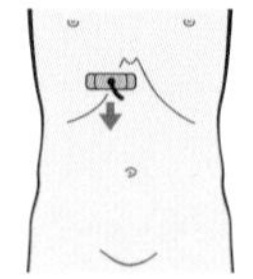

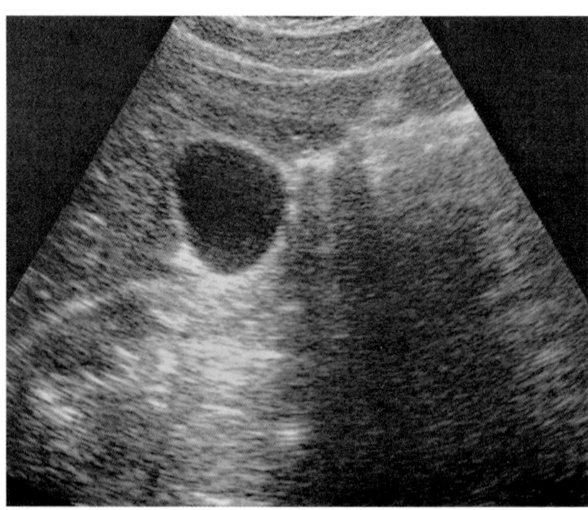

▶ **96** Inferior border of liver, kidney, gallbladder, ligamentum teres

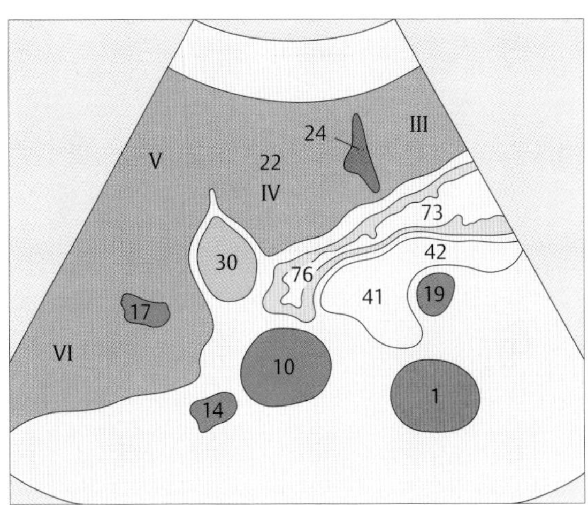

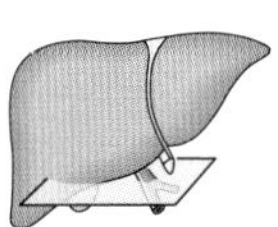

The vena cava–gallbladder plane marks the boundary between the right and left lobes of the liver based on functional criteria.

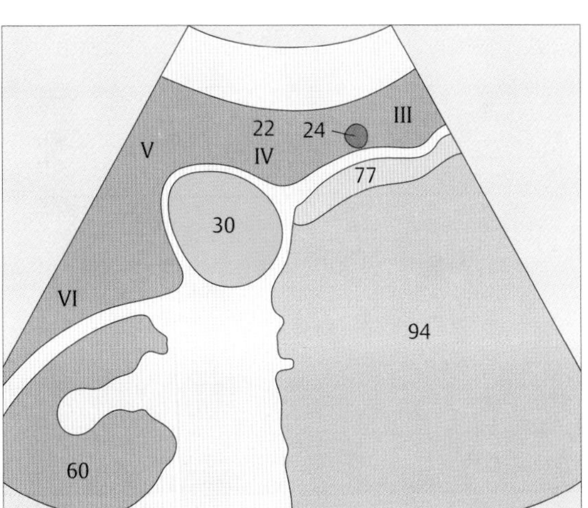

The shape of the inferior hepatic border is influenced by the kidney, the gallbladder, and the groove for ligamentum teres.

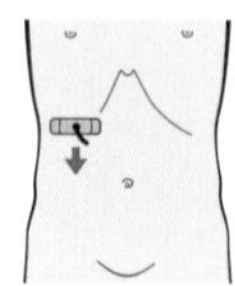

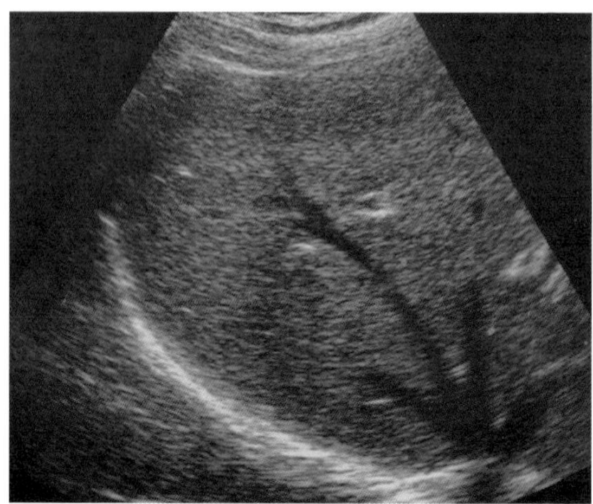

▶ **97** Posterior segment, upper subsegment

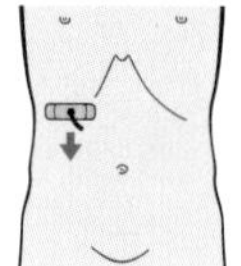

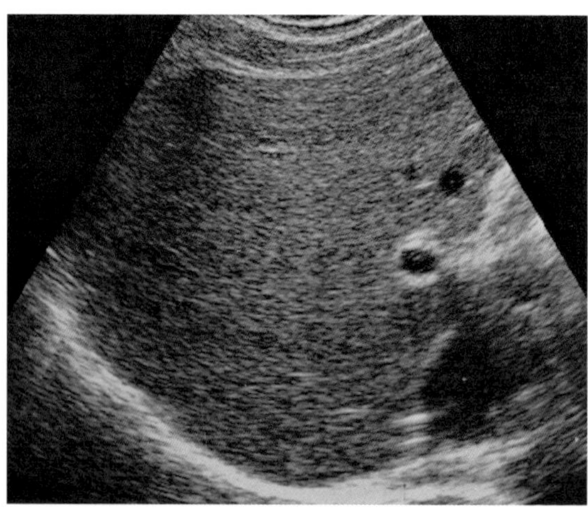

▶ **98** Posterior segment, portal vein

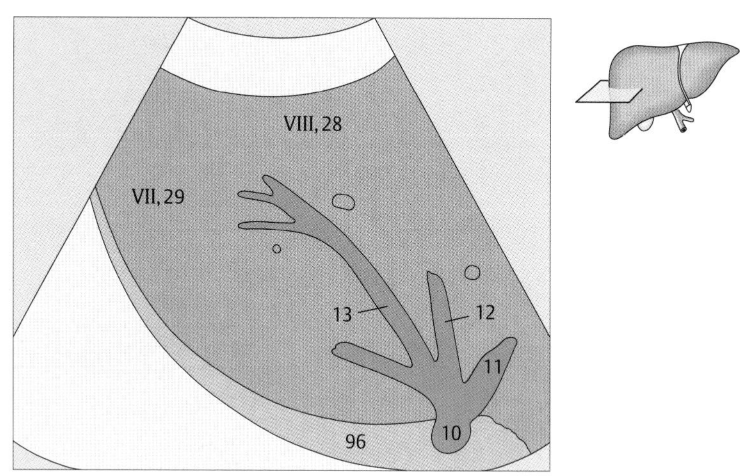

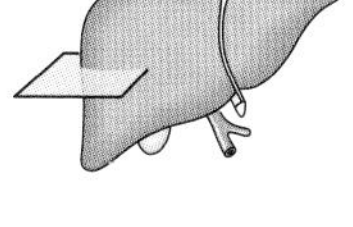

The upper subsegment of the posterior hepatic segment is designated as subsegment VII.

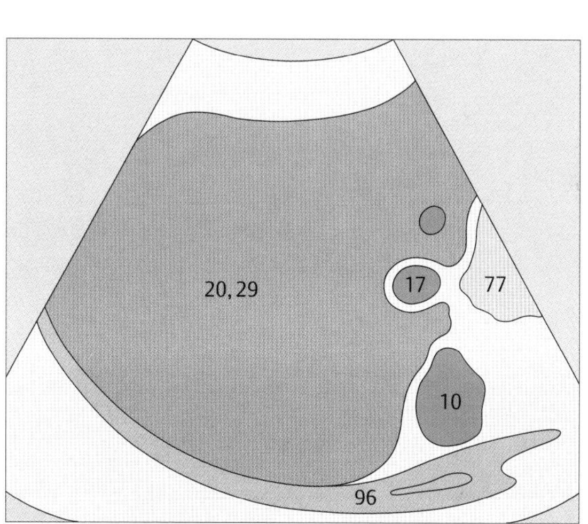

The right portal vein branch marks the approximate boundary between subsegment VII cranially and subsegment V caudally.

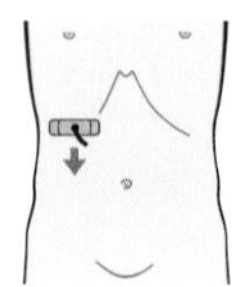

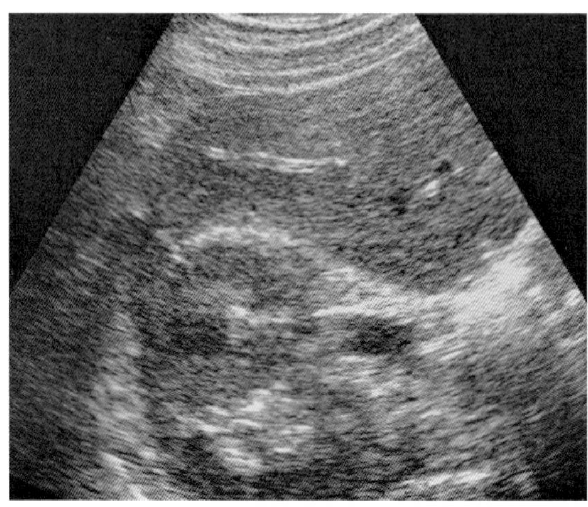

▶ **99** Posterior segment, lower subsegment, kidney

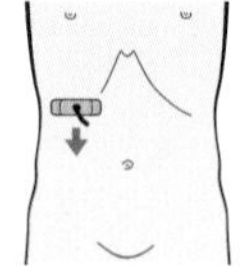

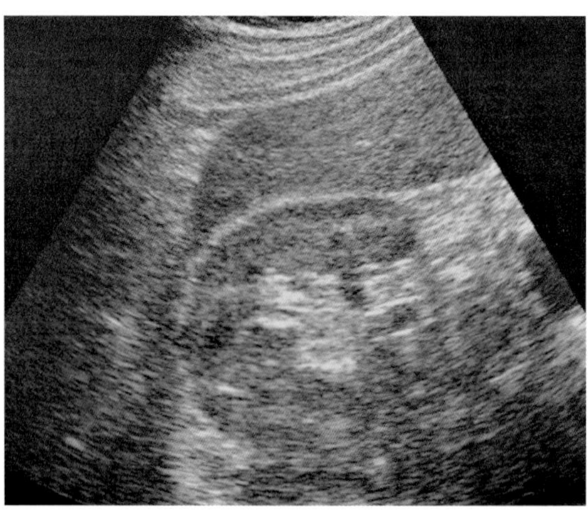

▶ **100** Posterior segment, inferior border

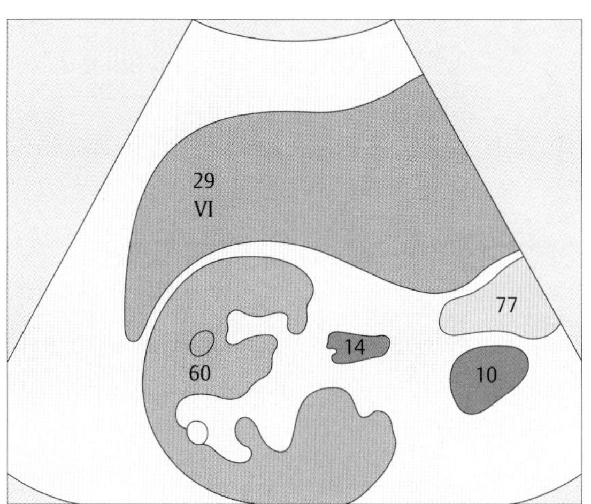

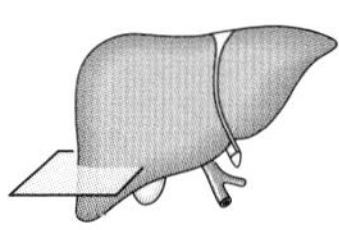

The lower subsegment of the posterior hepatic segment is designated as subsegment VI.

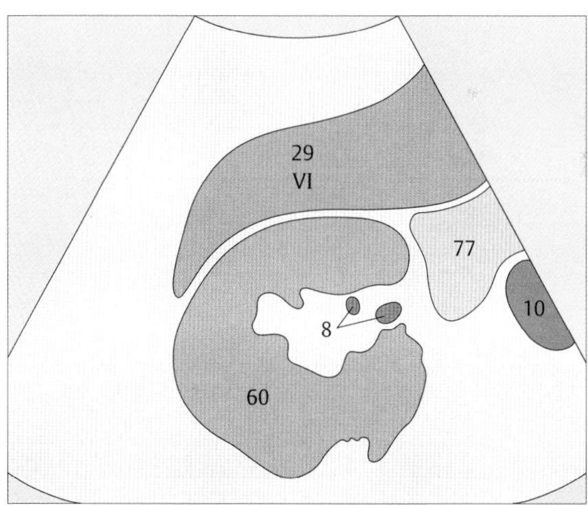

The right lobe of the liver is highly variable in its inferior extent.

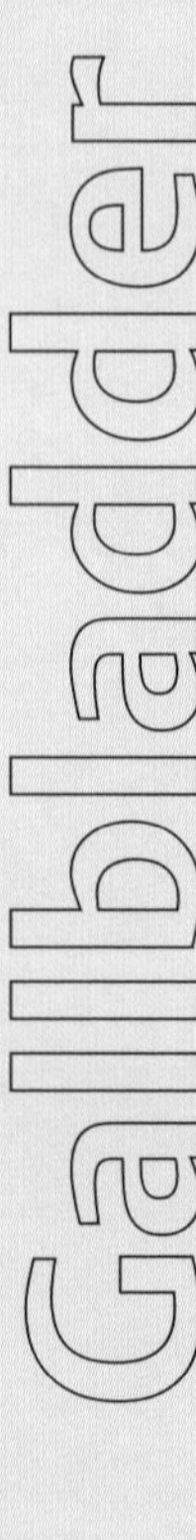

3 Gallbladder

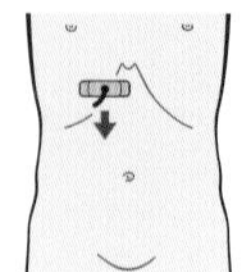

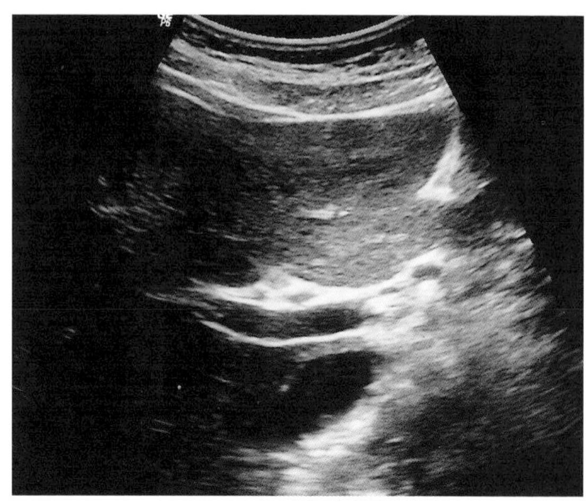

▶ **101** Right branch of the portal vein, ligamentum venosum

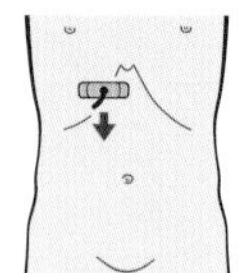

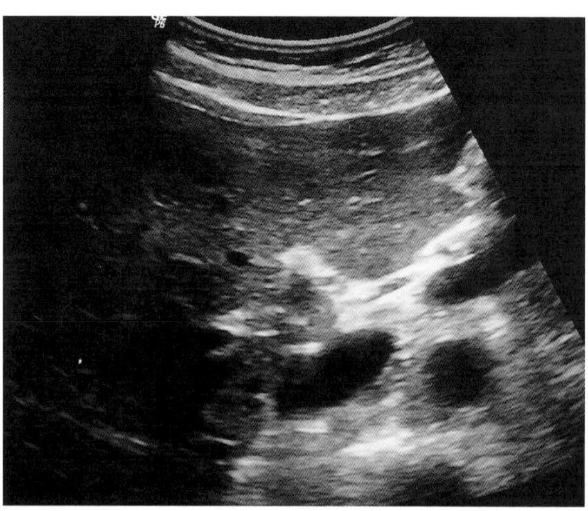

▶ **102** Portal vein, ligamentum venosum

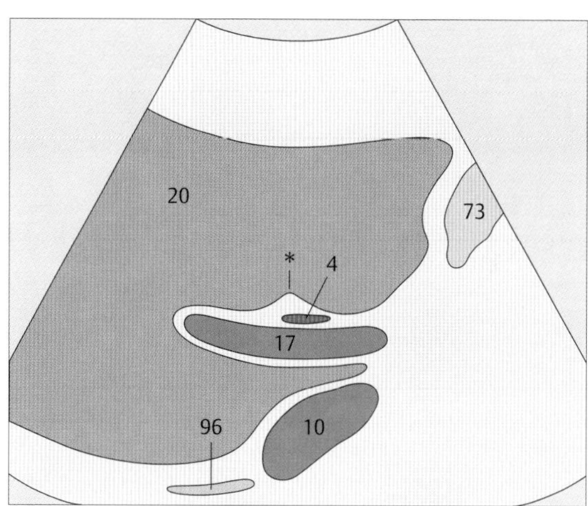

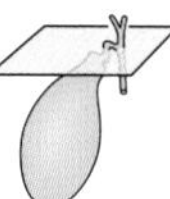

The interlobar fissure (*) anterior to the right branch of the portal vein is the key landmark for locating the gallbladder.

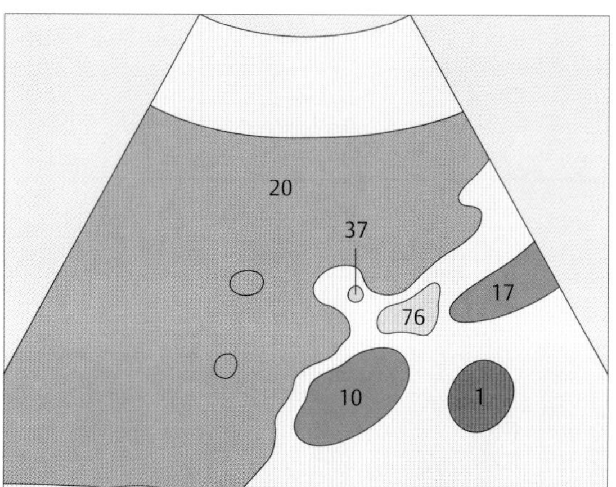

The gallbladder neck is located just caudal to the right portal vein branch and interlobar fissure.

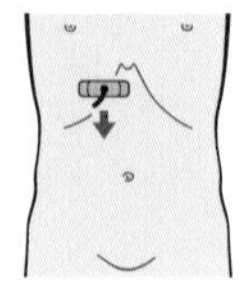

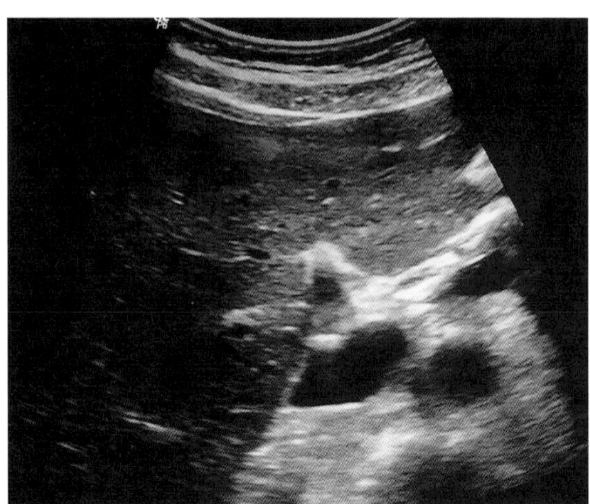

▶ **103** Neck of the gallbladder

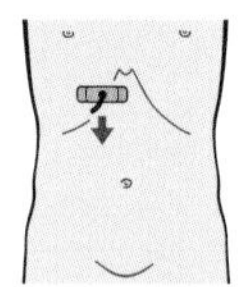

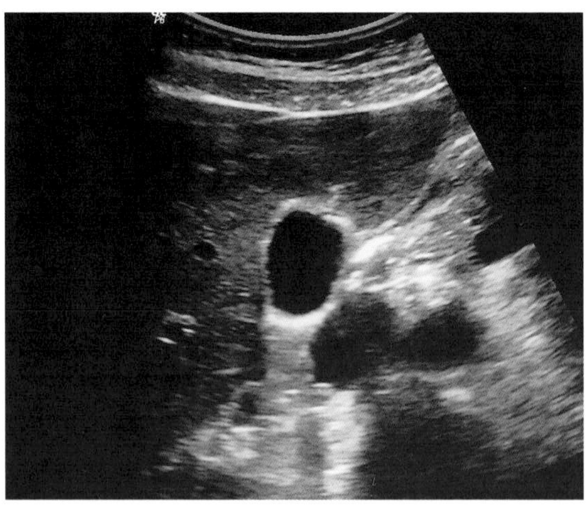

▶ **104** Junction of the neck and body of the gallbladder

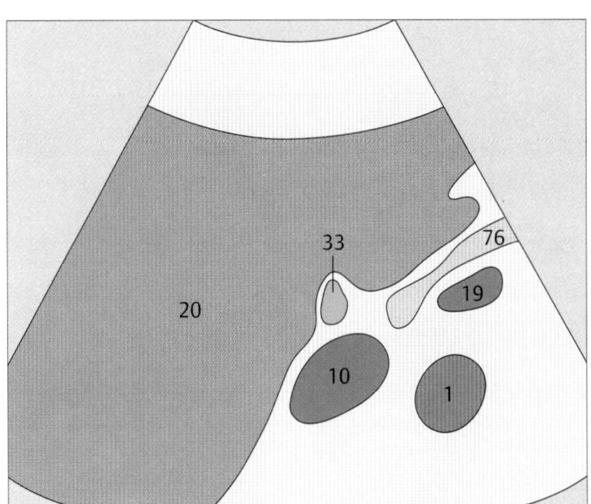

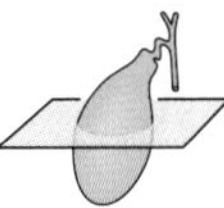

The duodenum is located medial to the neck of the gallbladder.

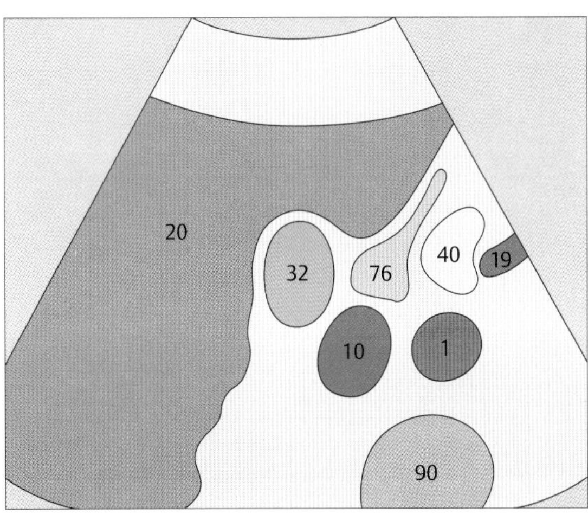

The duodenal bulb can be consistently identified on the free peritoneal side of the body or neck of the gallbladder.

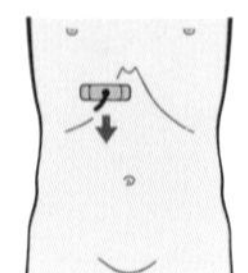

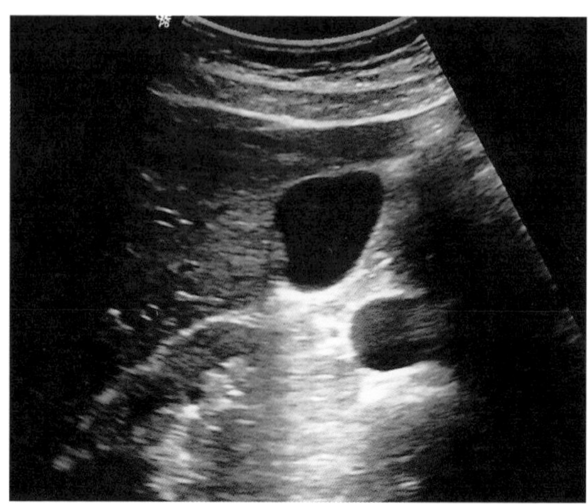

▶ **105** Body of the gallbladder

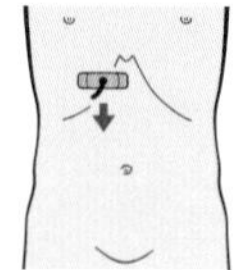

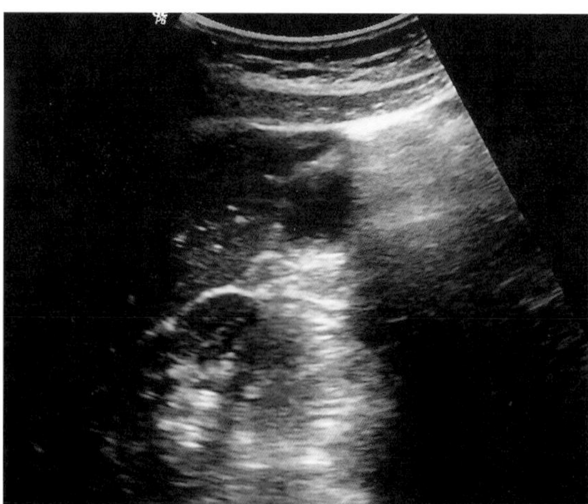

▶ **106** Gallbladder fundus

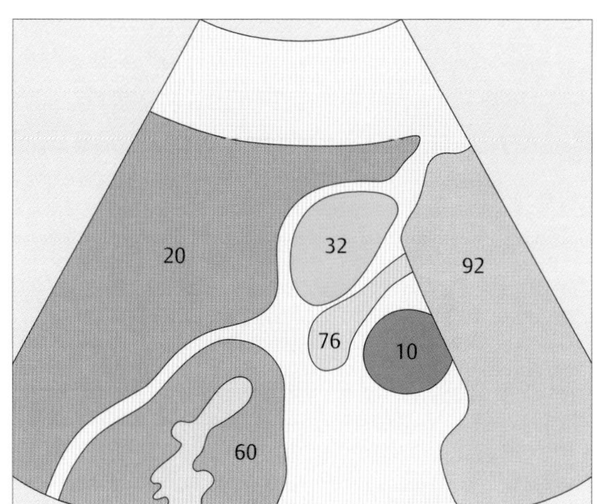

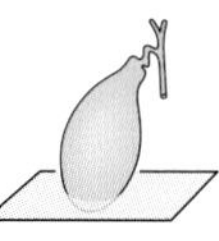

The duodenum passes between the body of the gallbladder and the vena cava.

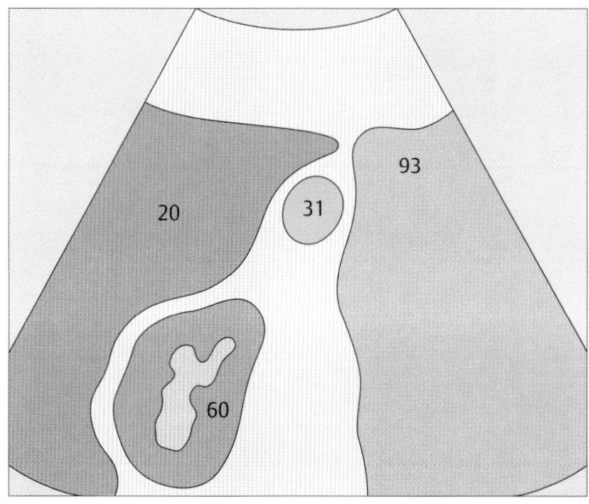

The gallbladder fundus may extend almost to the anterior wall of the trunk, or it may be situated very deeply behind the liver.

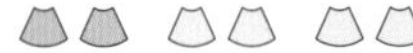

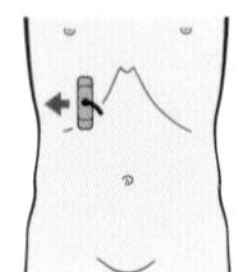

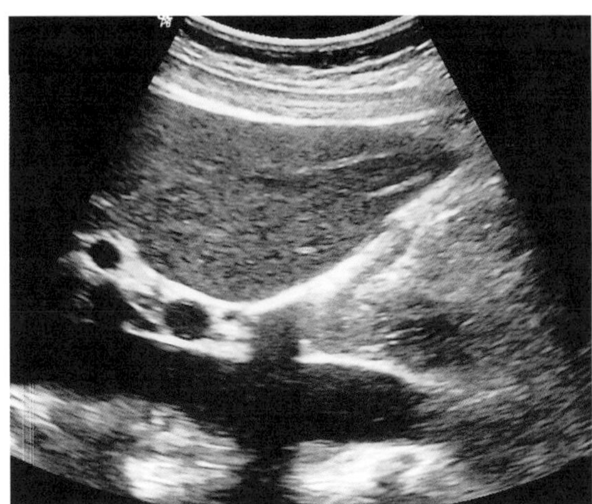

▶ **107** Vena cava, duodenum, portal vein bifurcation

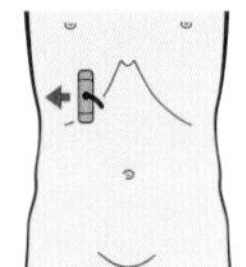

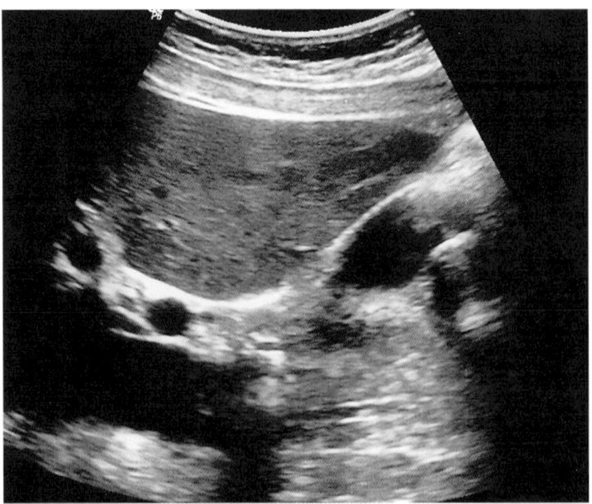

▶ **108** Body of the gallbladder, portal vein bifurcation

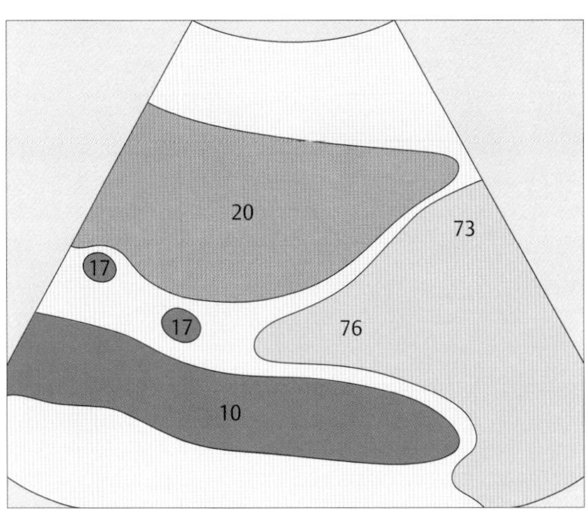

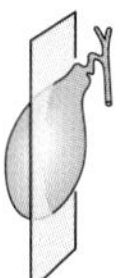

The vena cava, the portal vein bifurcation, and the echogenic band of the interlobar fissure are the principal landmarks for locating the gallbladder in longitudinal scans.

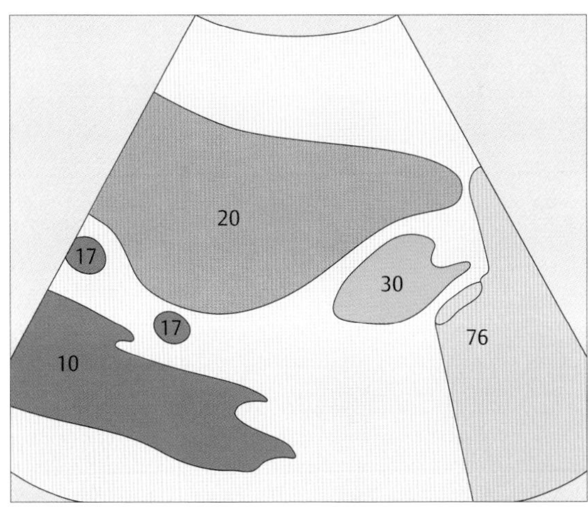

The duodenum is located posterior to the gallbladder and caudal to the right colic flexure.

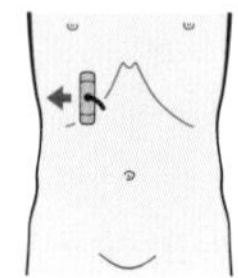

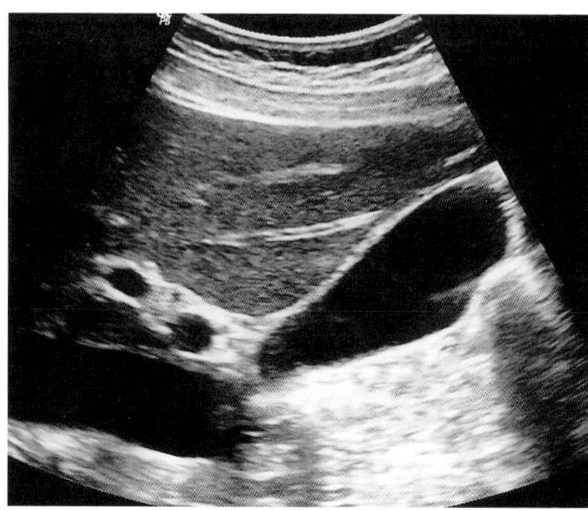

▶ **109** Gallbladder, portal vein

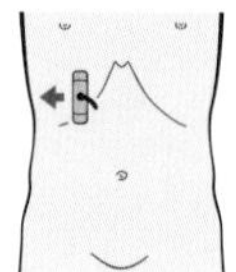

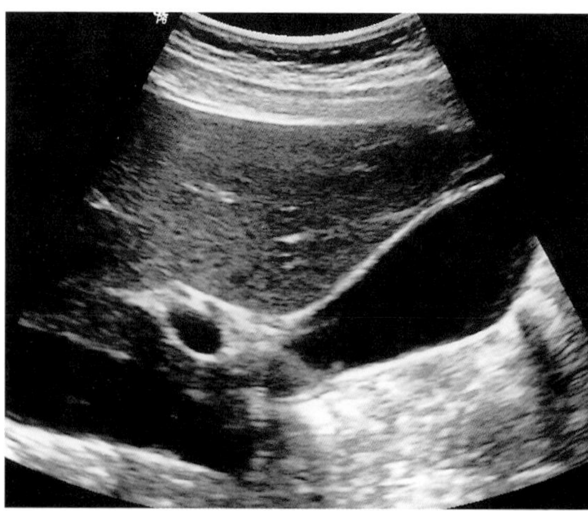

▶ **110** Gallbladder, portal vein

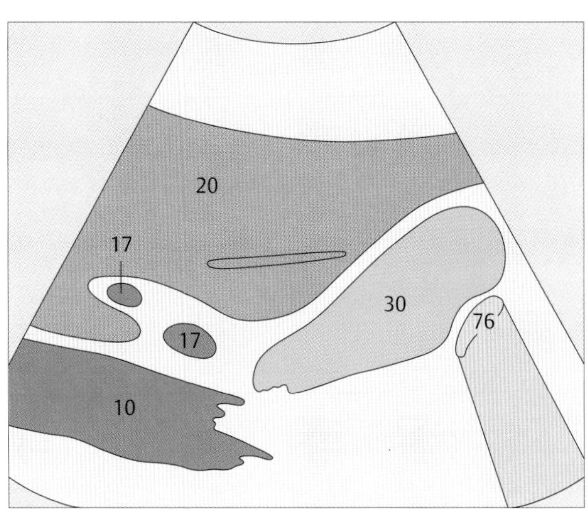

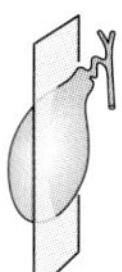

The shape and location of the gallbladder are highly variable. But the gallbladder neck is always located in the porta hepatis, caudal to the right branch of the portal vein.

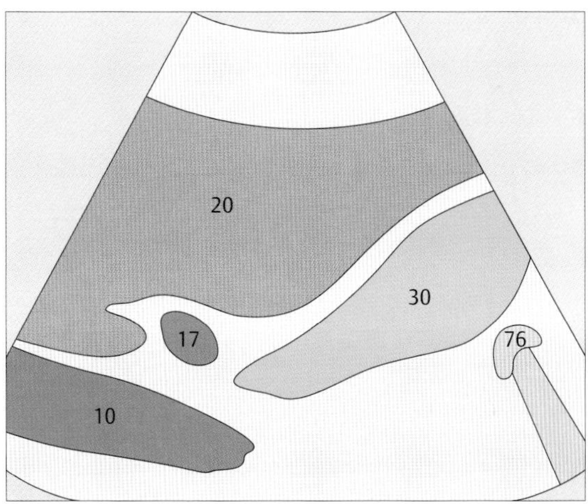

The healthy gallbladder is a fluid-filled organ, usually pear-shaped, that does not contain internal echoes.

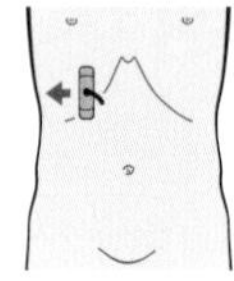

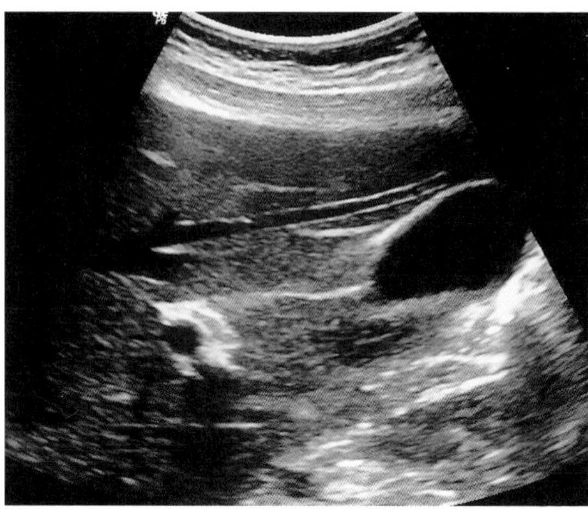

▶ **111** Gallbladder, portal vein, right kidney

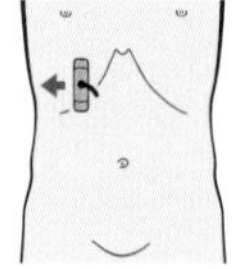

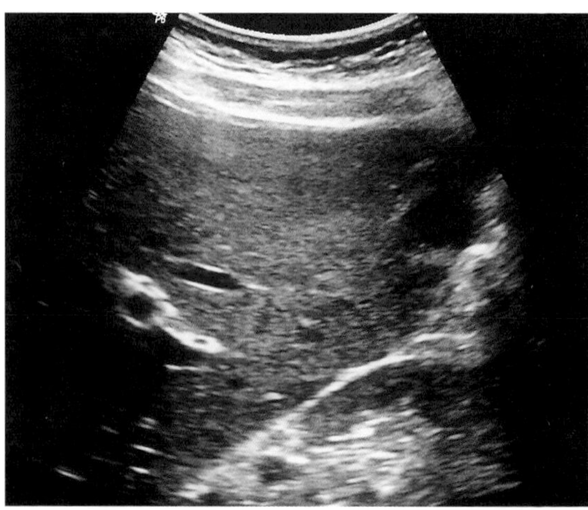

▶ **112** Gallbladder fundus, right kidney

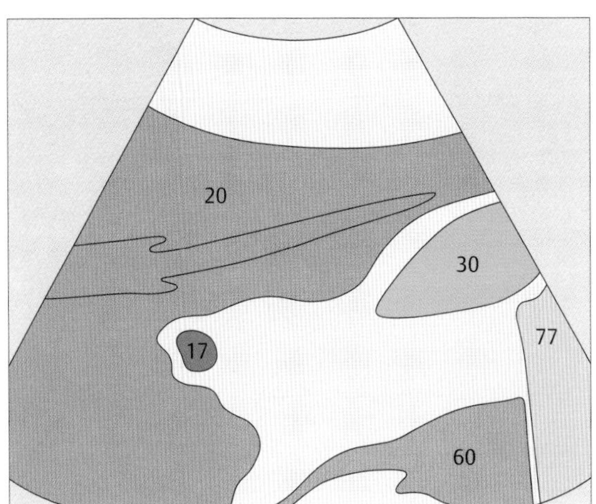

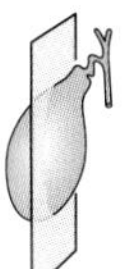

A variable-sized piece of liver is interposed between the gallbladder and kidney.

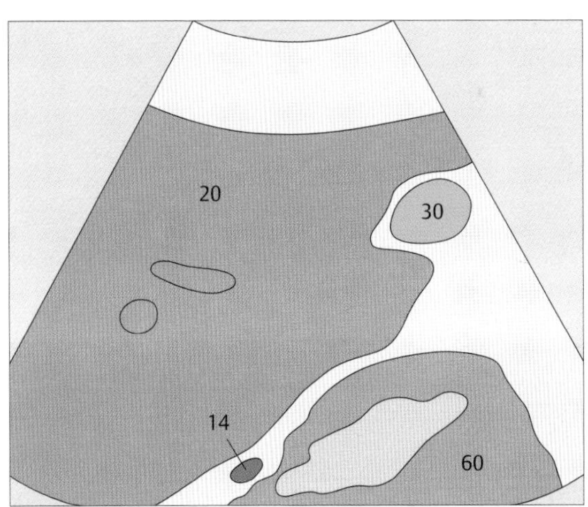

The gallbladder always borders directly on the right kidney, but it may appear separate from the kidney when scanned through its lateral portion.

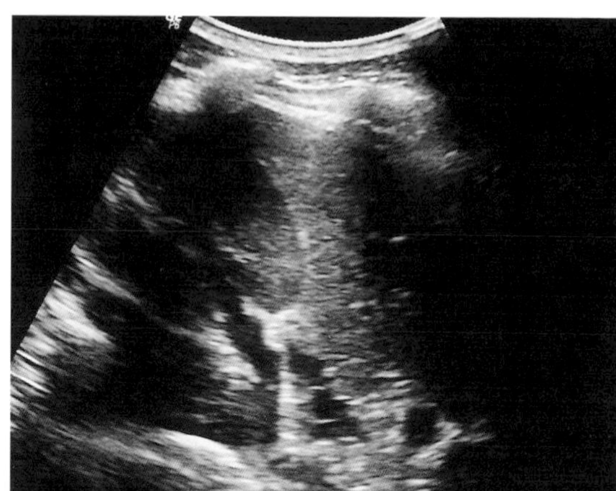

▶ **113** Gallbladder neck, duodenum, right kidney

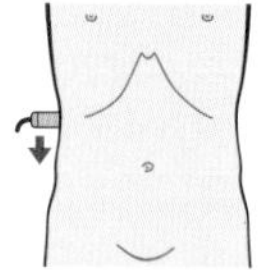

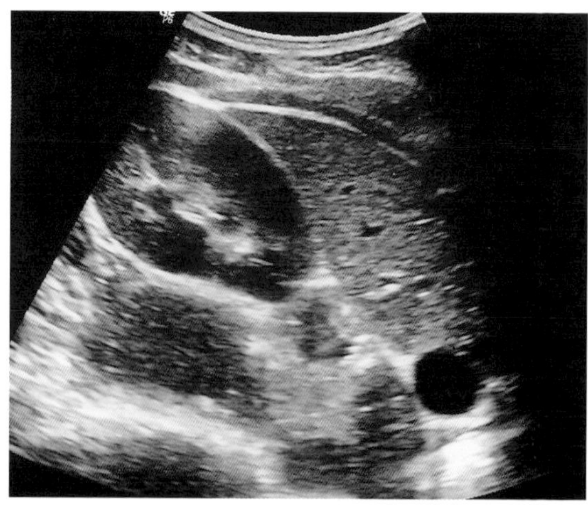

▶ **114** Gallbladder neck, small bowel, right kidney

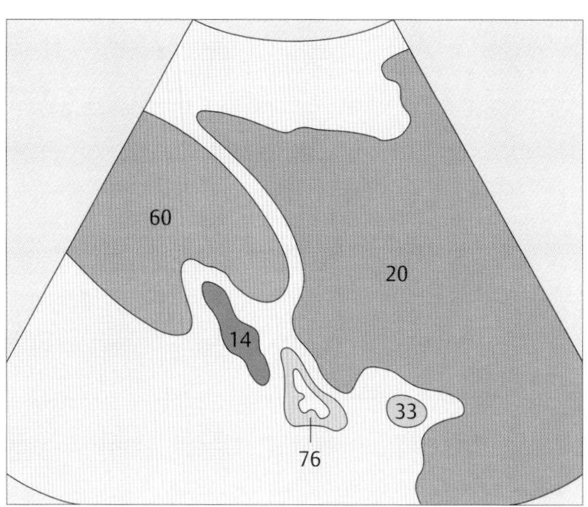

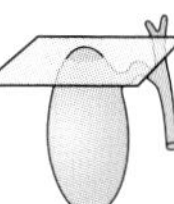

The gallbladder neck is identified at the level of the kidney in a high lateral transverse scan.

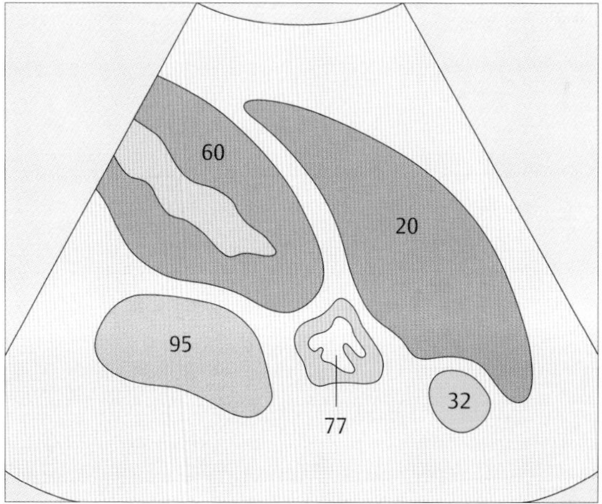

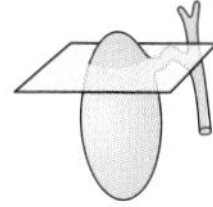

A scan through the gallbladder from the lateral side typically displays the triad of the gallbladder, kidney, and liver.

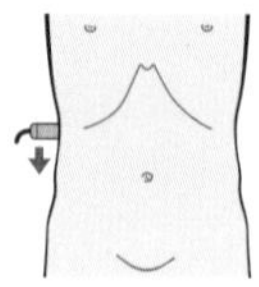

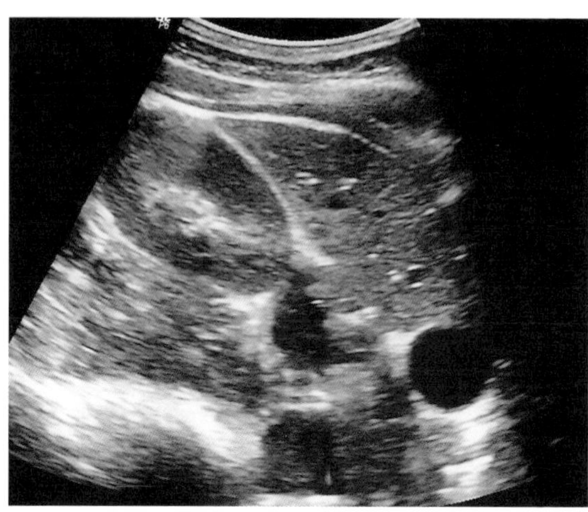

▶ **115** Gallbladder body, small bowel, right kidney

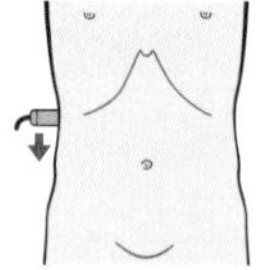

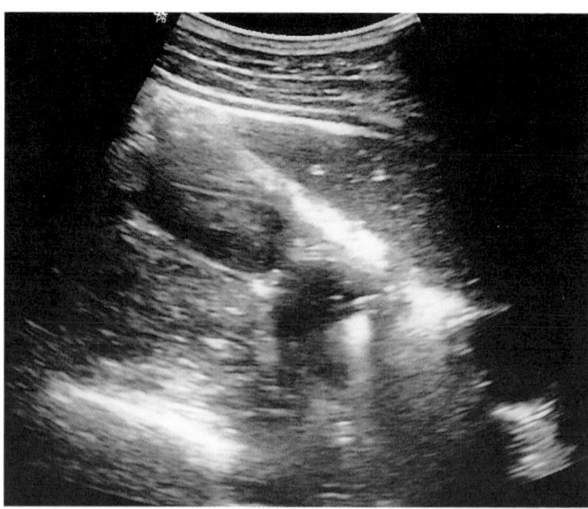

▶ **116** Gallbladder fundus, small bowel

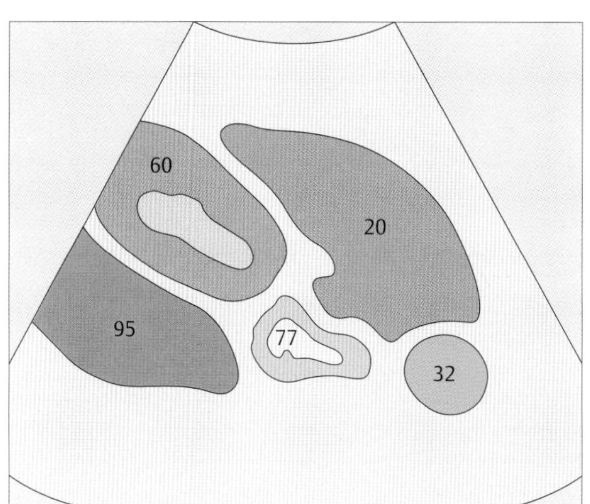

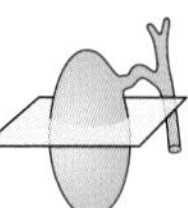

The gallbladder is often obscured by bowel gas when scanned from the lateral side.

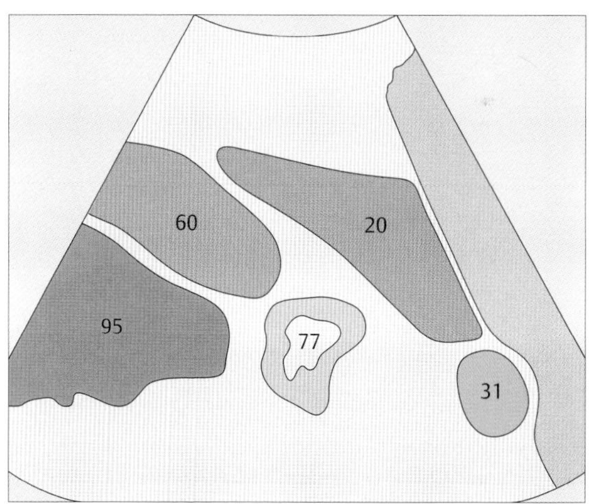

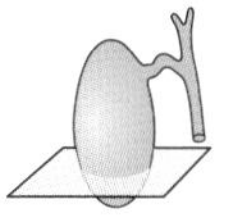

The gallbladder fundus may extend downward for some distance.

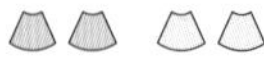

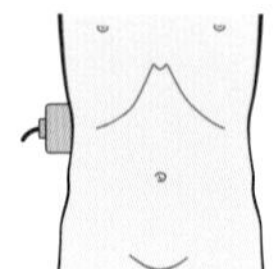

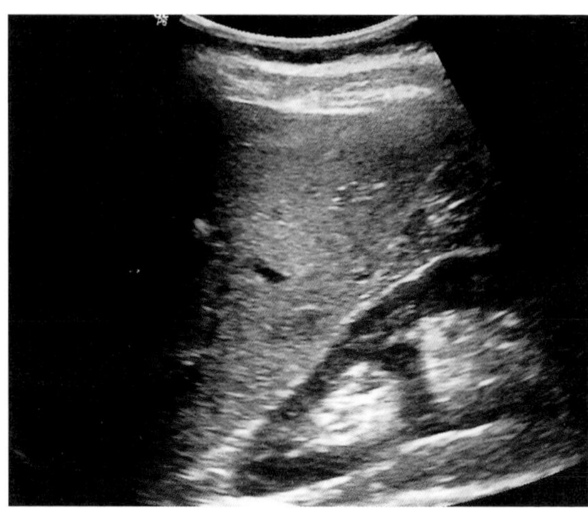

▶ **117** Right kidney, liver

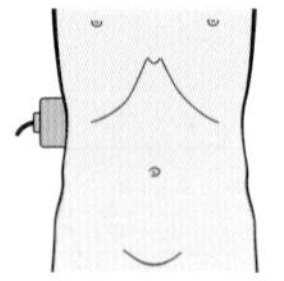

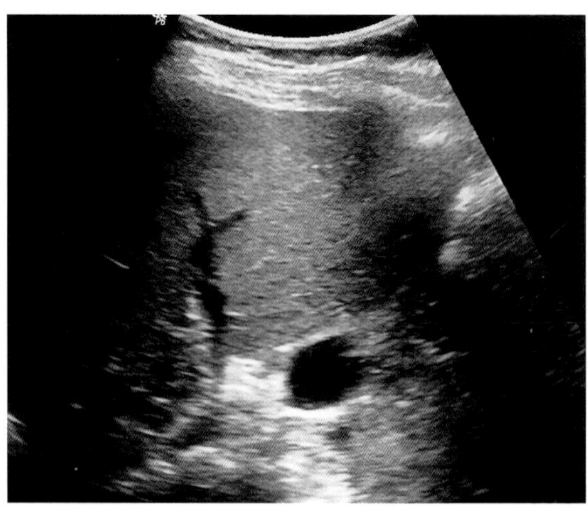

▶ **118** Gallbladder, liver

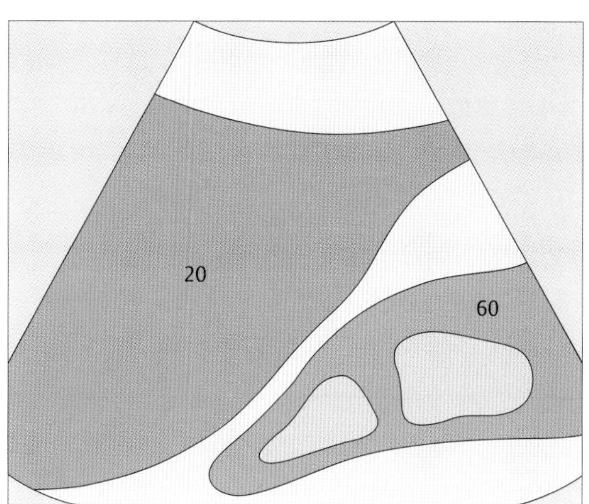

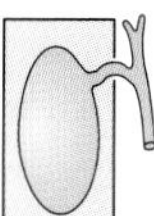

The kidney is the key landmark for locating the gallbladder in the lateral longitudinal scan.

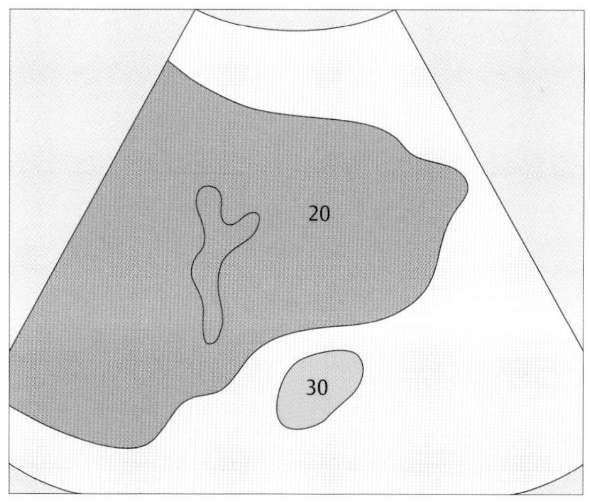

The gallbladder is consistently displayed anterior to the right kidney.

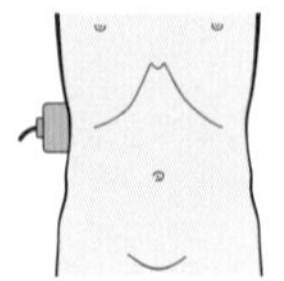

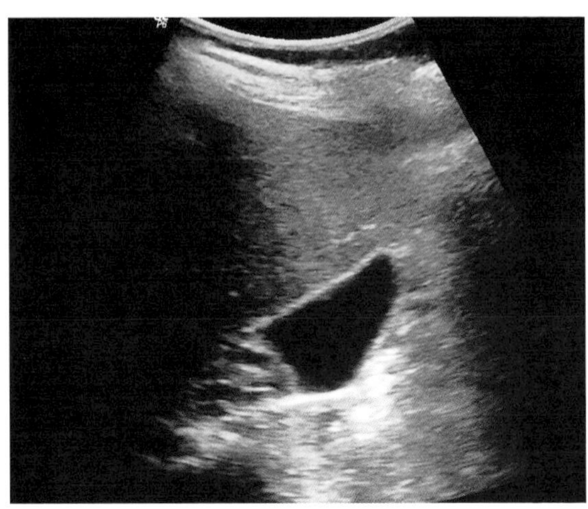

▶ **119** Gallbladder, liver

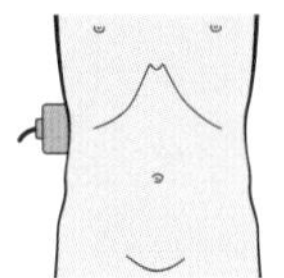

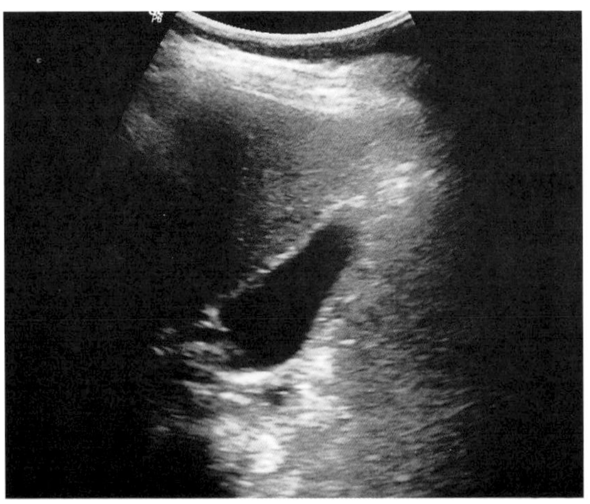

▶ **120** Gallbladder, liver

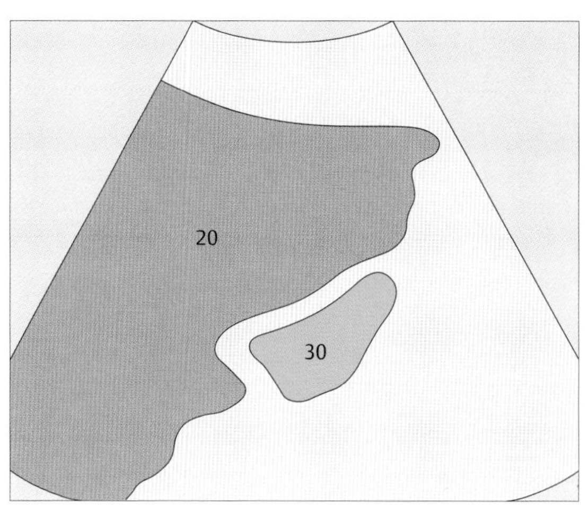

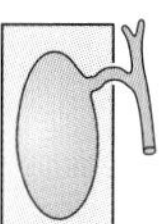

The gallbladder directly abuts the liver posteriorly.

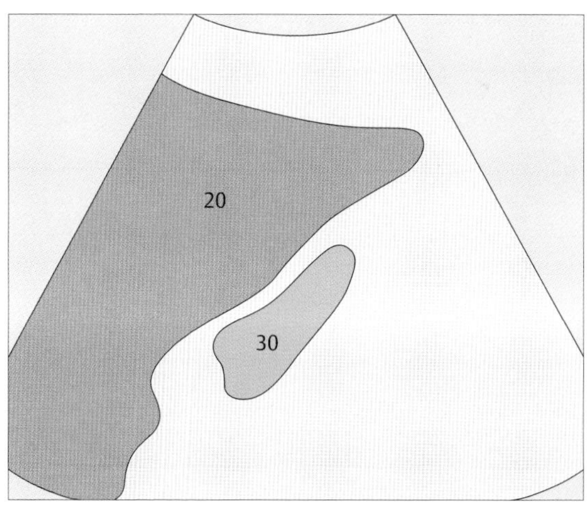

In most cases the gallbladder can be completely surveyed in a series of lateral longitudinal scans.

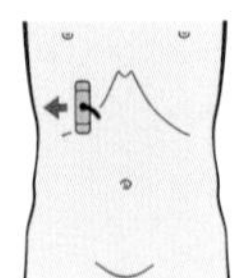

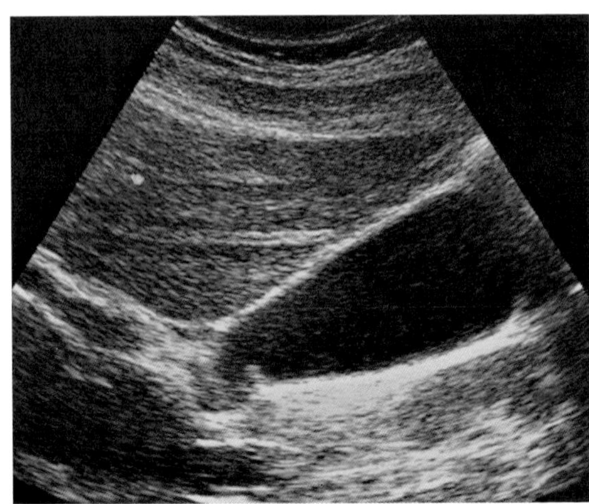

▶ **121** Regions of the gallbladder, Heister valves

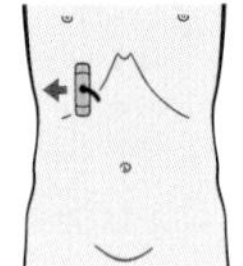

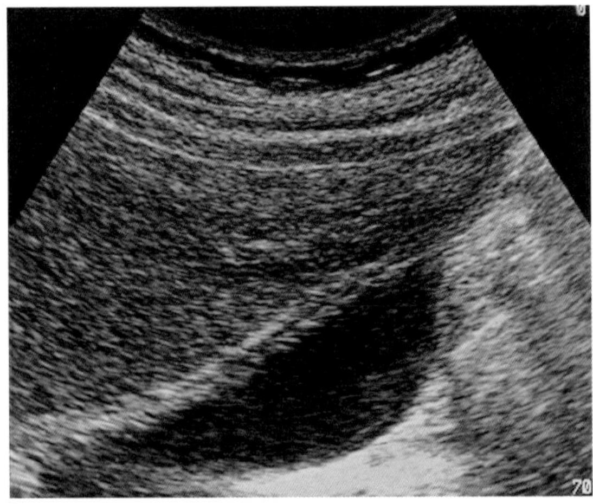

▶ **122** Layered structure of the gallbladder wall

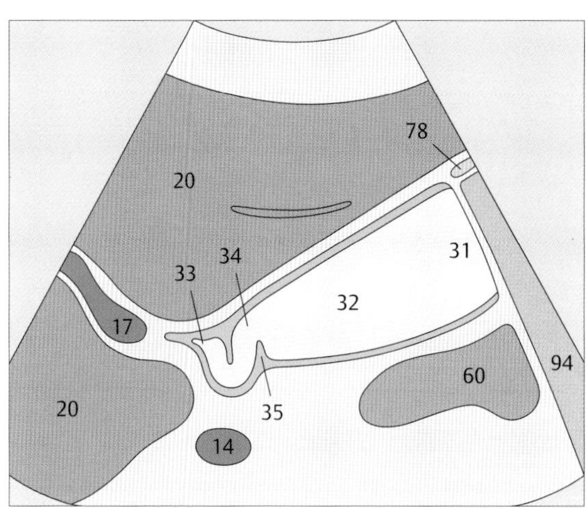

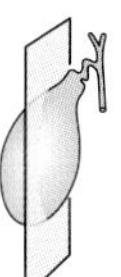

The Heister valves and gallbladder neck can often be clearly identified in a longitudinal scan over the gallbladder.

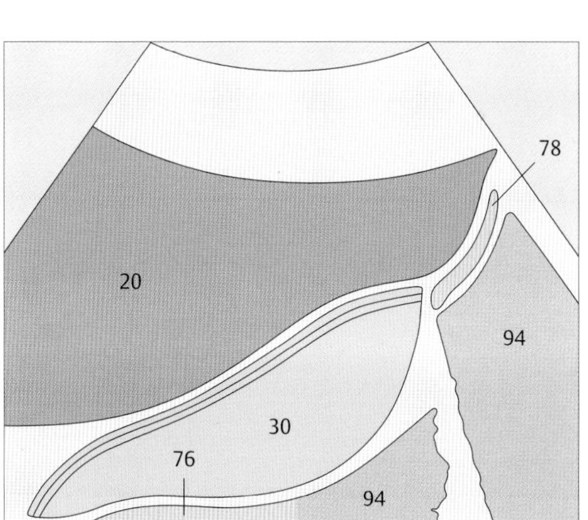

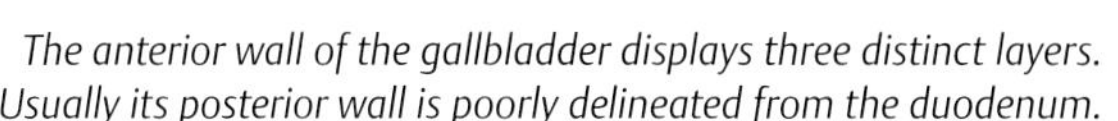

The anterior wall of the gallbladder displays three distinct layers. Usually its posterior wall is poorly delineated from the duodenum.

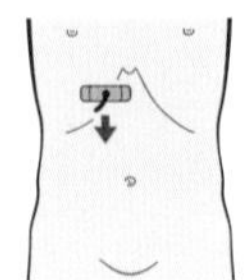

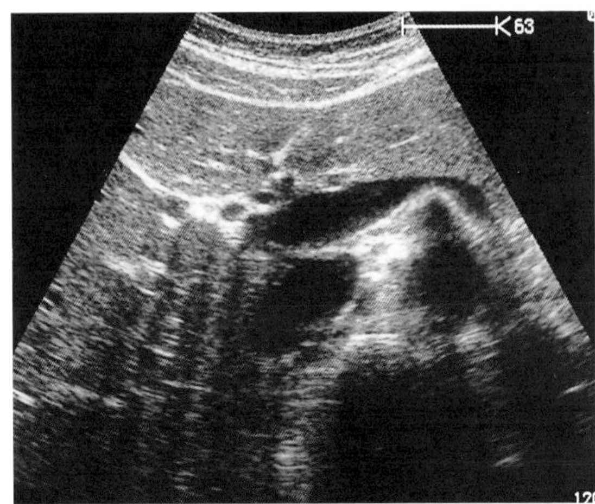

▶ **123** Common duct, hepatic artery, splenic vein

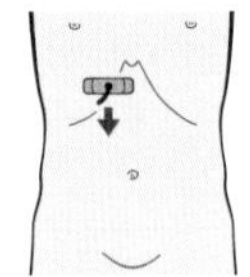

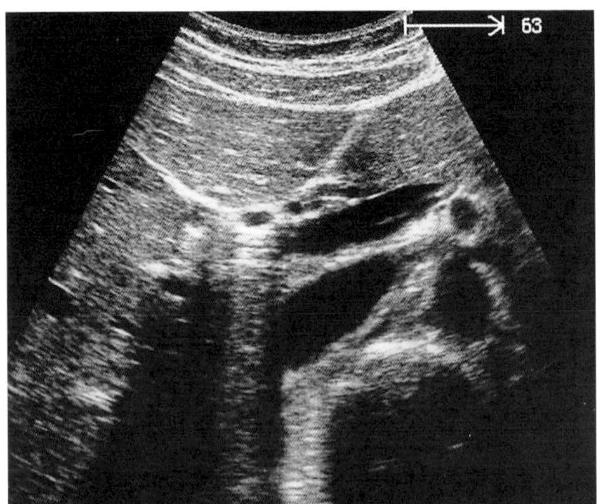

▶ **124** Common duct, hepatic artery, splenic vein

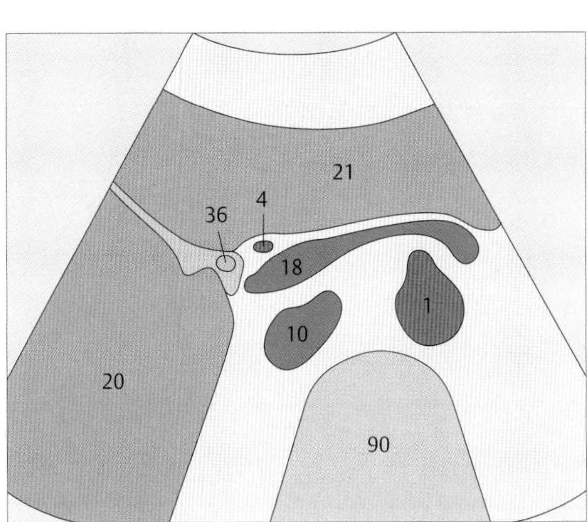

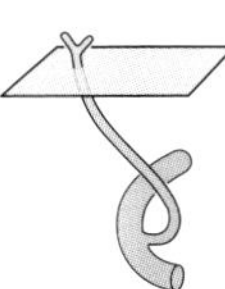

The common duct is located just anterior to the portal vein.

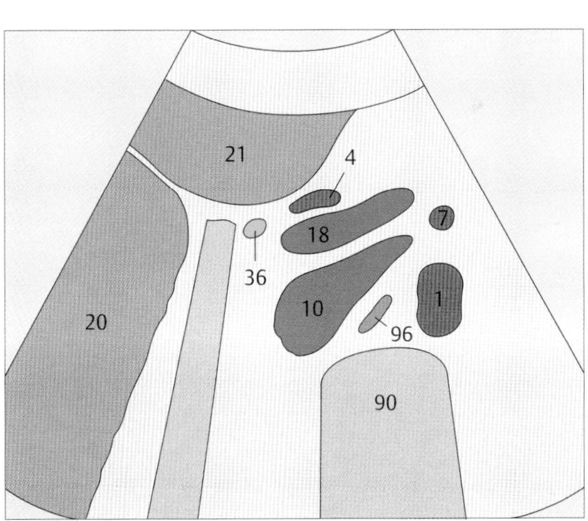

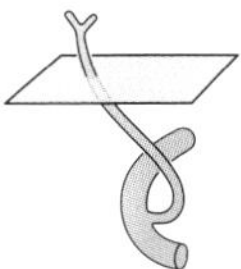

An upper abdominal longitudinal scan over the porta hepatis displays a longitudinal section of the common duct and a cross section of the hepatic artery.

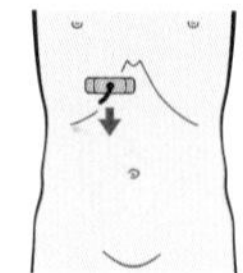

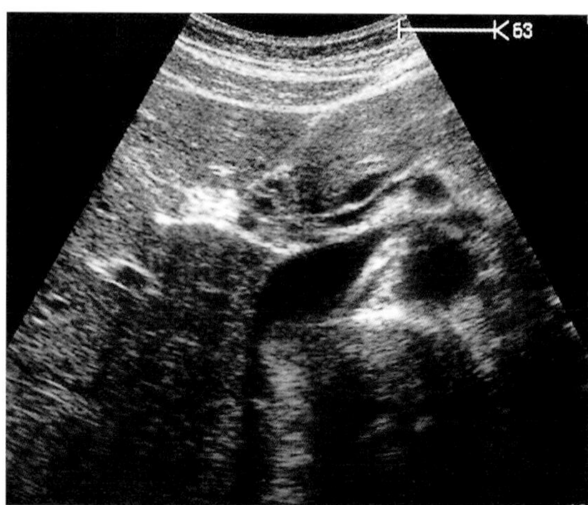

▶ **125** Common duct, hepatic artery

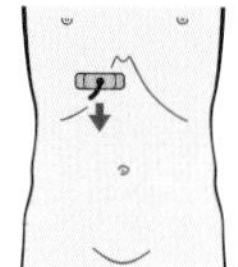

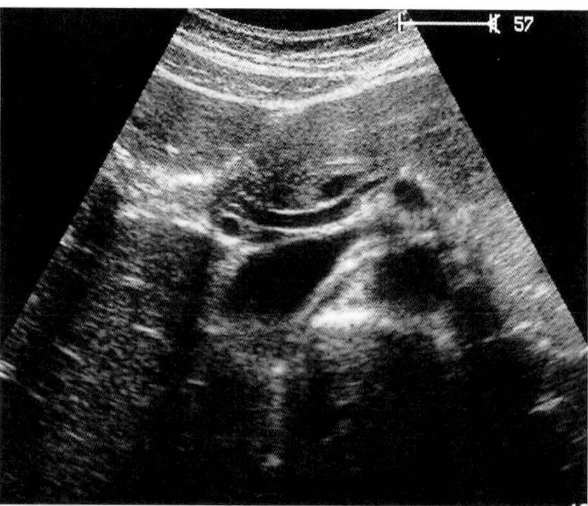

▶ **126** Common duct, hepatic artery

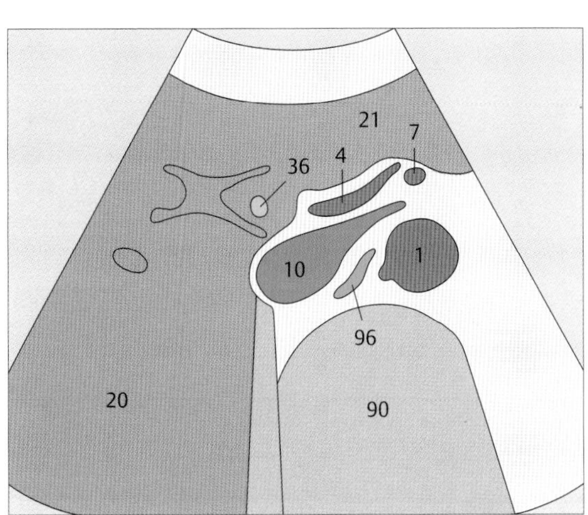

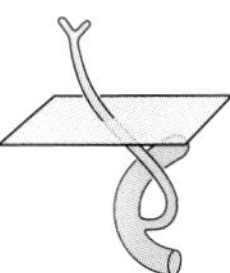

A portion of the common duct runs parallel and anterior to the vena cava.

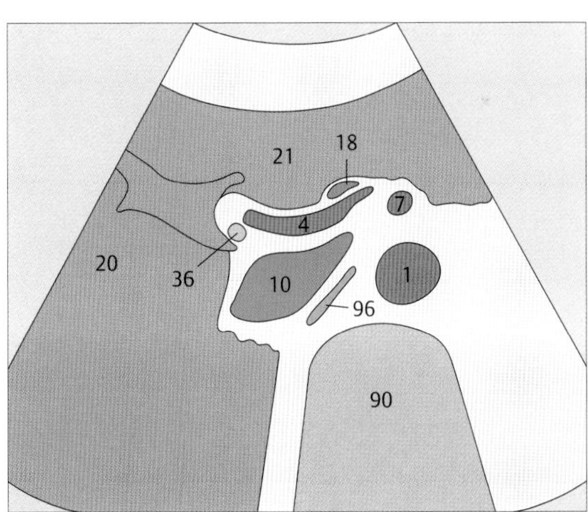

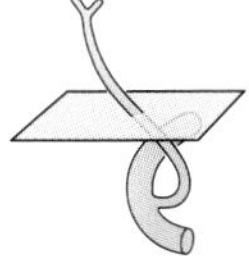

In most cases the common duct can be clearly traced into the head of the pancreas.

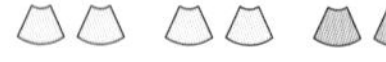

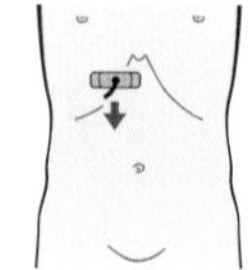

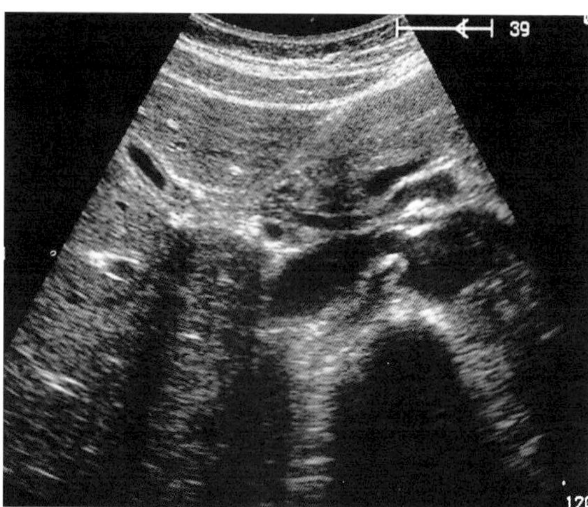

▶ **127** Common duct, hepatic artery

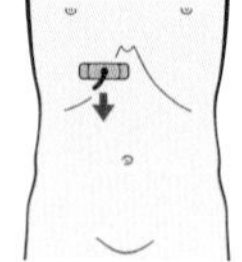

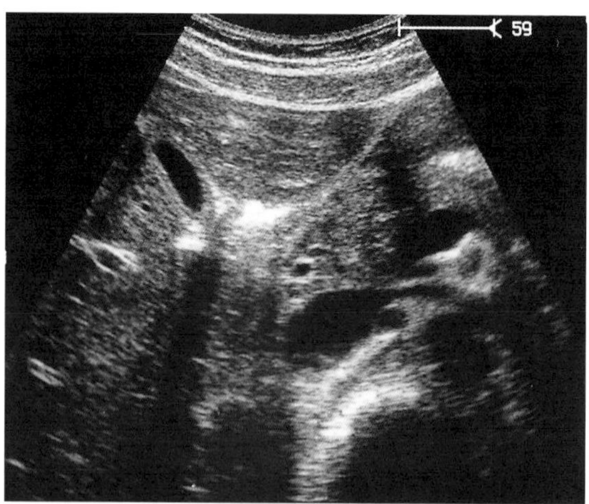

▶ **128** Common duct, head of pancreas

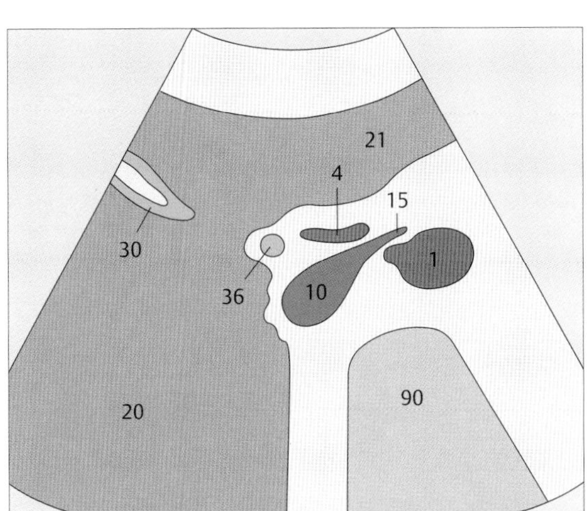

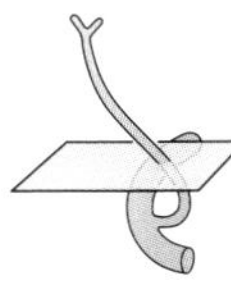

The common duct and hepatic artery are initially parallel to each other in the porta hepatis. The common duct is lateral, the artery medial.

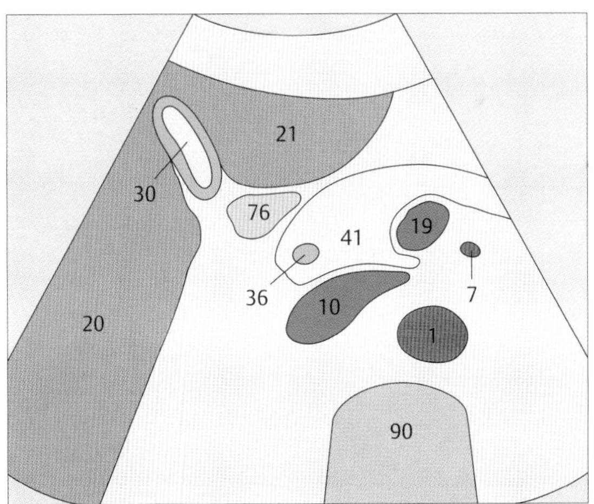

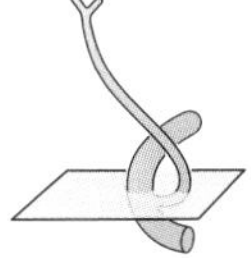

Below the porta hepatis, the common duct runs downward while the hepatic artery curves into the field from the medial side.

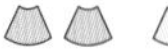

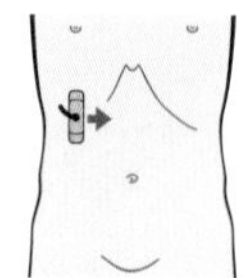

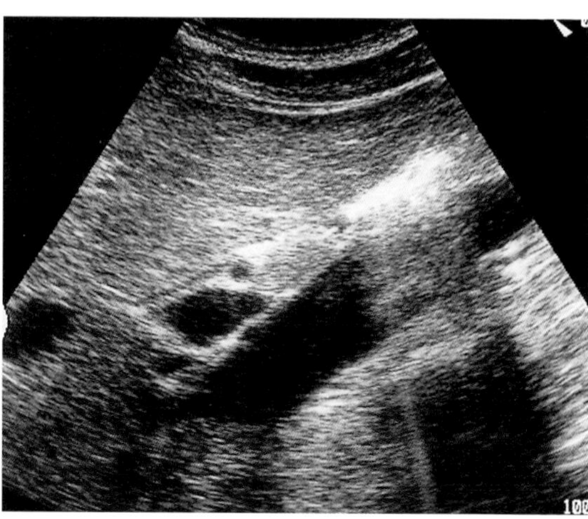

▶ **129** Common duct, portal vein, hepatic artery

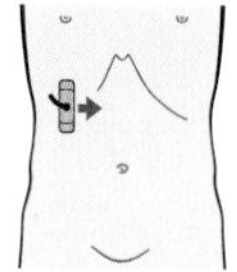

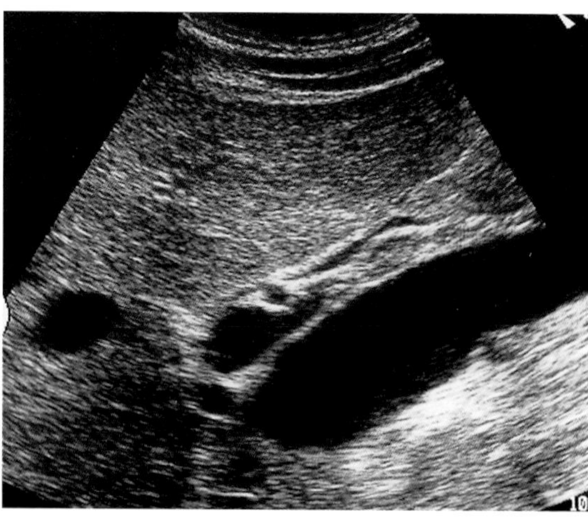

▶ **130** Common duct, hepatic artery, portal vein

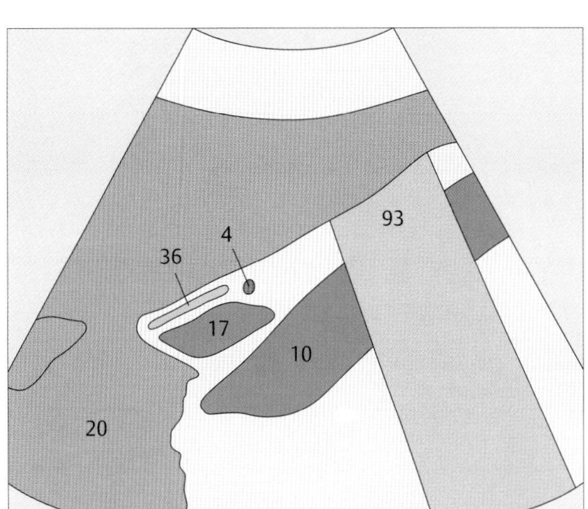

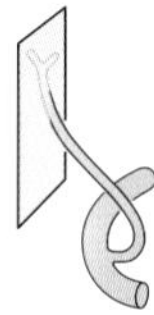

The common duct appears anterior and slightly lateral to the vena cava.

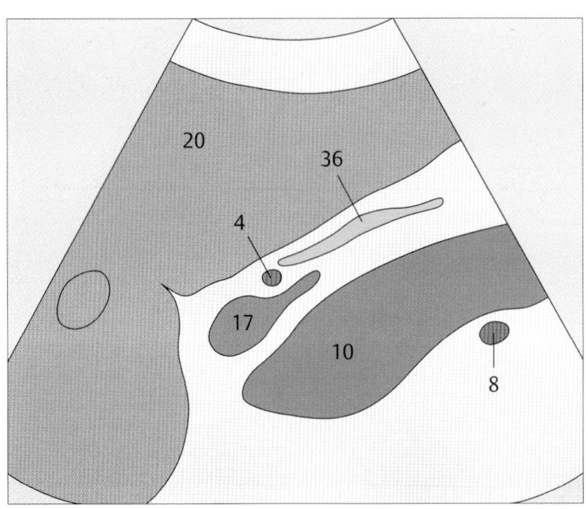

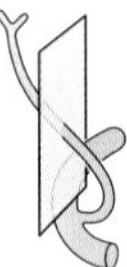

The common duct angles slightly toward the lateral side as it descends.

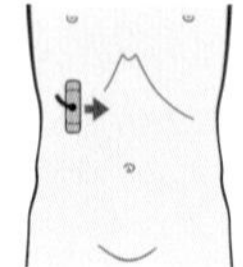

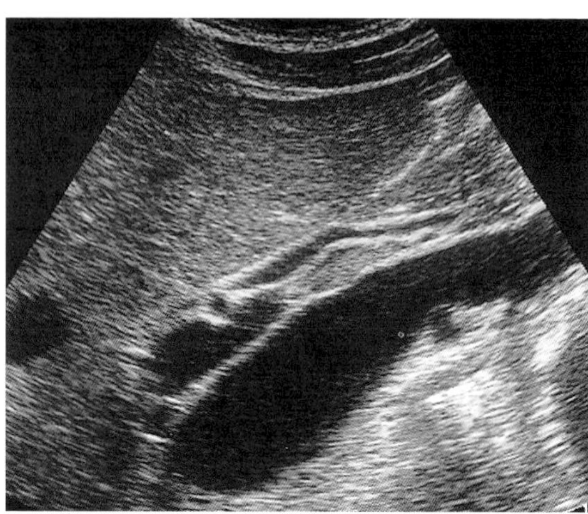

▶ **131** Common duct, hepatic artery, portal vein

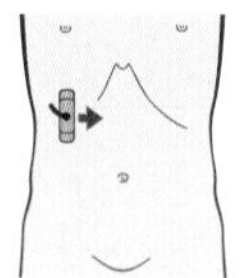

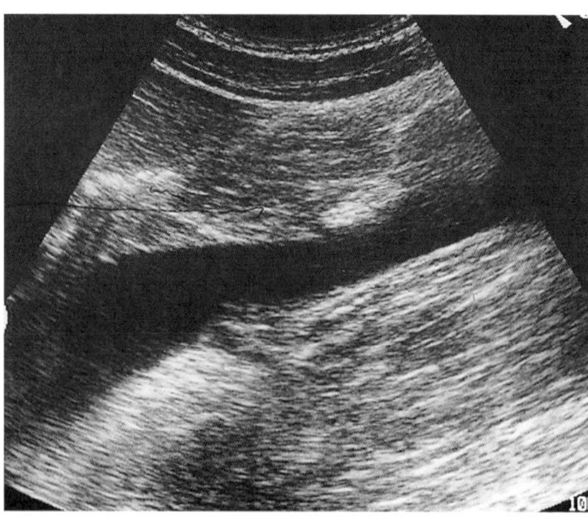

▶ **132** Common duct, head of pancreas

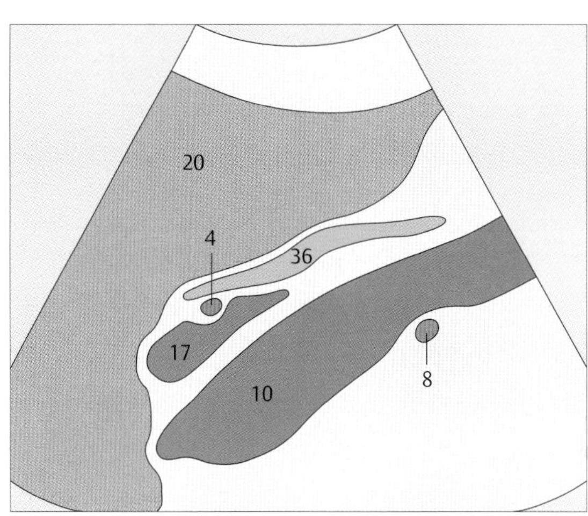

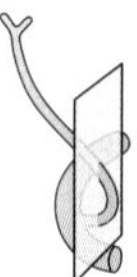

In most cases the rounded cross section of the common duct can be clearly identified above the pancreatic head.

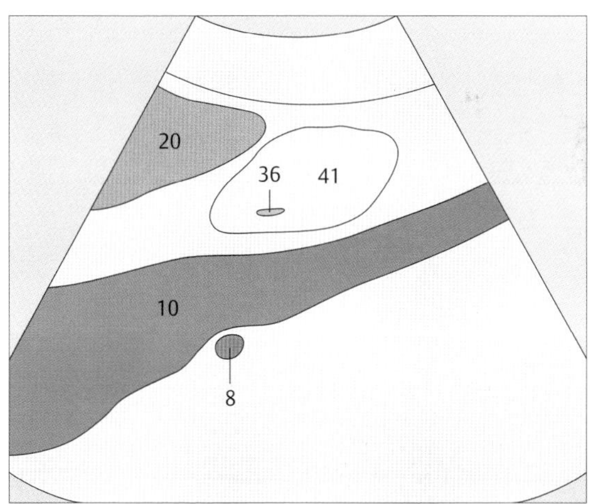

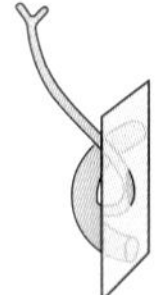

The common duct is clearly visible anterior to the vena cava at the level of the pancreatic head.

4 Pancreas

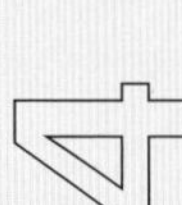

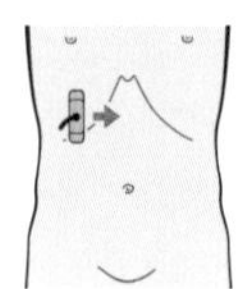

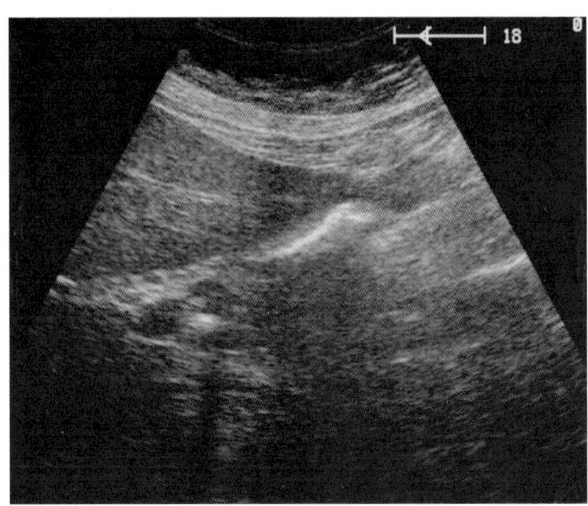

▶ **133** Duodenum lateral to head of pancreas

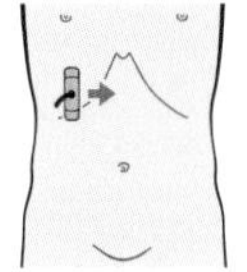

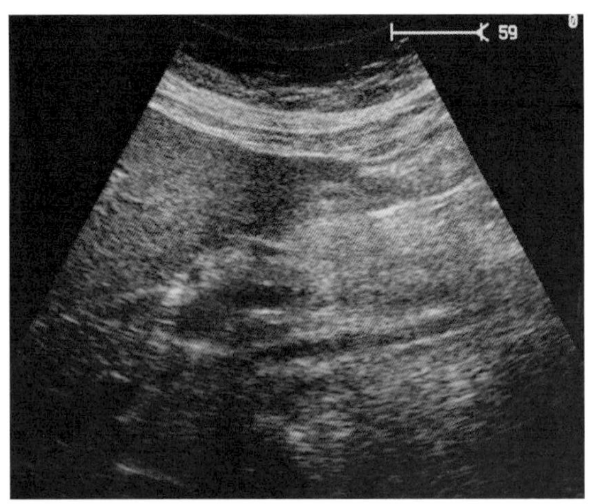

▶ **134** Head of pancreas, bile duct

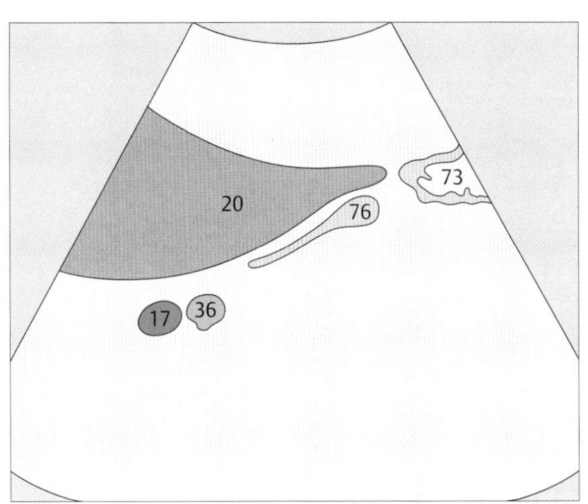

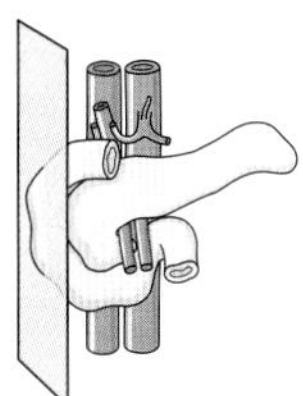

The head of the pancreas lies in the duodenal loop of the duodenum and is bounded laterally by the duodenum.

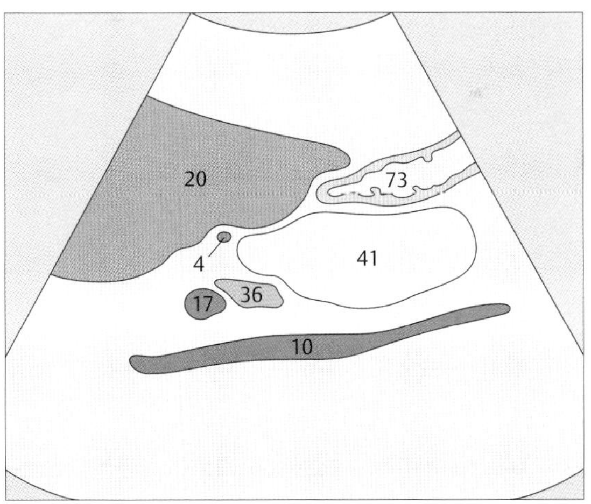

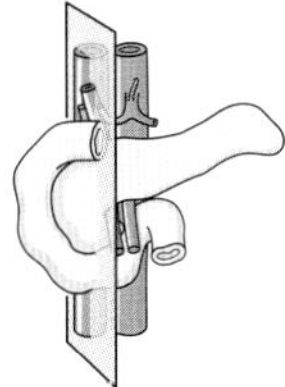

The bile duct, hepatic artery, and portal vein are located cranial to the head of the pancreas.

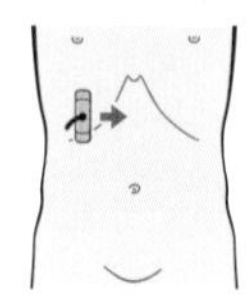

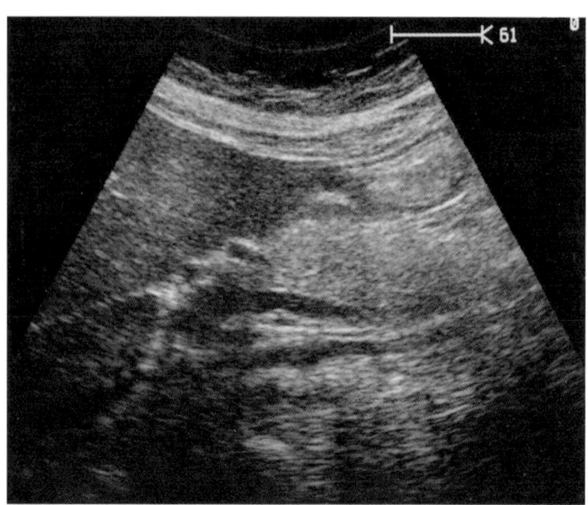

▶ **135** Head of pancreas, bile duct

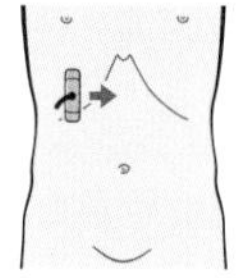

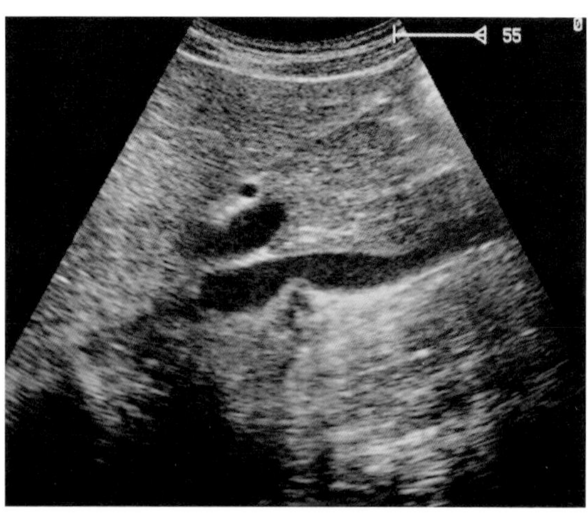

▶ **136** Head of pancreas, hilar vessels, vena cava

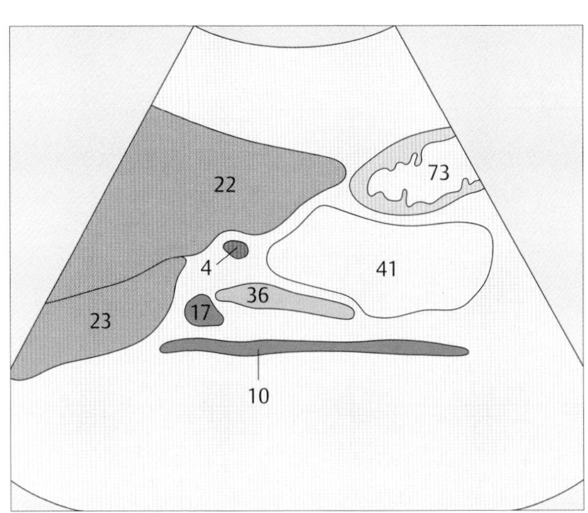

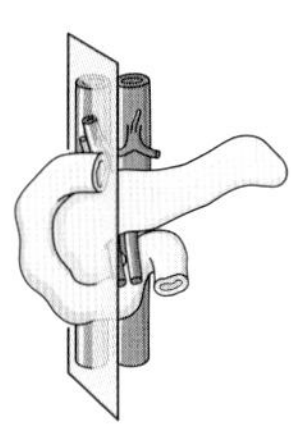

The bile duct runs posteriorly in the head of the pancreas to the papilla, which usually cannot be visualized with ultrasound.

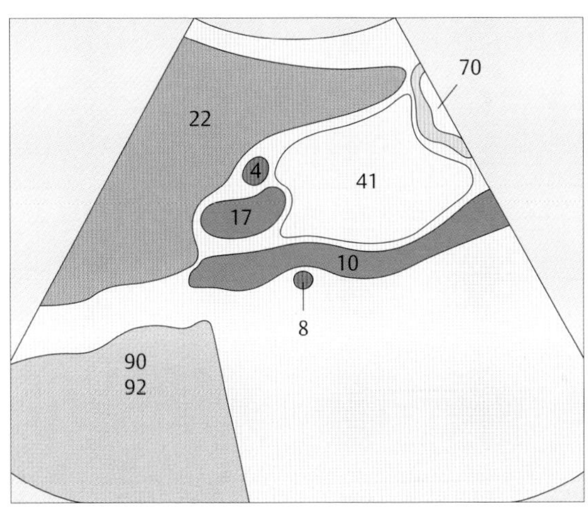

The head of the pancreas lies against the anterior surface of the vena cava and is bordered cranially by the main trunk of the portal vein.

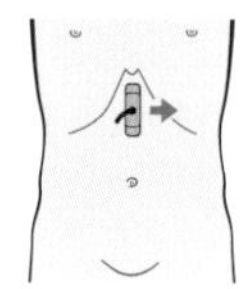

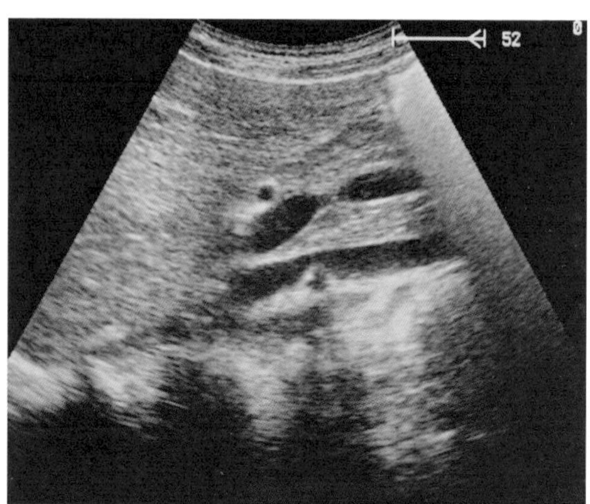

▶ **137** Head of pancreas, superior mesenteric vein, uncinate process

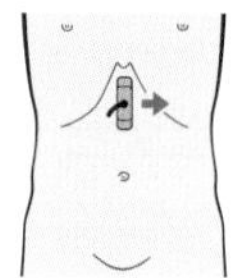

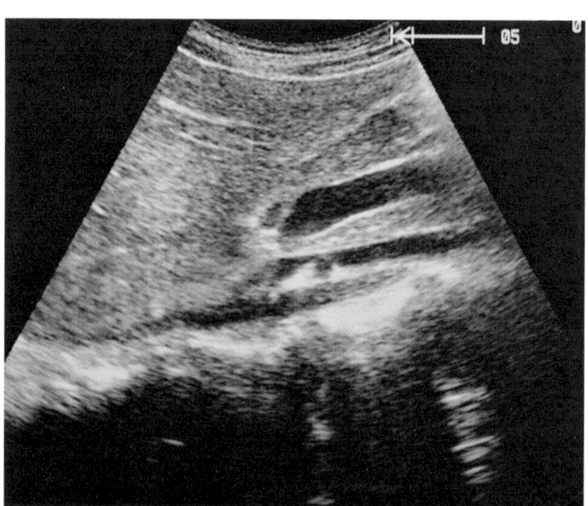

▶ **138** Head of pancreas, superior mesenteric vein, uncinate process

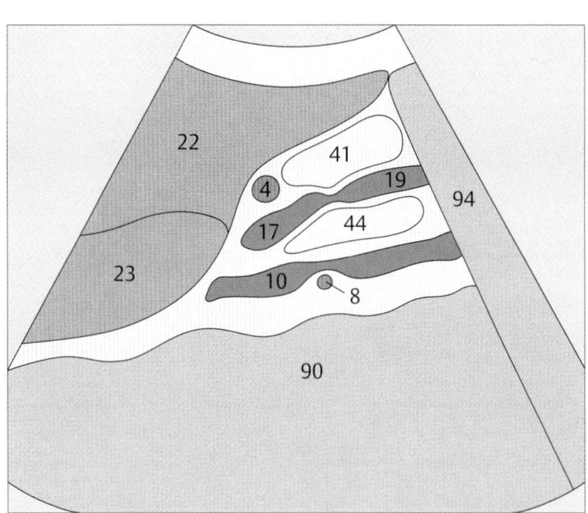

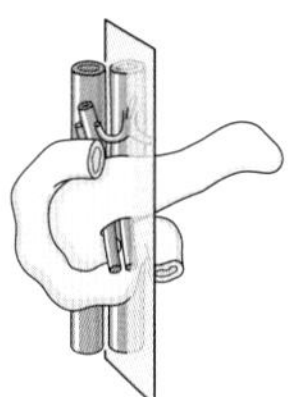

The uncinate process runs posteriorly around the mesenteric vein, coming between that vessel and the vena cava.

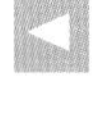

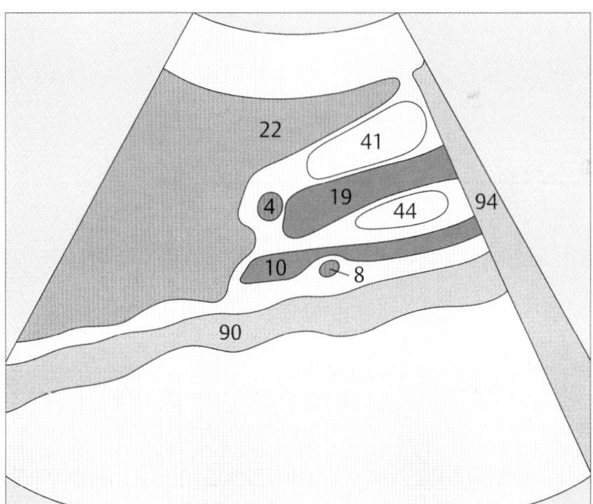

The superior mesenteric vein marks the boundary between the head and body of the pancreas.

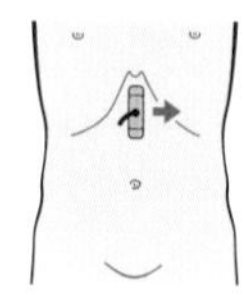

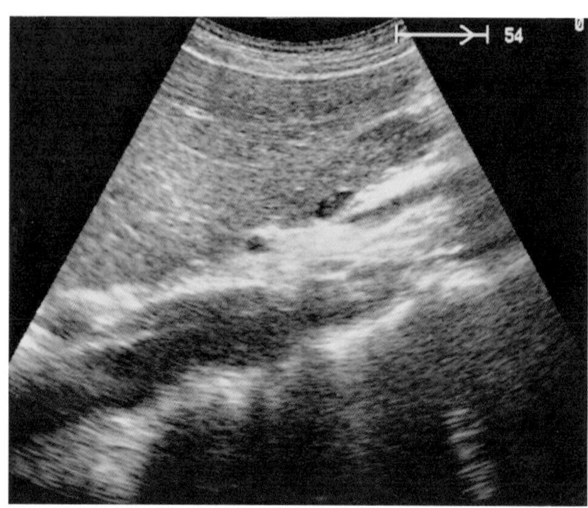

▶ **139** Body of pancreas, splenic vein

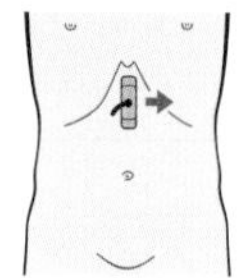

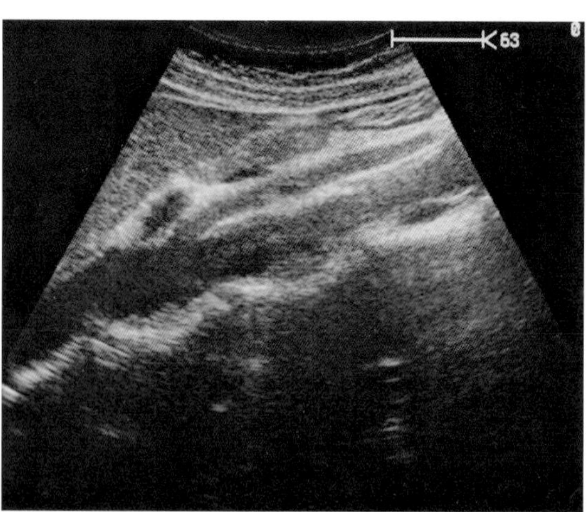

▶ **140** ody of pancreas, splenic vein, superior mesenteric artery, aorta

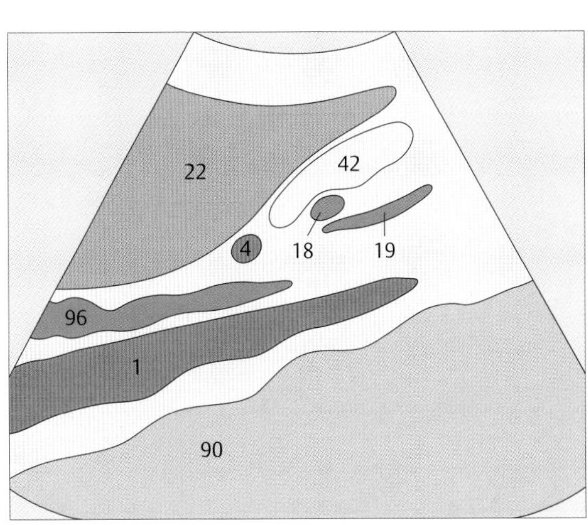

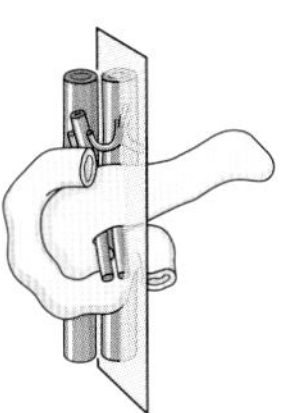

The body of the pancreas is the narrowest part of the organ in its ventrodorsal dimension.

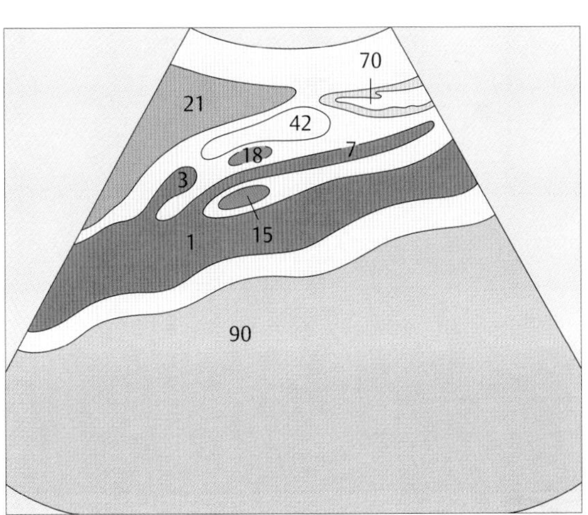

The celiac trunk is cranially adjacent to the body of the pancreas. The splenic vein and body of the pancreas cross over the superior mesenteric artery.

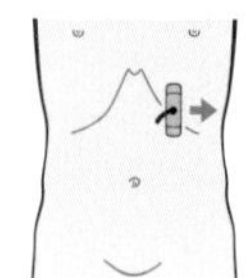

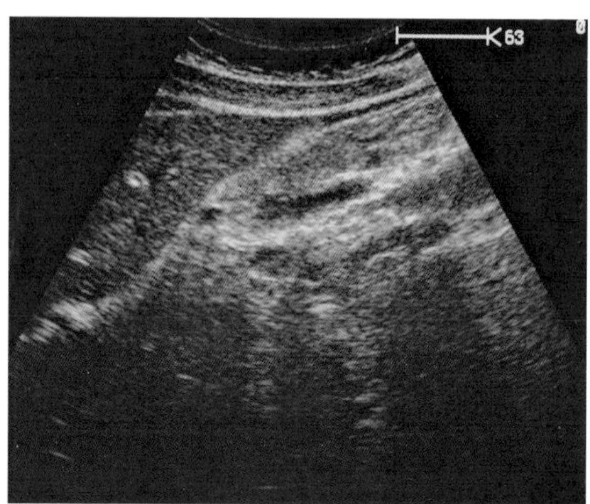

▶ **141** Body of pancreas, splenic vein

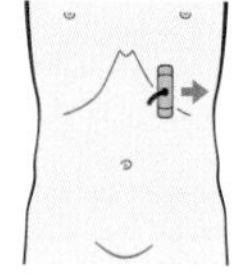

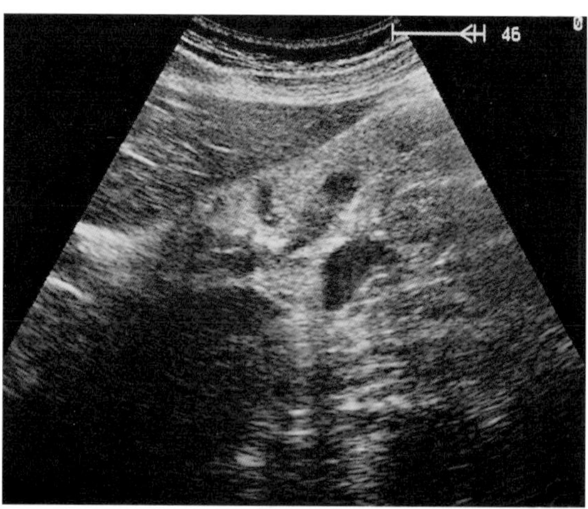

▶ **142** Tail of pancreas, splenic artery and vein, renal artery and vein

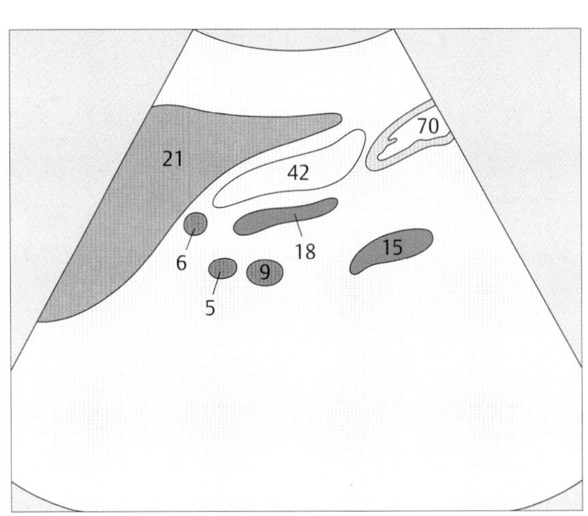

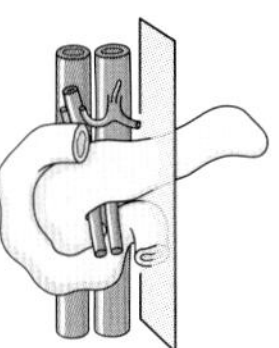

The left margin of the aorta marks the junction between the body and tail of the pancreas.

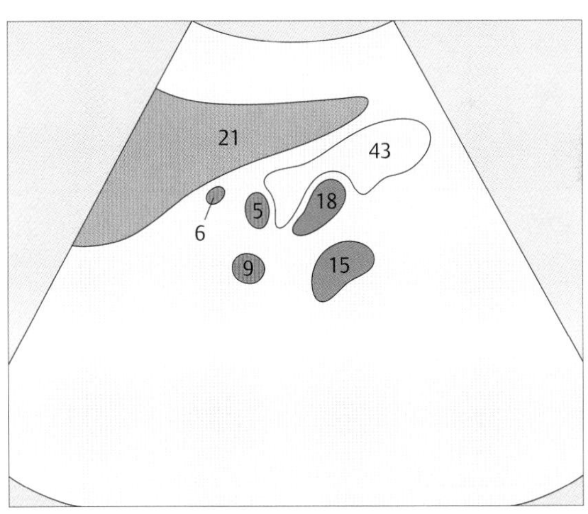

A longitudinal scan at the junction of the body and tail of the pancreas displays four vessels in cross section: the splenic artery, splenic vein, renal artery, and renal vein.

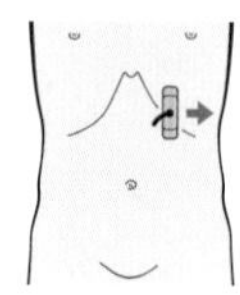

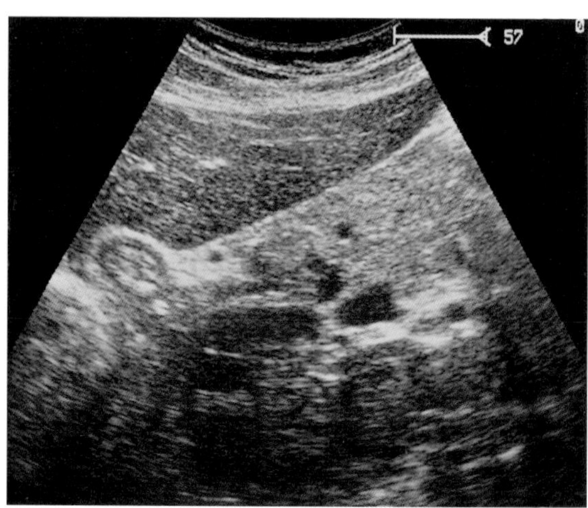

▶ **143** Tail of pancreas, splenic artery and vein, renal artery and vein

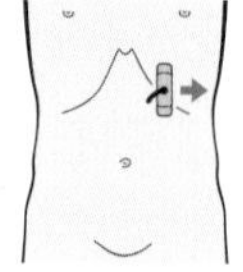

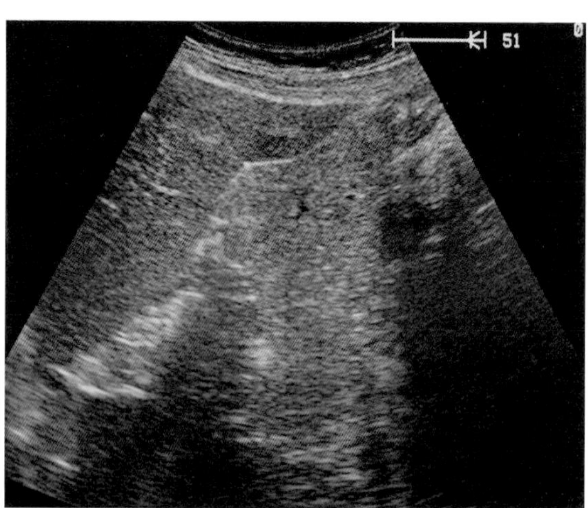

▶ **144** Tail of pancreas

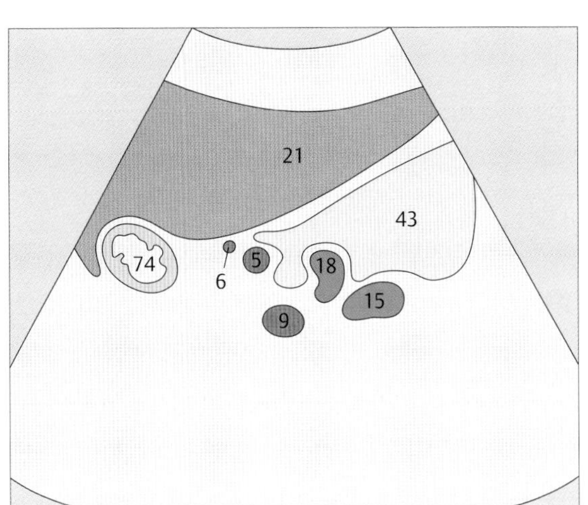

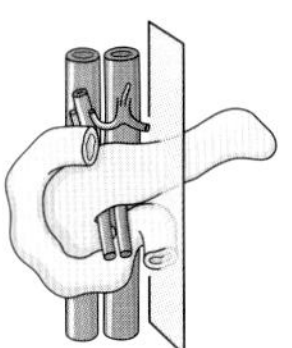

The tail of the pancreas often has a plump appearance in cross section.

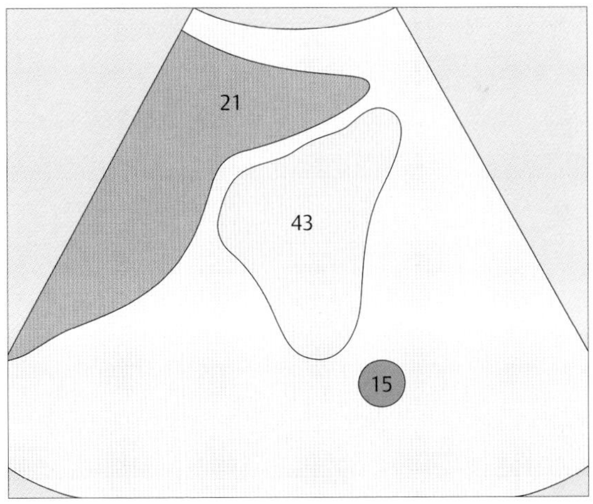

The tail of the pancreas can be completely visualized in an anterior scan only if acoustic conditions are good.

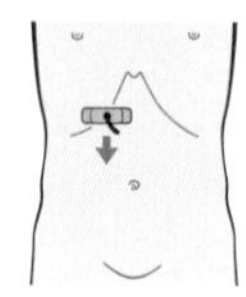

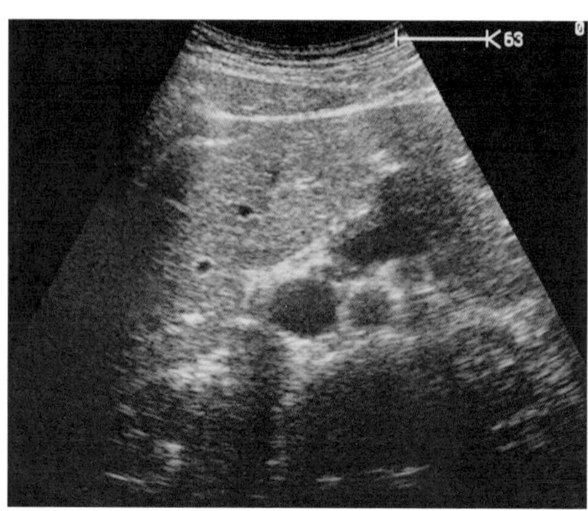

▶ **145** Section cranial to head of pancreas, vena cava, splenic vein

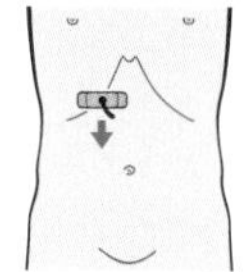

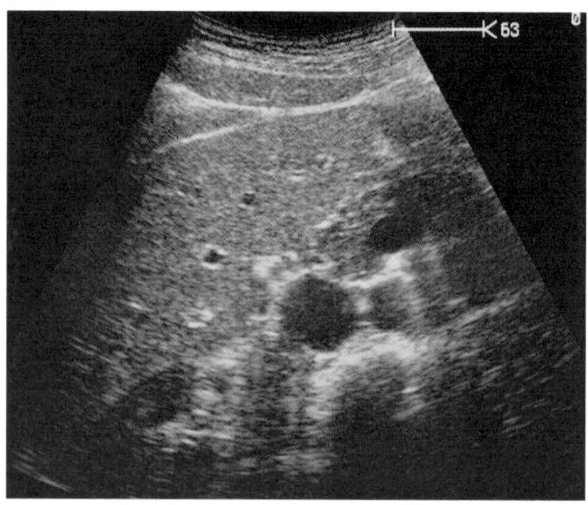

▶ **146** Head of pancreas, vena cava, superior mesenteric vein

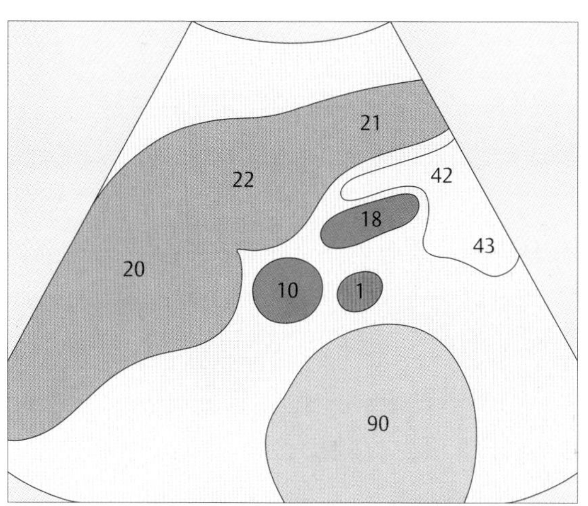

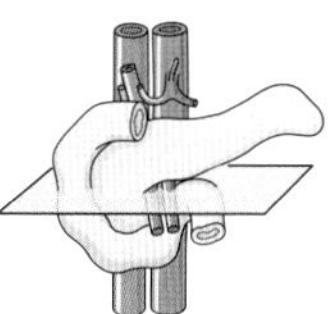

The body of the pancreas overlies the superior mesenteric vein. All parts of the gland that lie to the right of the superior mesenteric vein are designated as the head of the pancreas.

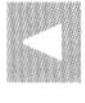

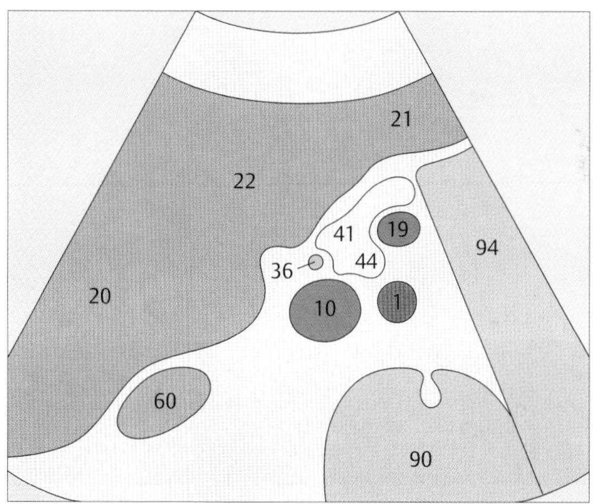

The uncinate process extends between the vena cava and superior mesenteric vein.

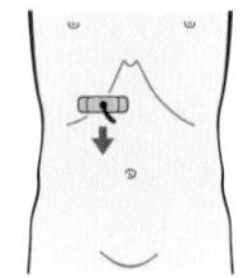

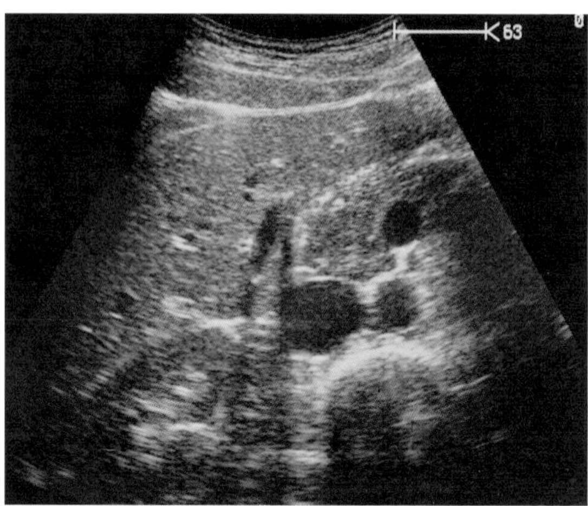

▶ **147** Head of pancreas, vena cava, superior mesenteric vein, uncinate process, common bile duct

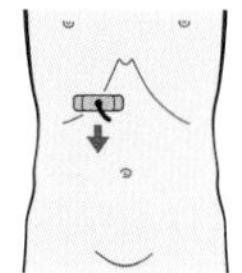

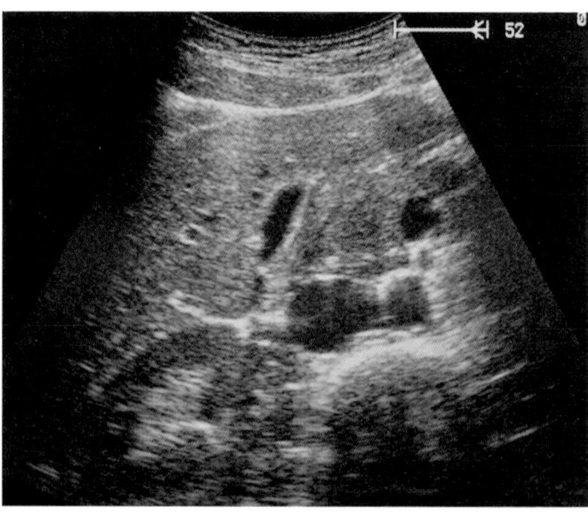

▶ **148** Head of pancreas, vena cava, superior mesenteric vein, uncinate process, gallbladder

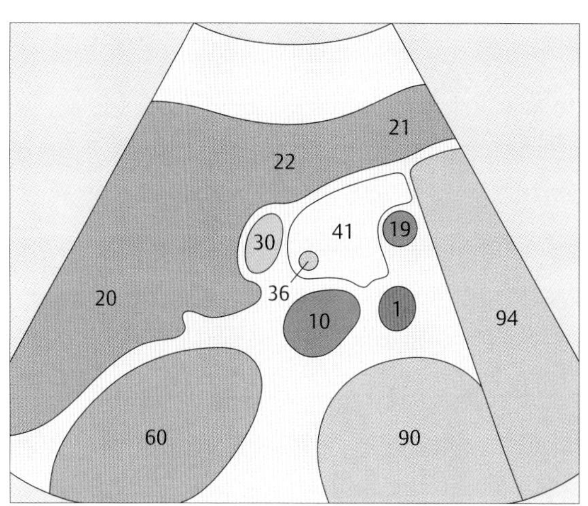

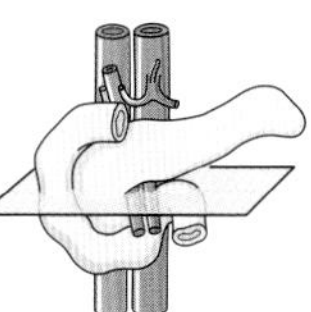

The common bile duct is visible at the right border of the pancreatic head in transverse section.

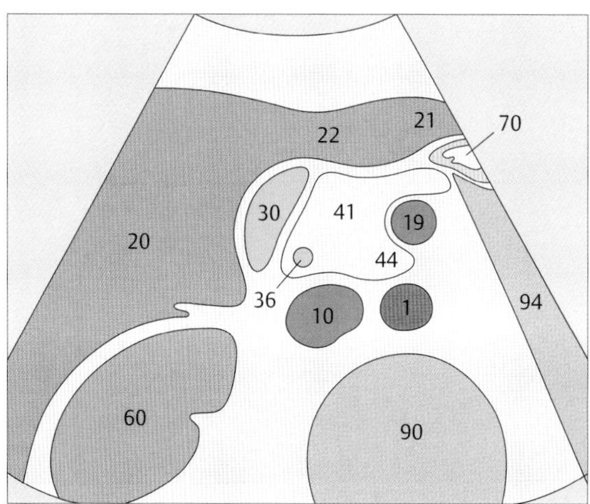

The head of the pancreas lies between the liver, gallbladder, vena cava, and superior mesenteric vein.

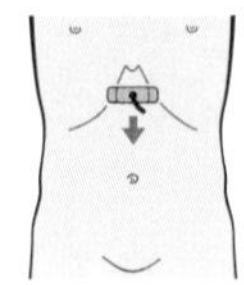

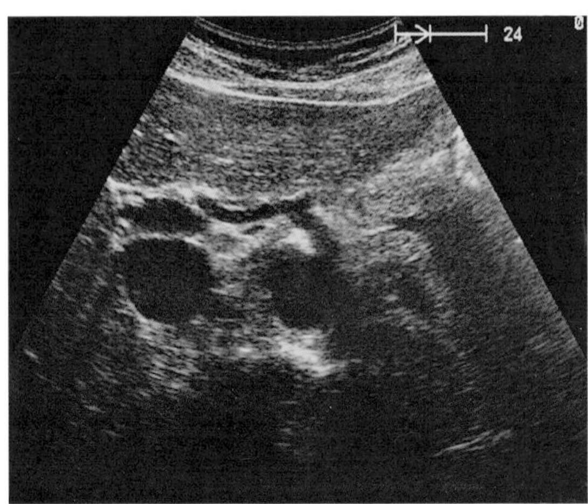

▶ **149** Scan cranial to body of pancreas, celiac trunk

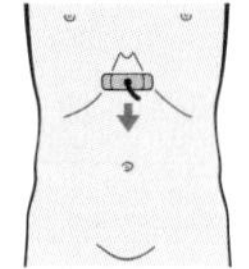

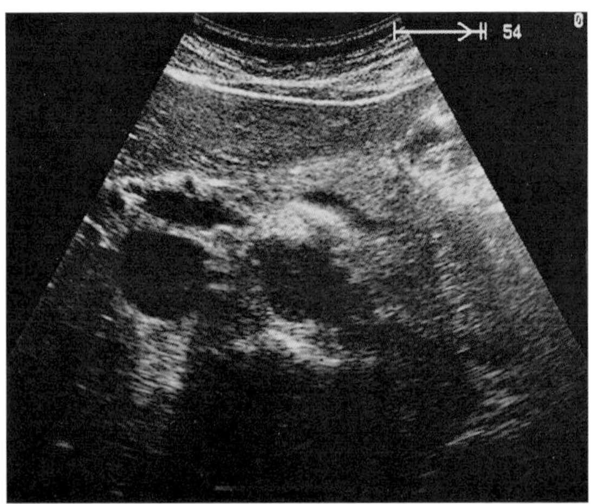

▶ **150** Body of pancreas, splenic vein

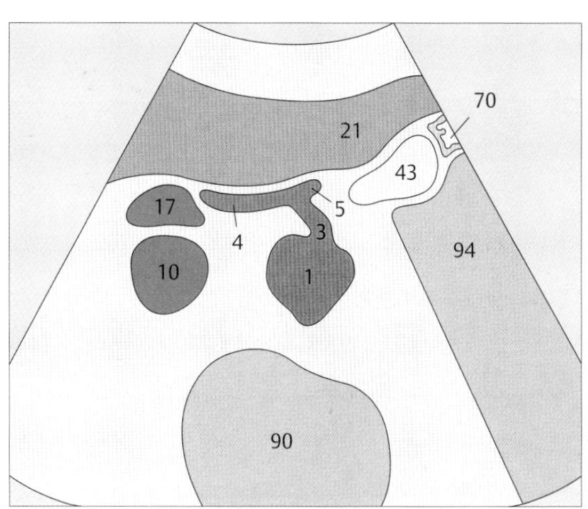

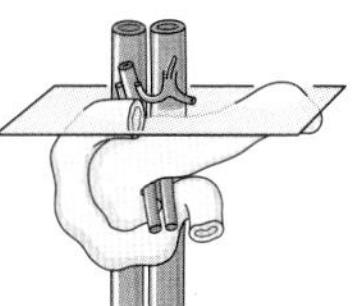

The body of the pancreas is bounded cranially by the celiac trunk and its two branches, the hepatic artery and splenic artery.

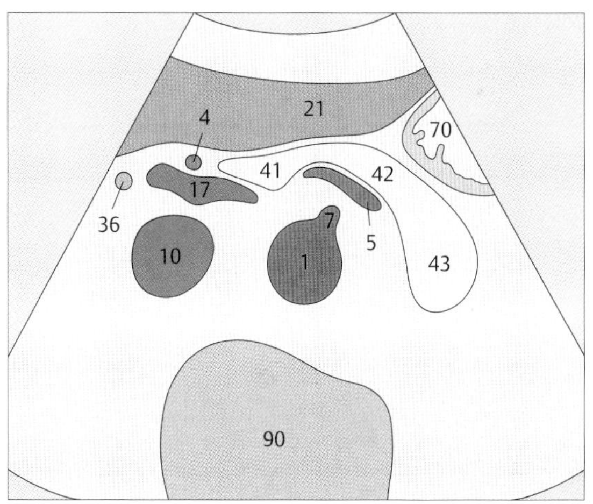

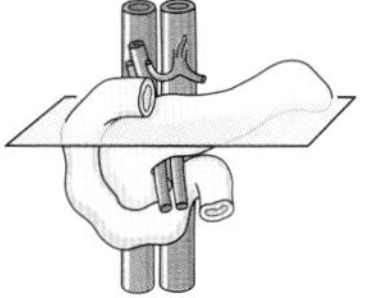

The borders of the healthy pancreas form a continuous outline from head to body to tail.

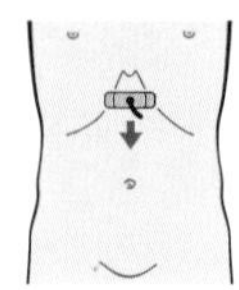

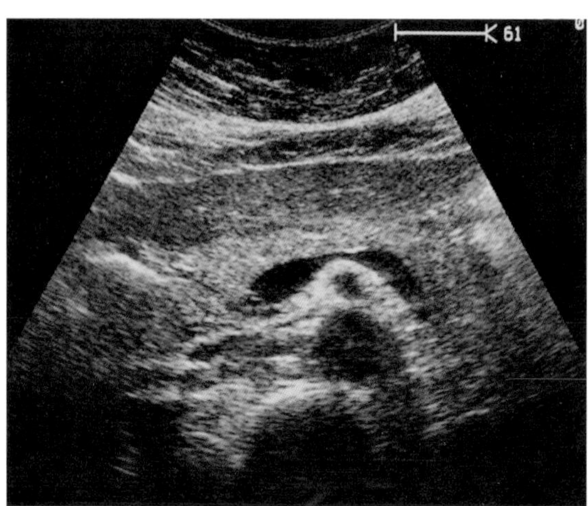

▶ **151** Body of pancreas, splenic vein, superior mesenteric artery, aorta

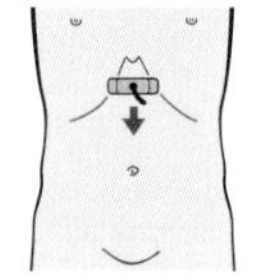

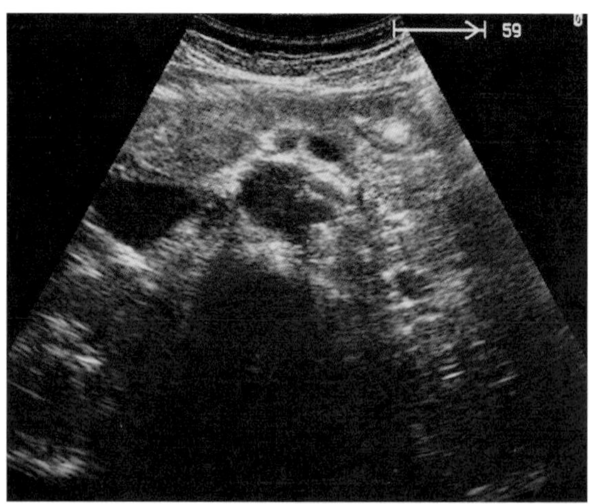

▶ **152** Left renal artery and vein, superior mesenteric artery and vein, aorta

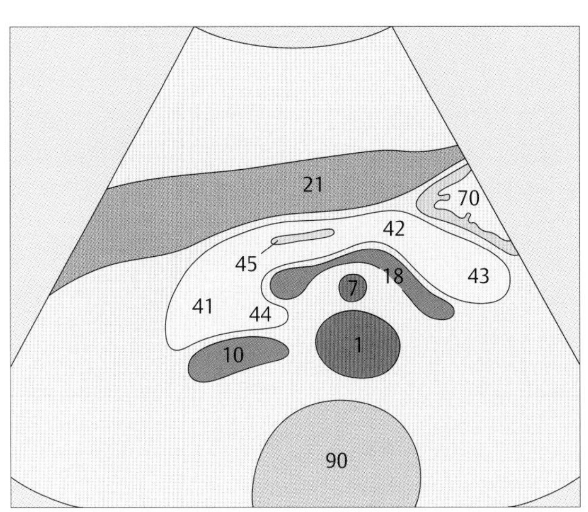

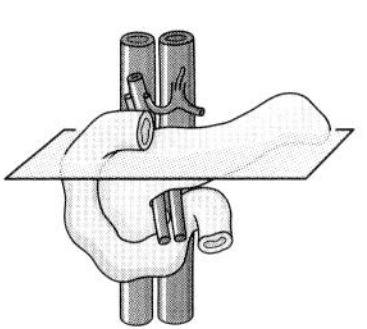

The splenic vein is the landmark for locating the pancreas.
The superior mesenteric artery lies between the splenic vein and the aorta, appearing as an echo-free spot surrounded by bright echoes.

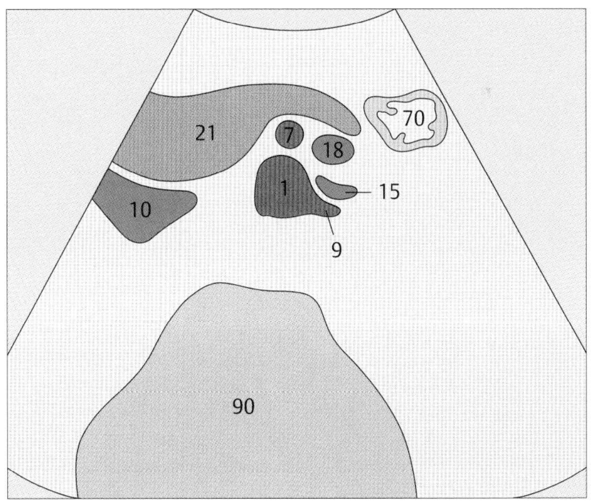

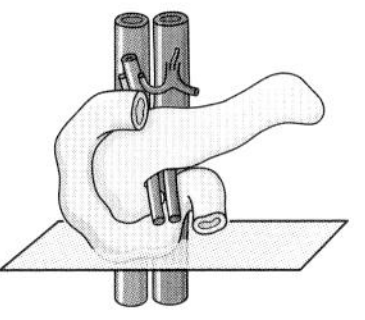

When the renal vessels are displayed in a transverse scan, usually the pancreas is no longer visualized.

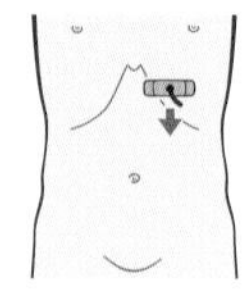

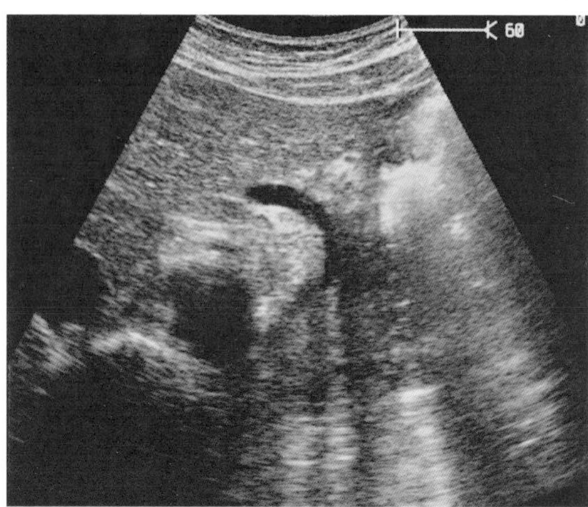

▶ **153** Tail of pancreas, splenic artery

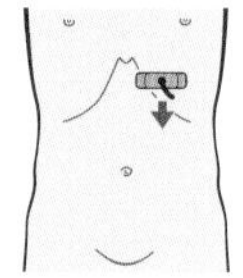

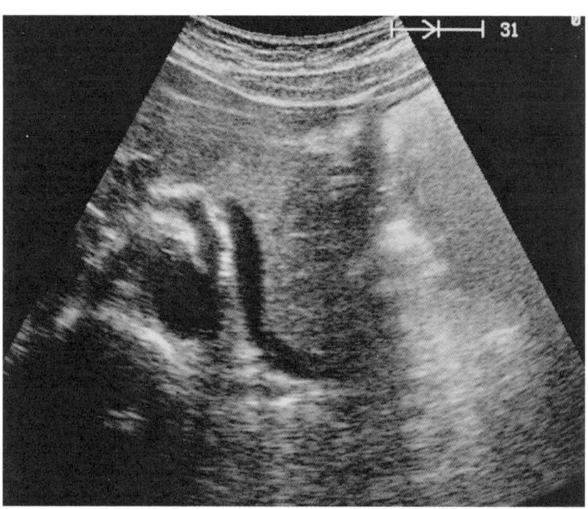

▶ **154** Tail of pancreas, splenic vein

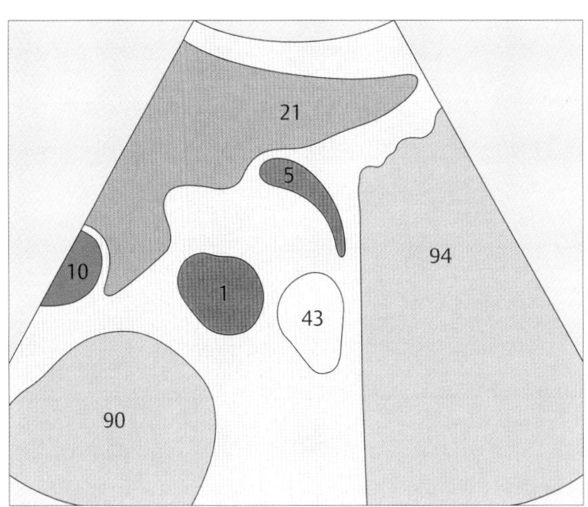

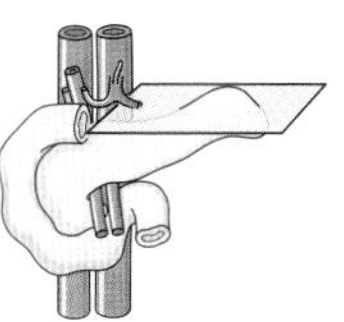

The tail of the pancreas is located well posteriorly, on the left side of the aorta.

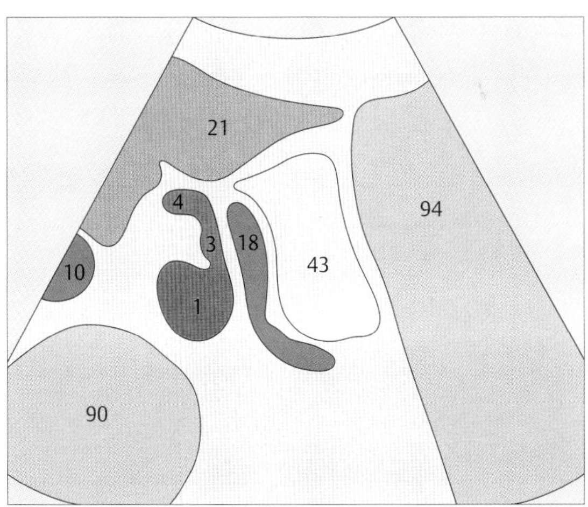

The tail of the pancreas is angled sharply posterior from the body and extends a variable distance between the stomach and the upper renal pole toward the splenic hilum.

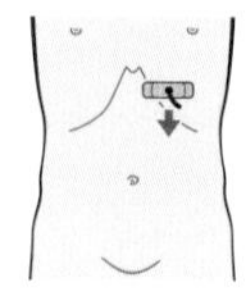

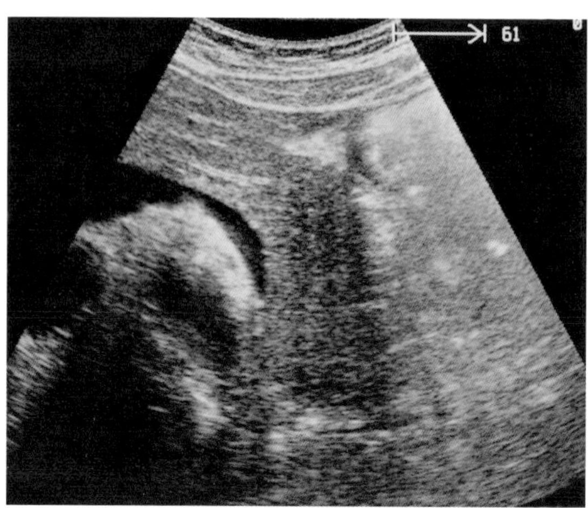

▶ **155** Tail of pancreas, gas in stomach

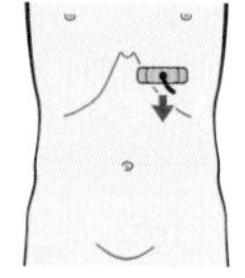

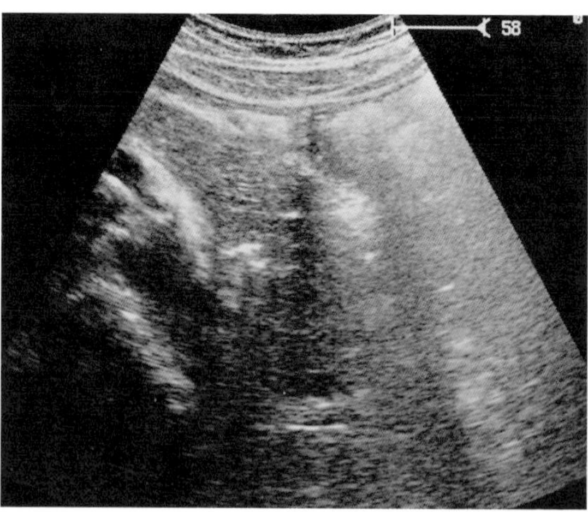

▶ **156** Tail of pancreas

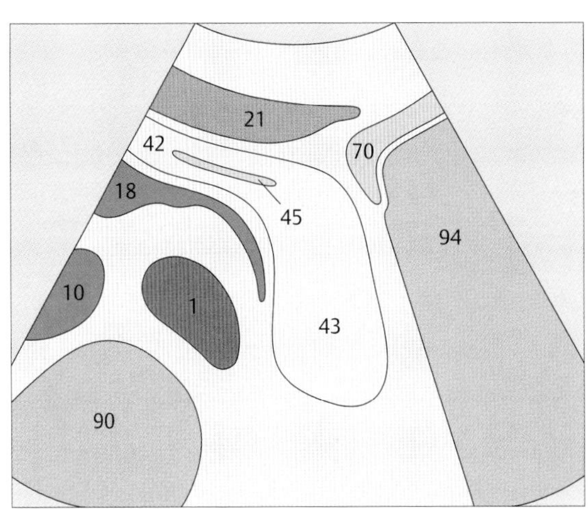

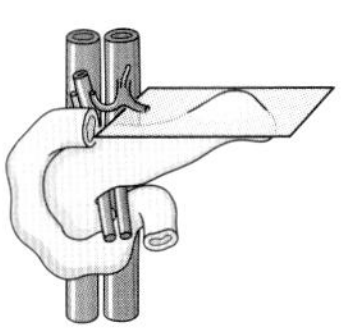

The junction between the body and tail of the pancreas is located at the level of the left aortic margin.

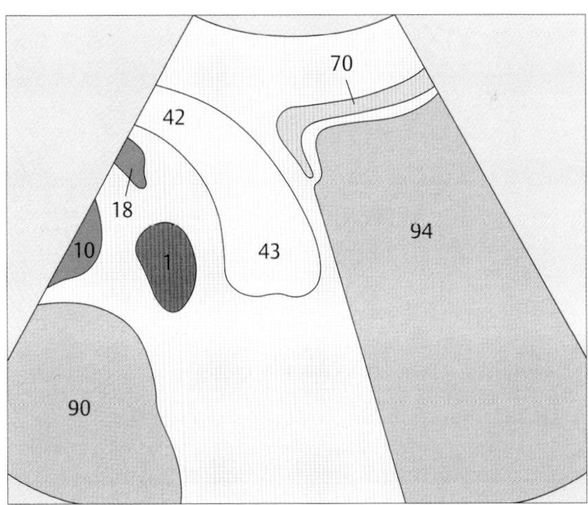

The tail of the pancreas is the most difficult part of the gland to evaluate with ultrasound.

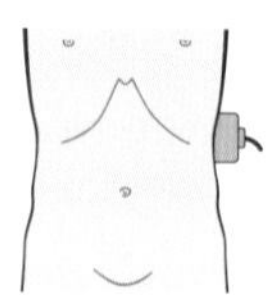

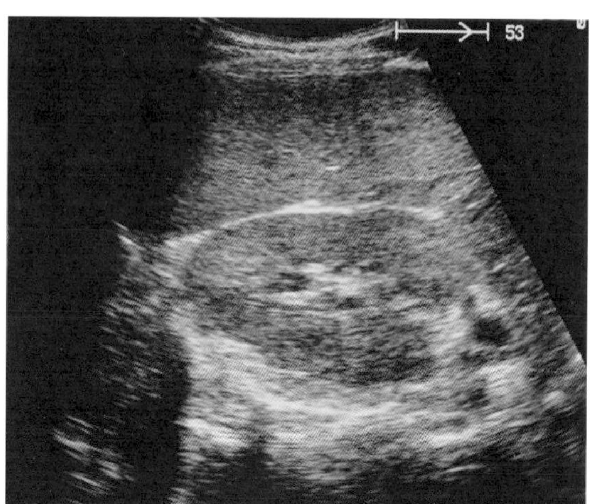

▶ **157** Scan posterior to tail of pancreas, spleen, kidney

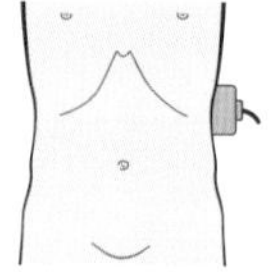

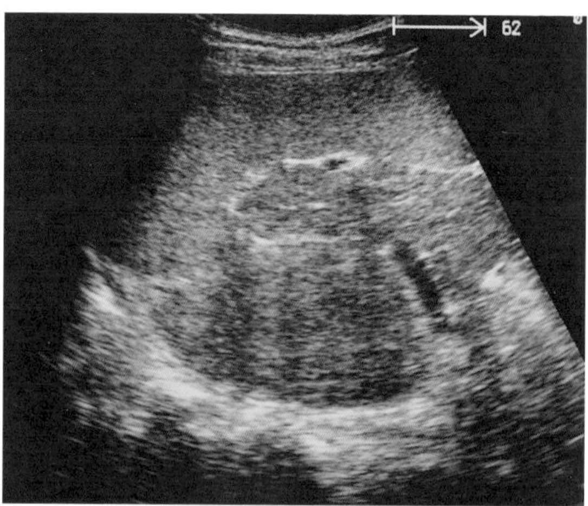

▶ **158** Spleen, tail of pancreas, kidney

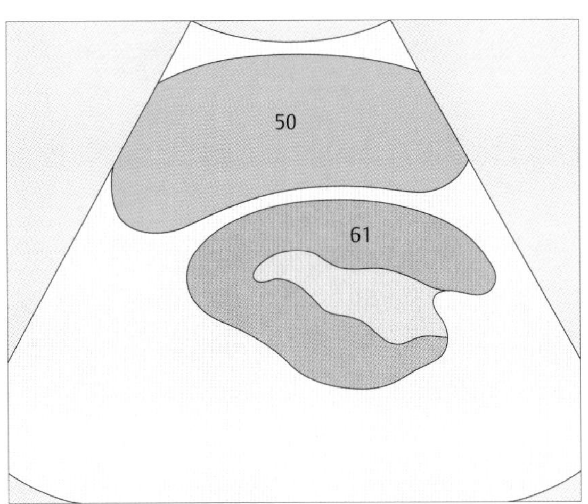

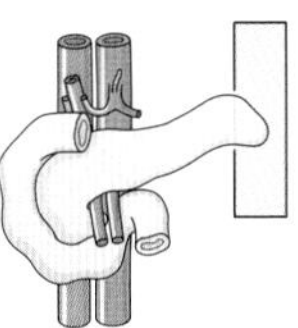

The tail of the pancreas is scanned intercostally through the spleen. Kidney and spleen serve as landmarks.

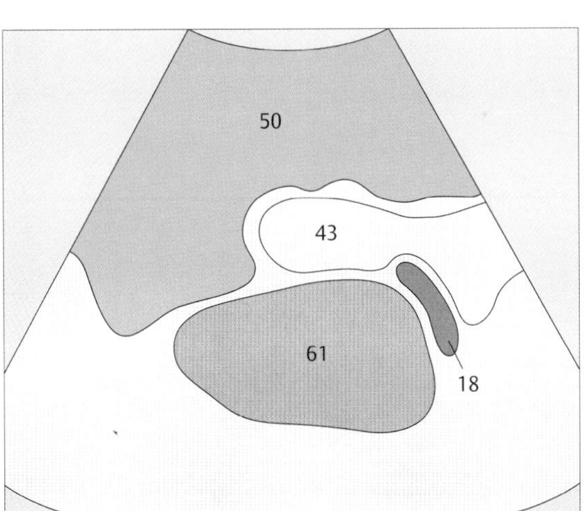

The tail of the pancreas is located in the splenic hilum between the spleen and the kidney.

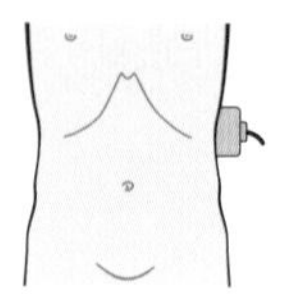

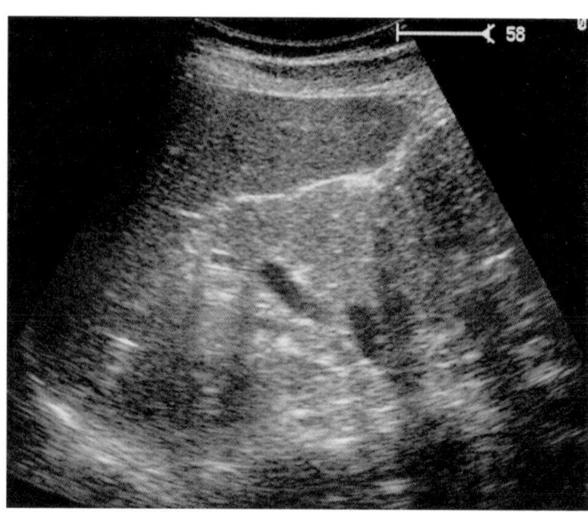

▶ **159** Spleen, tail of pancreas, kidney

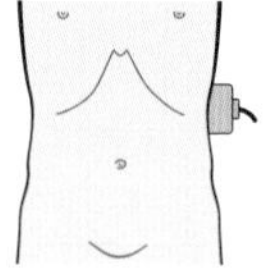

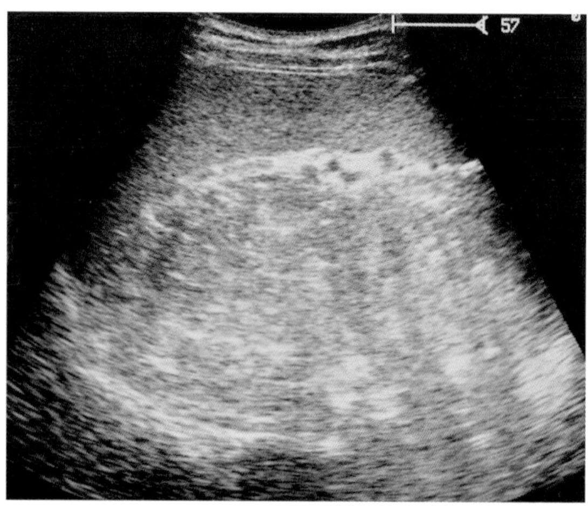

▶ **160** Scan anterior to tail of pancreas, spleen, stomach

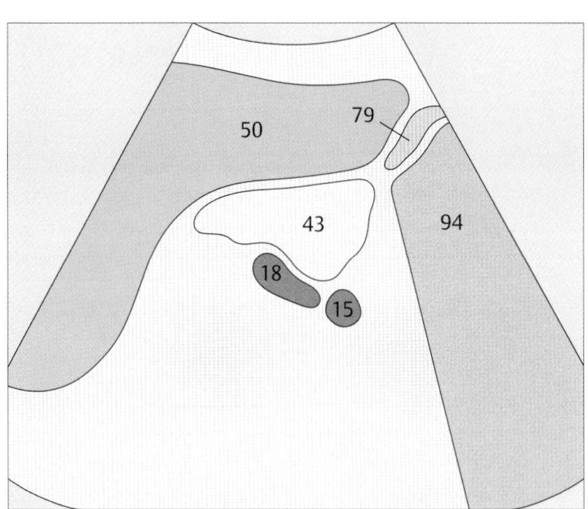

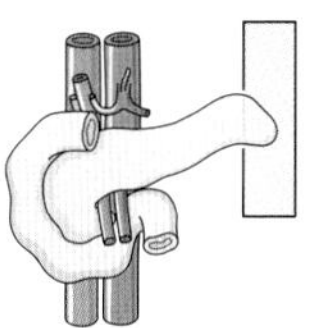

Interference from bowel gas is often encountered caudal to the tail of the pancreas.

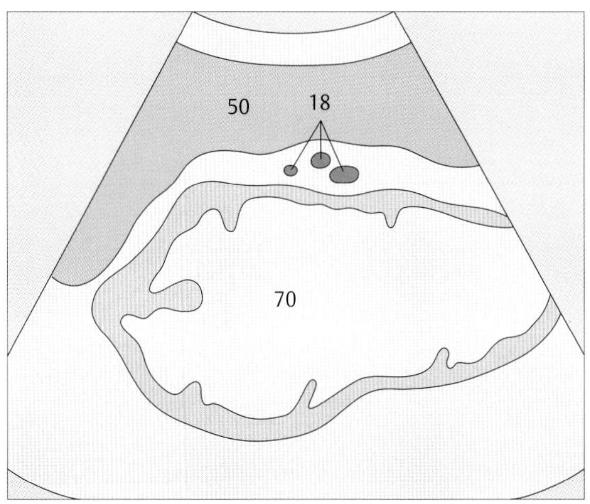

The stomach is a source of numerous artifacts anterior to the tail of the pancreas.

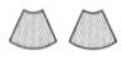

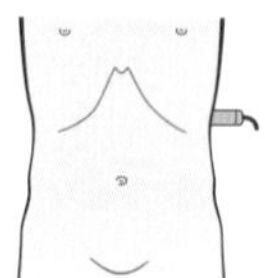

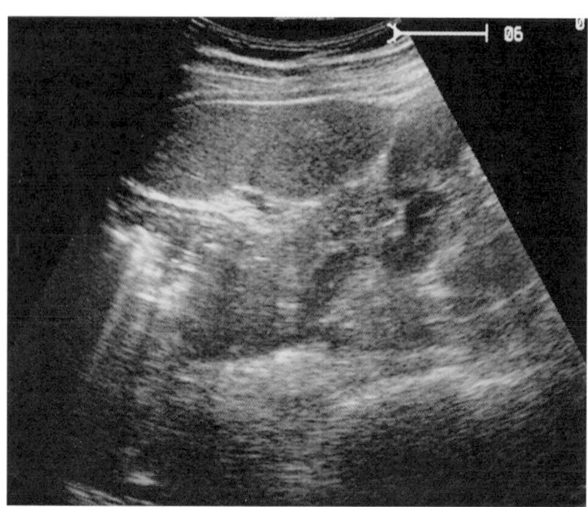

▶ **161** Spleen, tail of pancreas, kidney

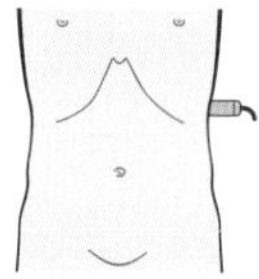

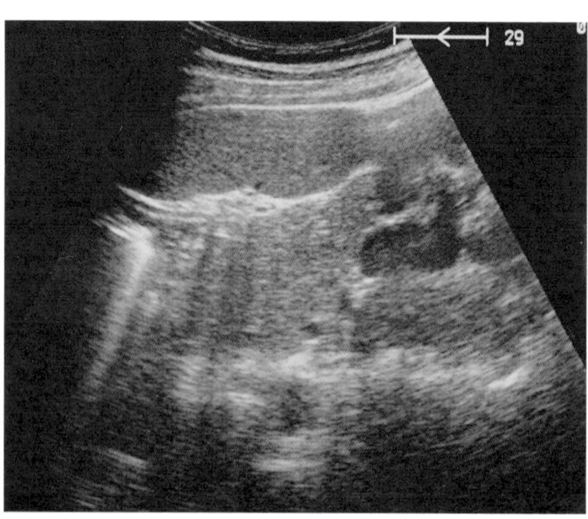

▶ **162** Spleen, tail of pancreas, kidney

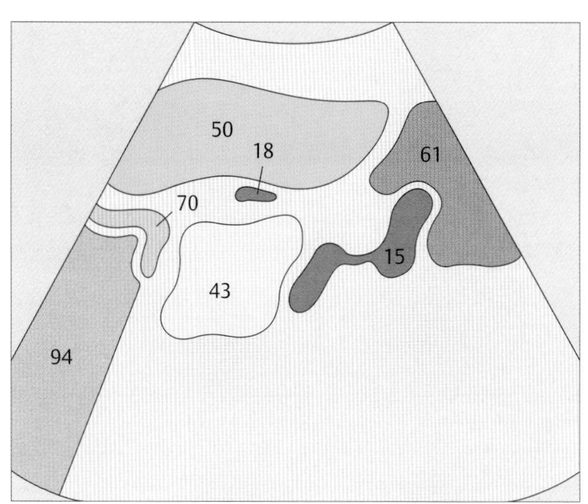

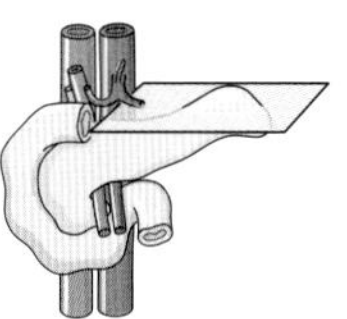

In transverse sections as well, the spleen is used as an acoustic window for scanning the tail of the pancreas.

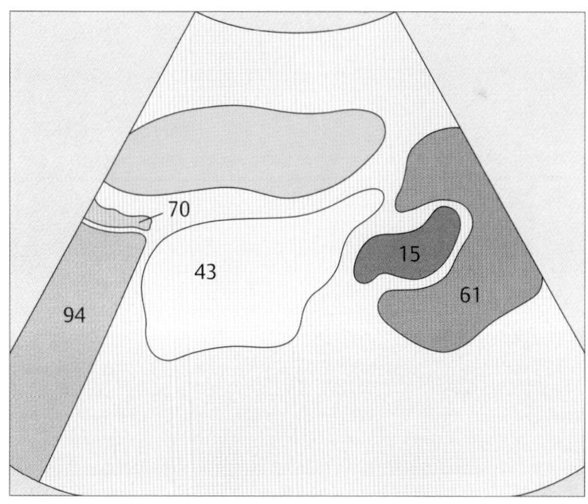

The tail of the pancreas lies in an angle between the spleen and the kidney.

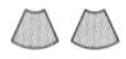

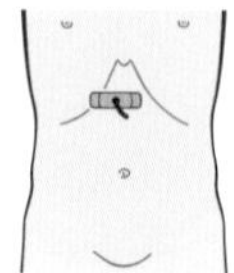

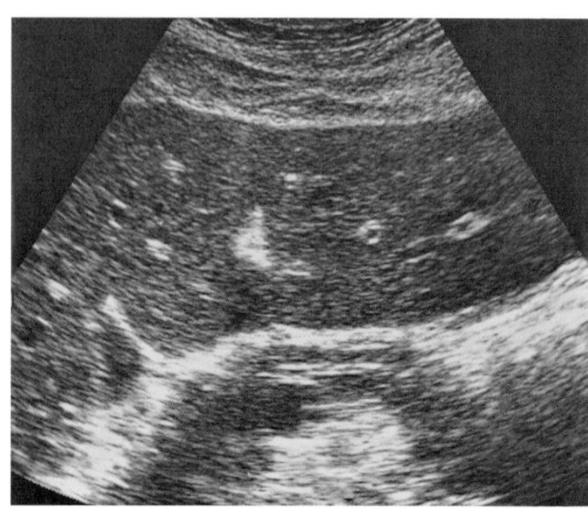

▶ **163** Transverse scan of pancreatic duct

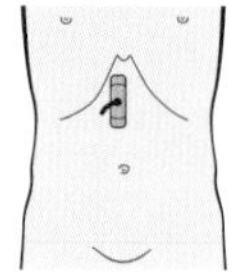

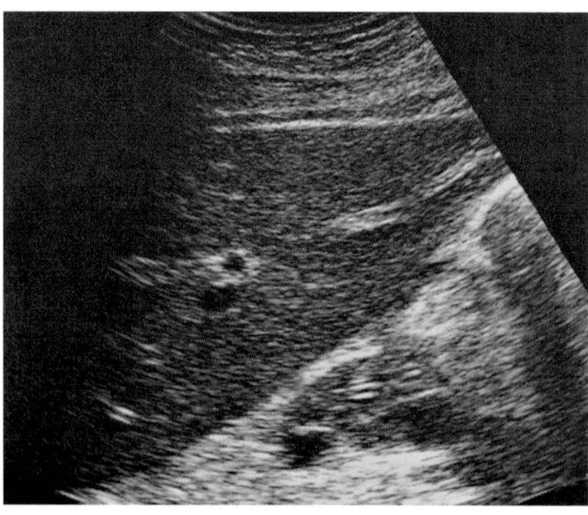

▶ **164** Longitudinal scan of pancreatic duct

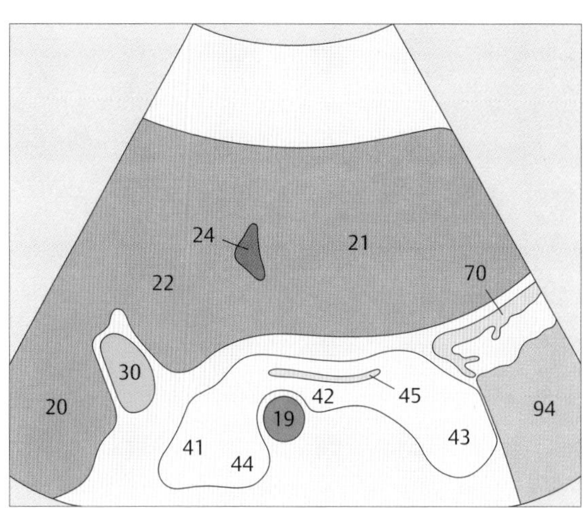

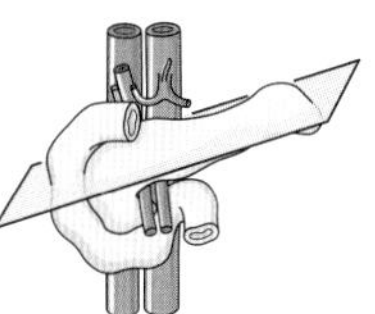

The pancreatic duct has a variable course. It usually runs in the ventrocranial part of the parenchyma, appearing sonographically as two parallel echogenic lines.

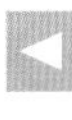

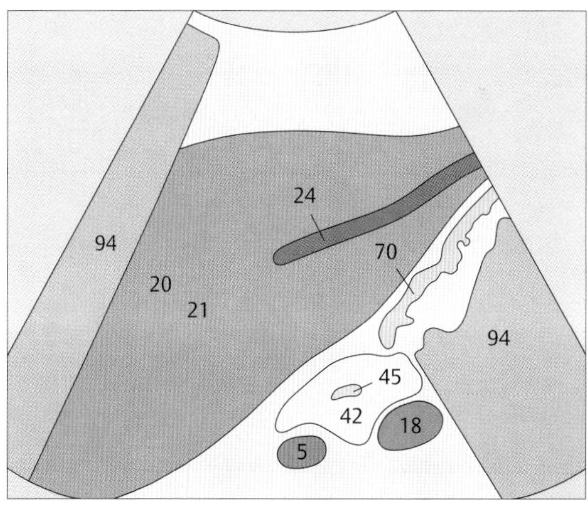

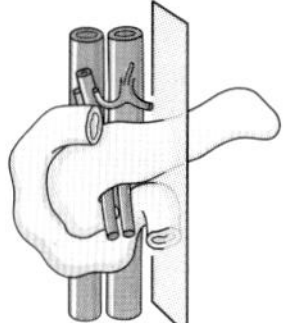

In this plane the pancreatic duct appears as a fine, tubular structure with a luminal diameter up to 3 mm. It is located slightly anterior to the center of the gland.

5 Spleen

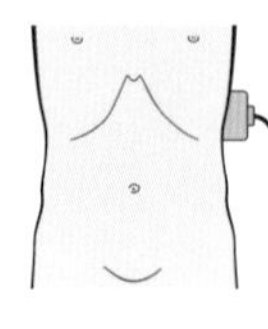

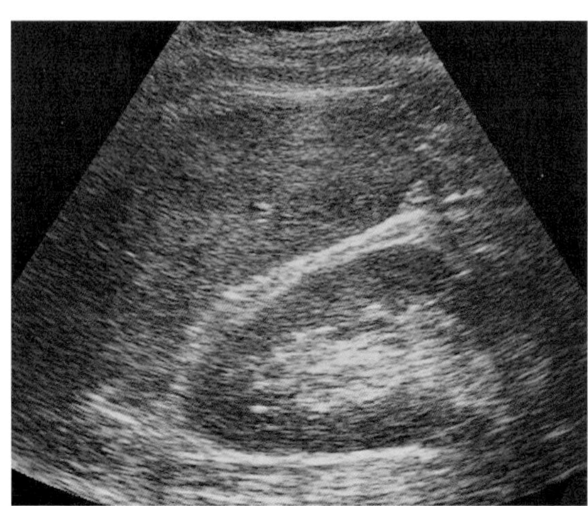

▶ **165** Spleen, kidney

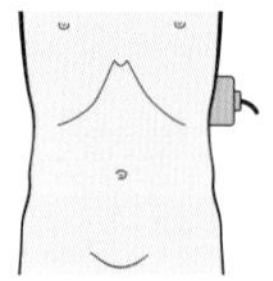

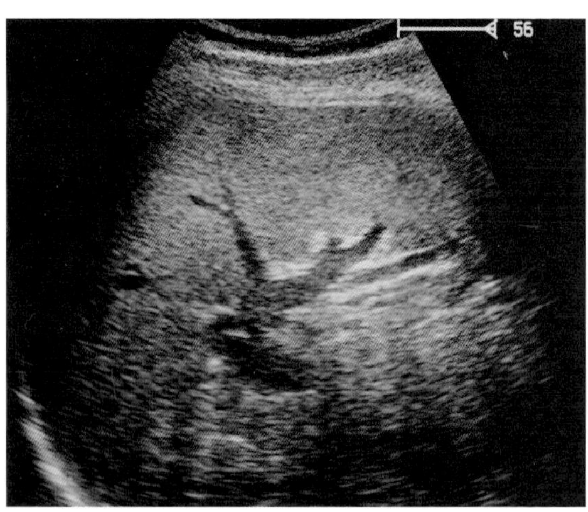

▶ **166** Splenic hilum, splenic vein

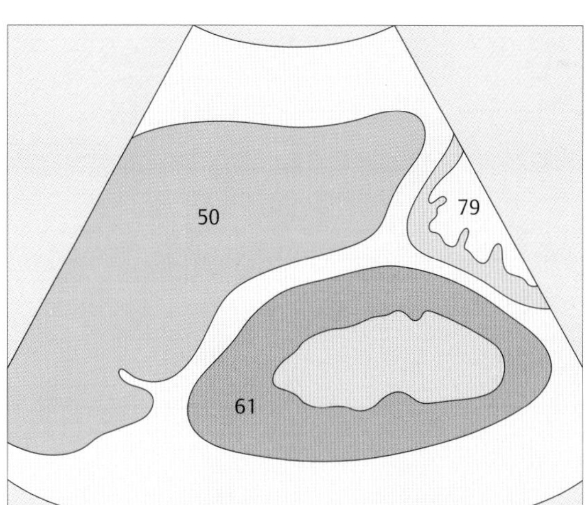

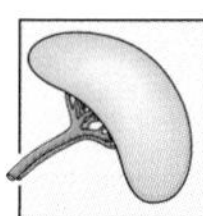

The spleen is identified in the longitudinal flank scan as a rounded triangle between the upper renal pole and the diaphragm.

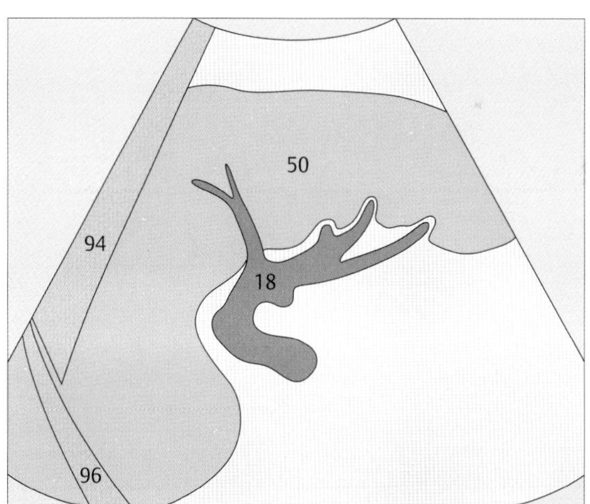

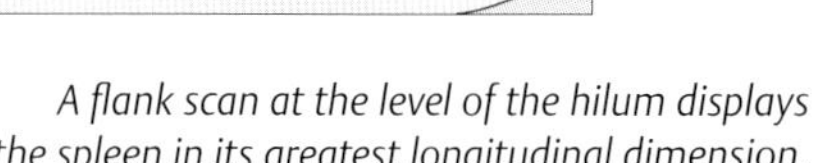

A flank scan at the level of the hilum displays the spleen in its greatest longitudinal dimension.

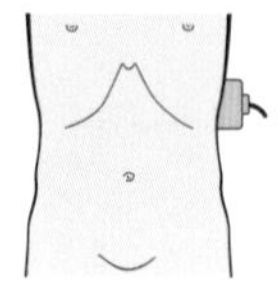

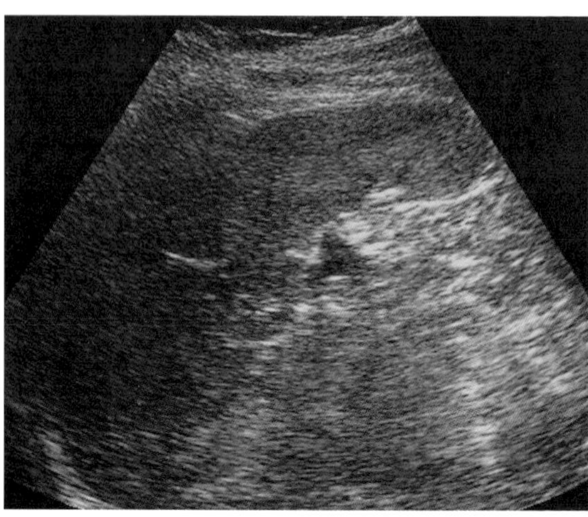

▶ **167** Spleen, stomach

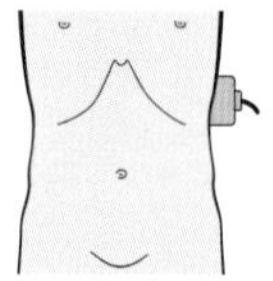

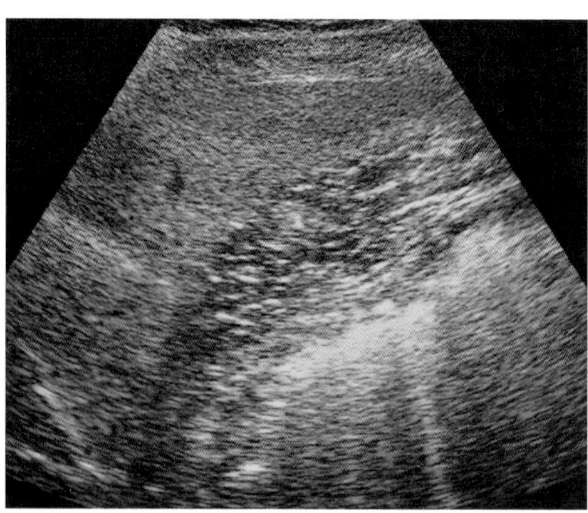

▶ **168** Spleen, stomach

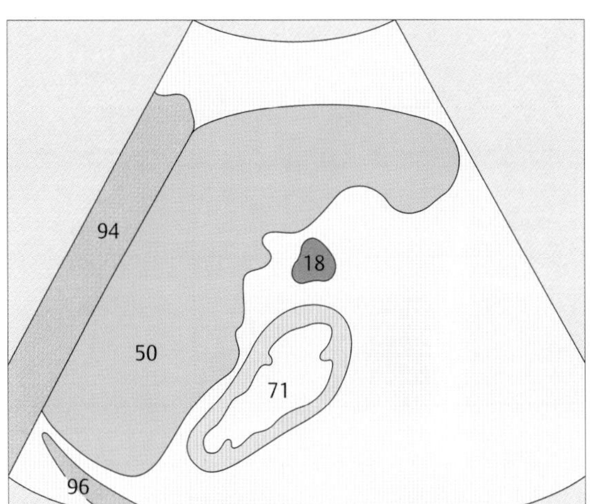

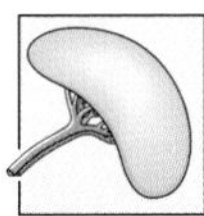

The spleen lies against the stomach anteriorly and medially.

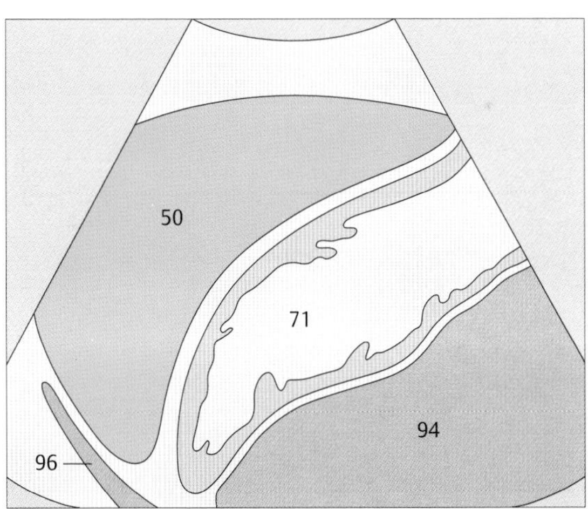

The spleen exhibits a typical crescent shape in an anterior flank scan.

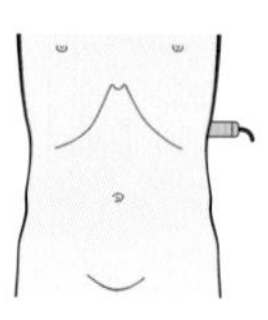

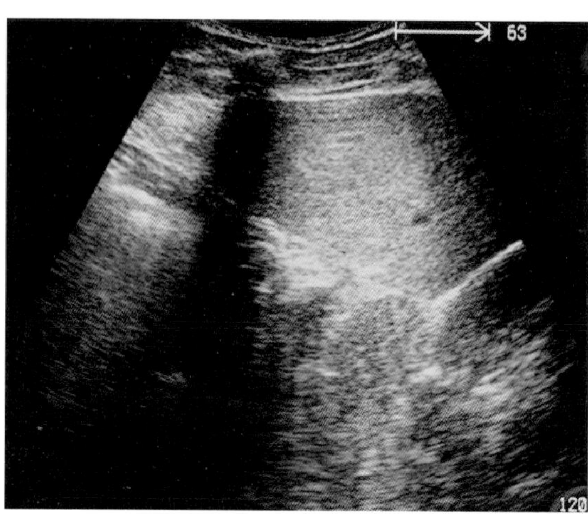

▶ **169** Spleen, kidney, stomach

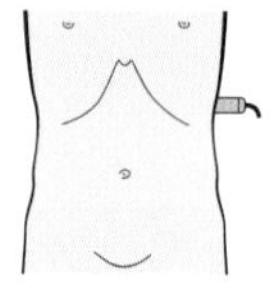

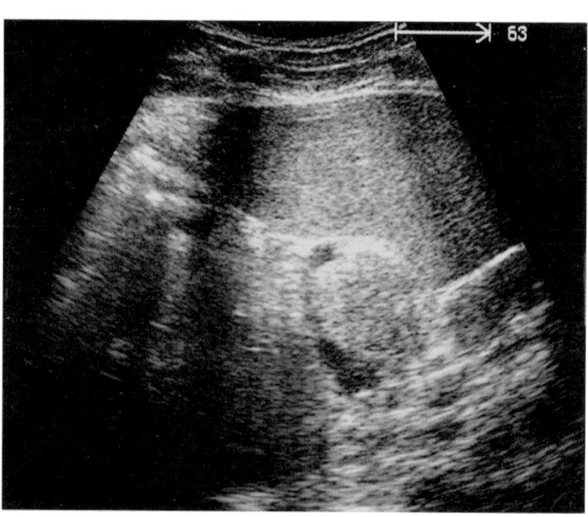

▶ **170** Spleen, kidney, pancreas

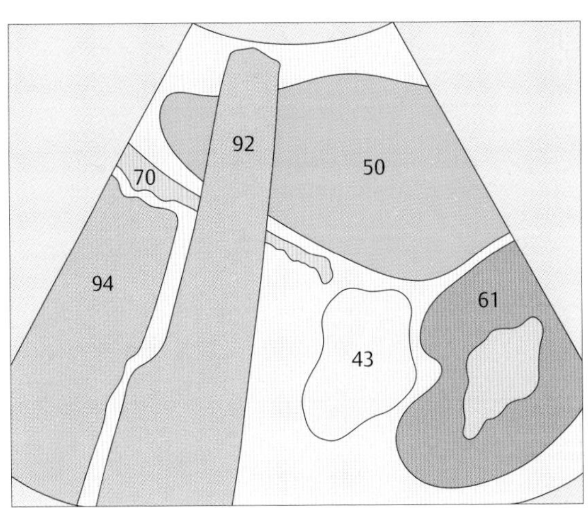

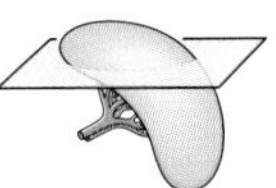

A high transverse flank scan demonstrates the typical triad of the spleen, kidney, and stomach.

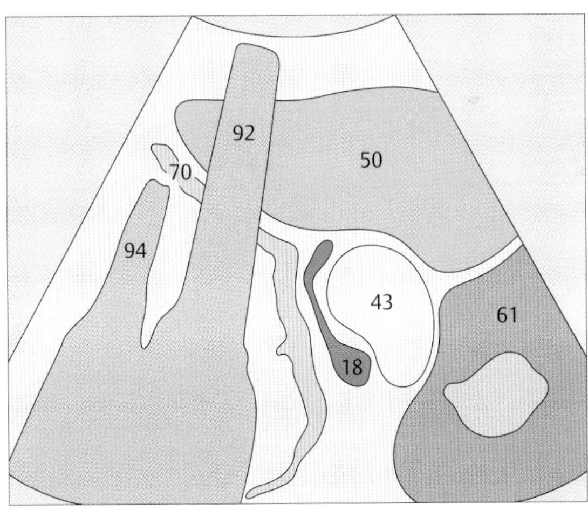

The tail of the pancreas can usually be identified in the splenic hilum next to the splenic vessels.

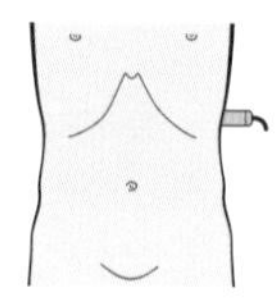

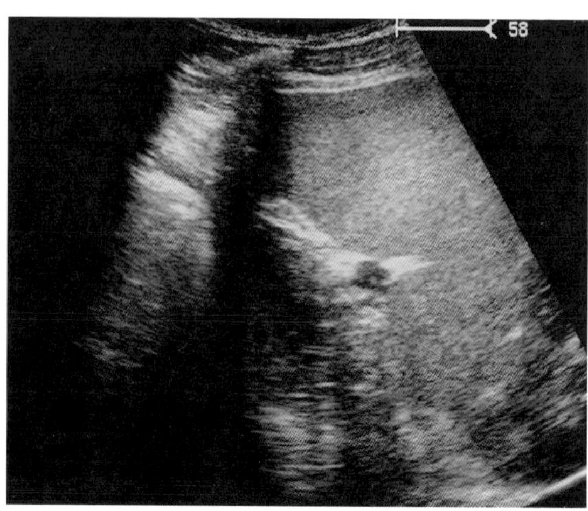

▶ **171** Spleen, stomach

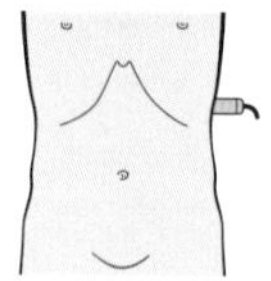

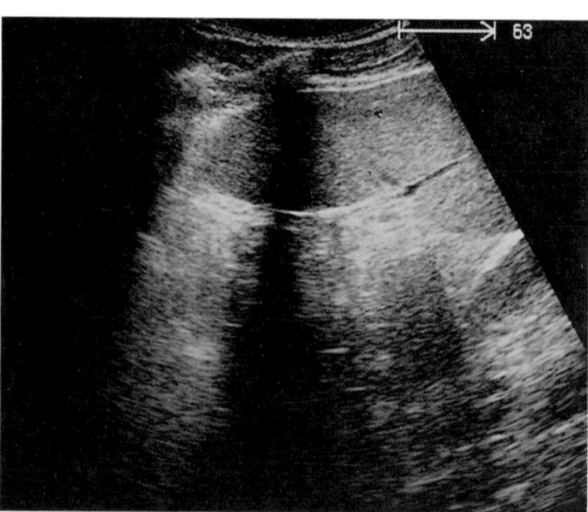

▶ **172** Spleen, small bowel

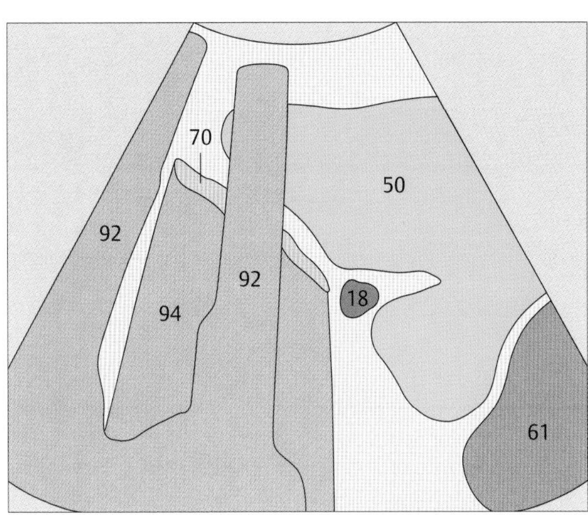

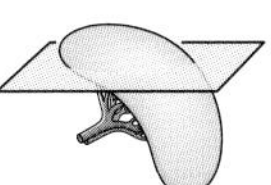

The spleen may be deeply lobulated by septa.

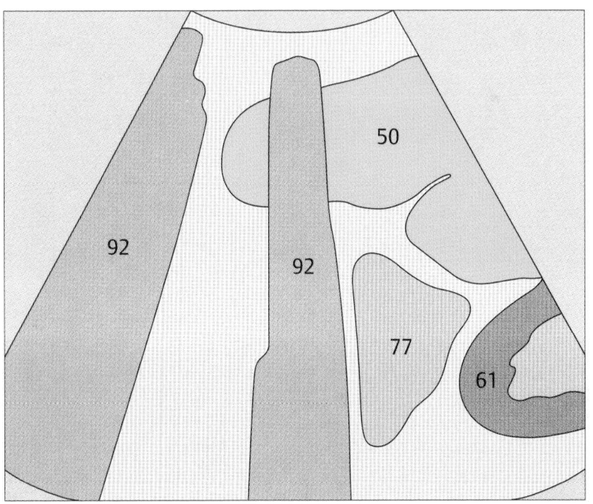

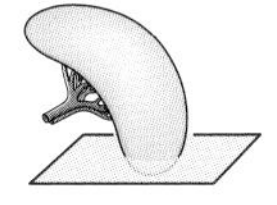

Loops of small bowel are located medial to the lower pole of the spleen.

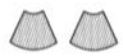

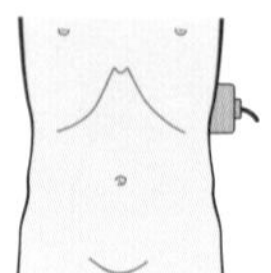

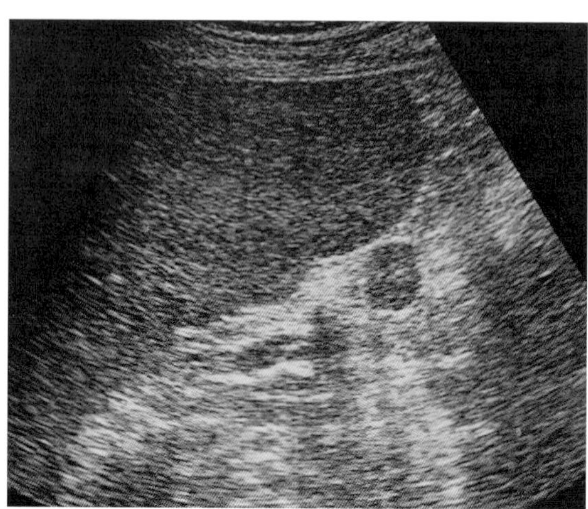

▶ **173** Accessory spleen

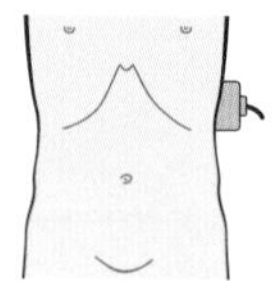

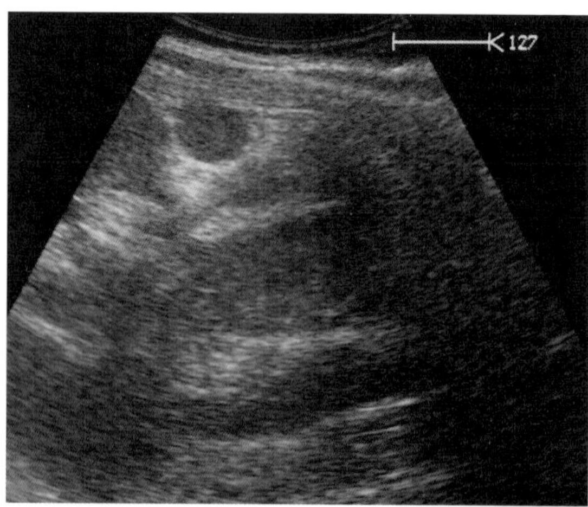

▶ **174** Accessory spleen

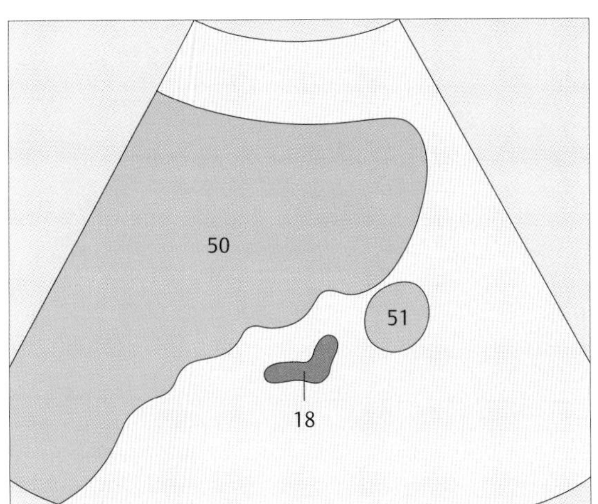

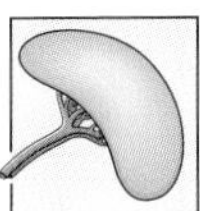

Accessory spleens are most commonly found in the hilar region.

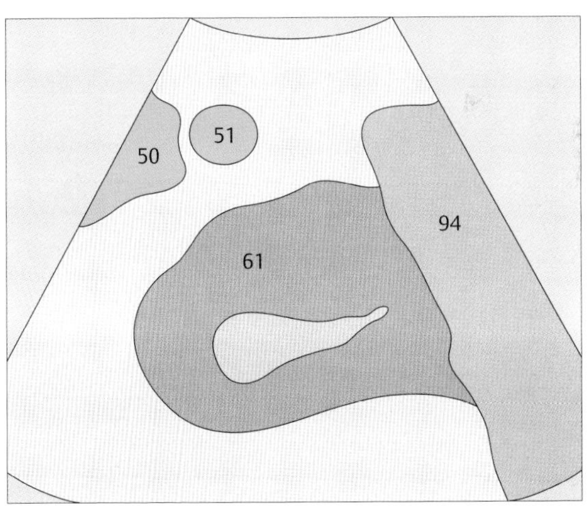

An accessory spleen is occasionally found at the lower pole.

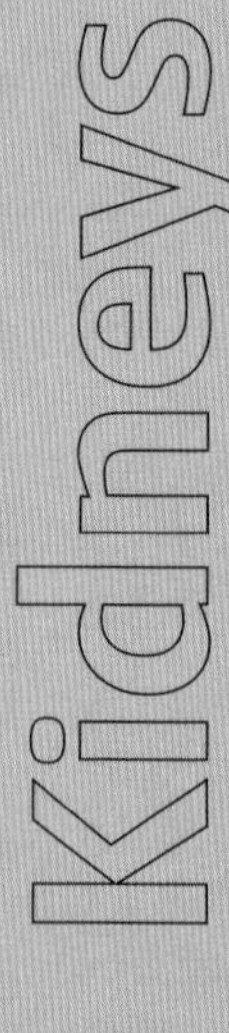
6 Kidneys

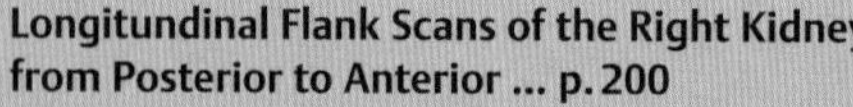

Longitudinal Flank Scans of the Left Kidney from Posterior to Anterior ... p. 216

Transverse Flank Scans of the Left Kidney from Above Downward ... p. 220

Details of the Kidneys ... p. 224

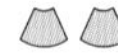

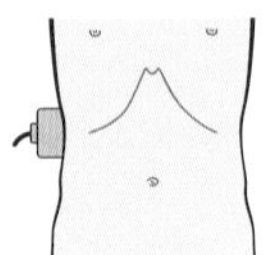

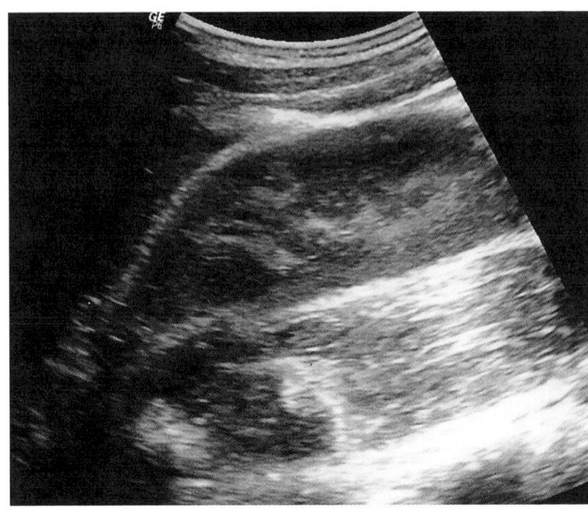

▶ **175** Kidney, liver, psoas muscle

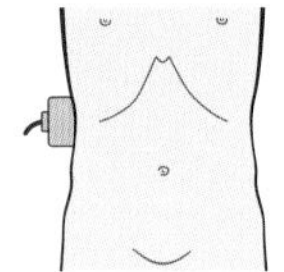

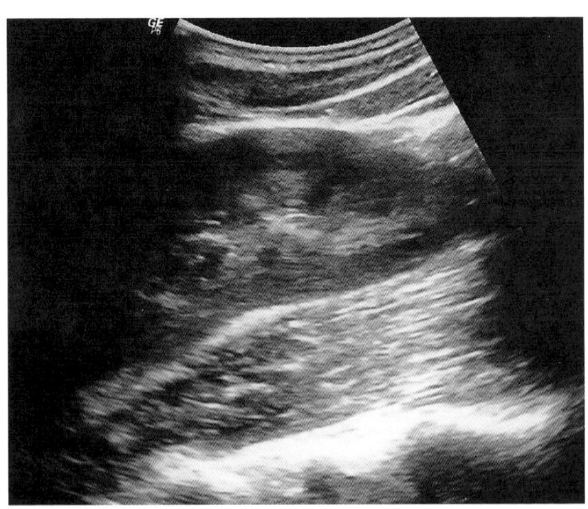

▶ **176** Kidney, liver, psoas muscle

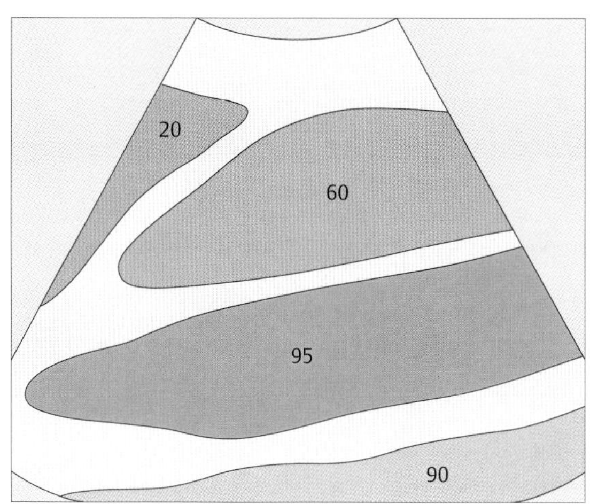

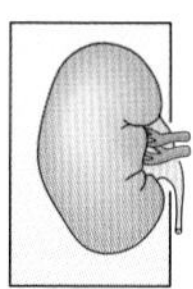

The right kidney is clearly demonstrated through the acoustic window of the liver.

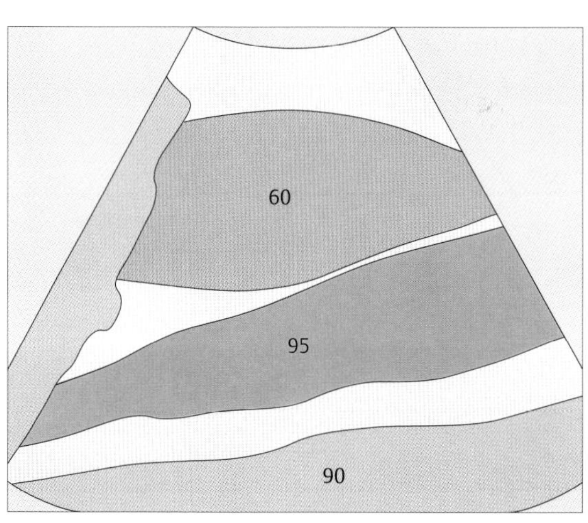

The kidneys slide downward along the lumbar muscles during respiratory excursions.

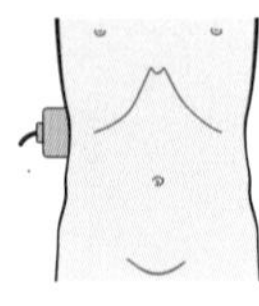

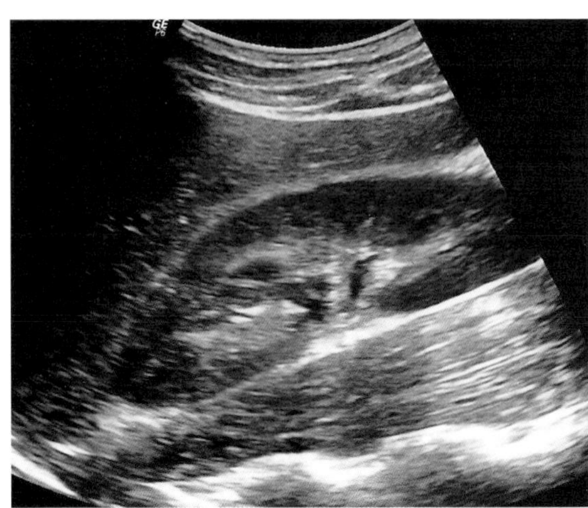

▶ **177** Kidney, liver, psoas muscle

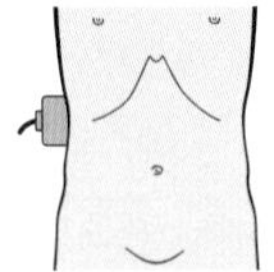

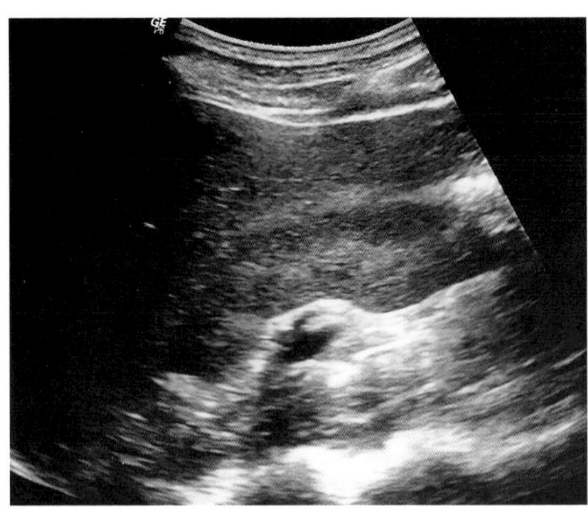

▶ **178** Kidney, right renal vein

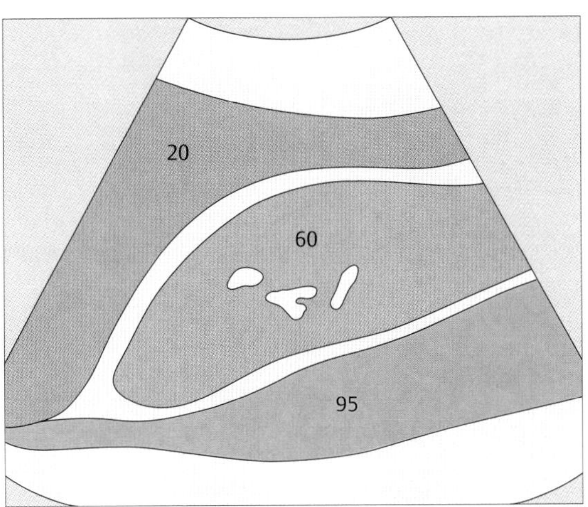

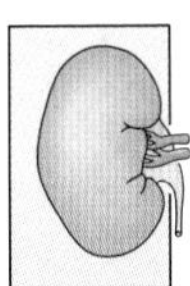

The summation of portions of the pelvicalyceal system, blood vessels, lymphatics, fatty tissue, and renal sinus form an echogenic complex at the center of the kidney.

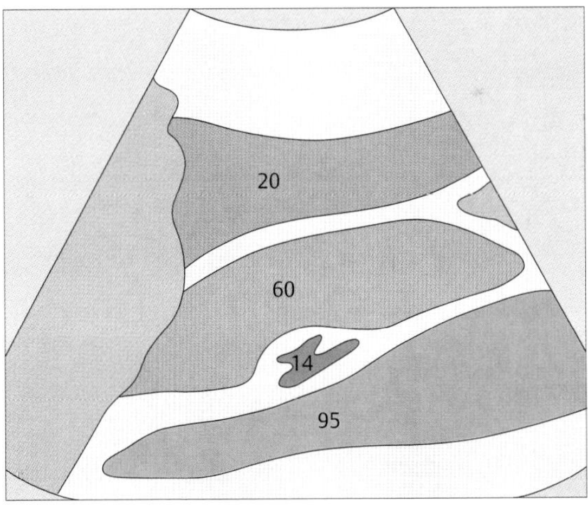

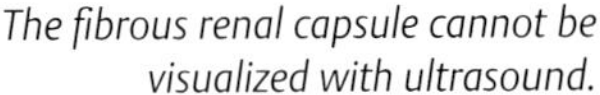

The fibrous renal capsule cannot be visualized with ultrasound.

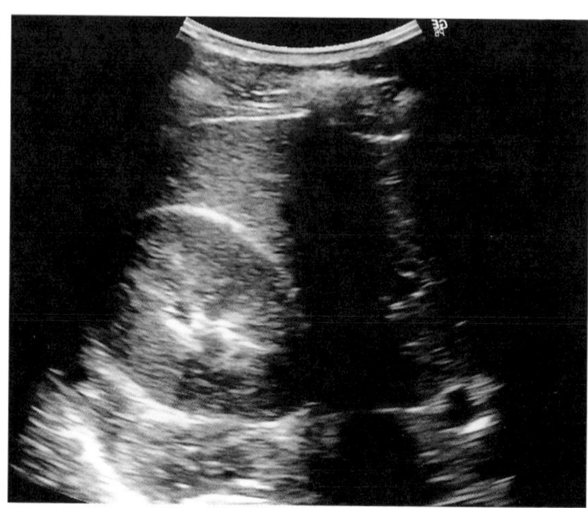

▶ **179** Kidney, liver

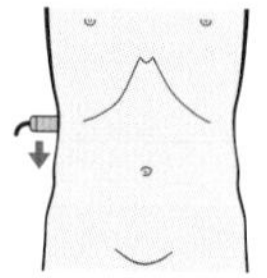

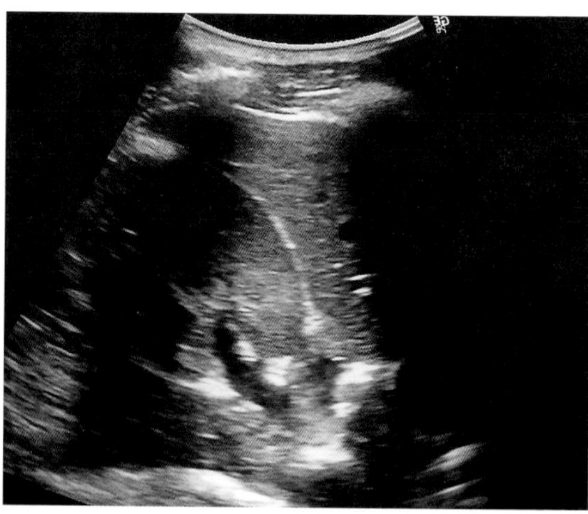

▶ **180** Kidney, liver, right renal vein

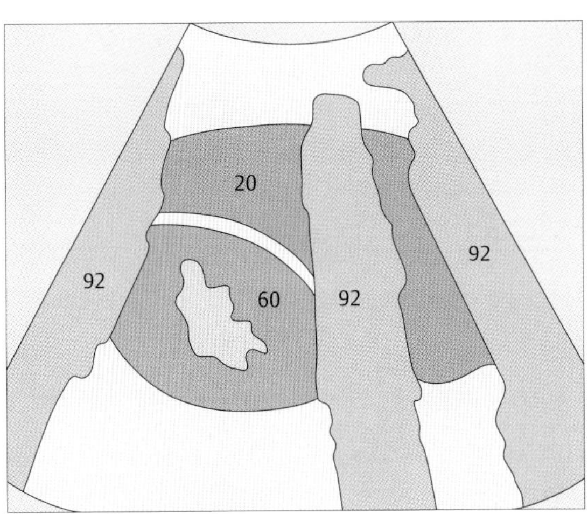

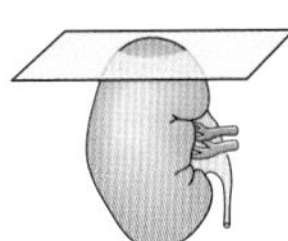

The right kidney occupies a posterior site in the angle between the spinal column, muscles, and right lobe of the liver.

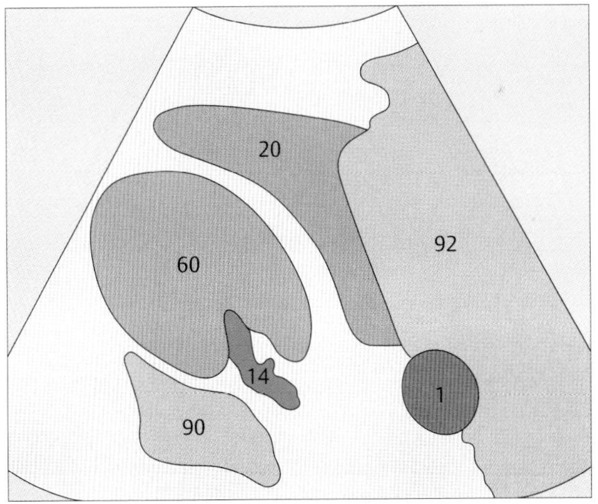

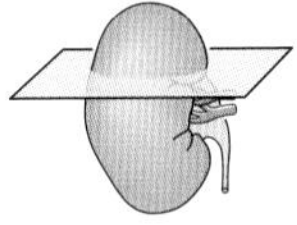

Generally the renal hilar vessels can be clearly defined.

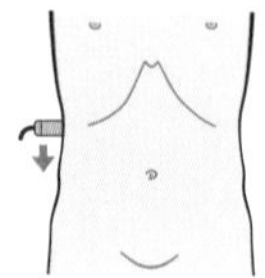

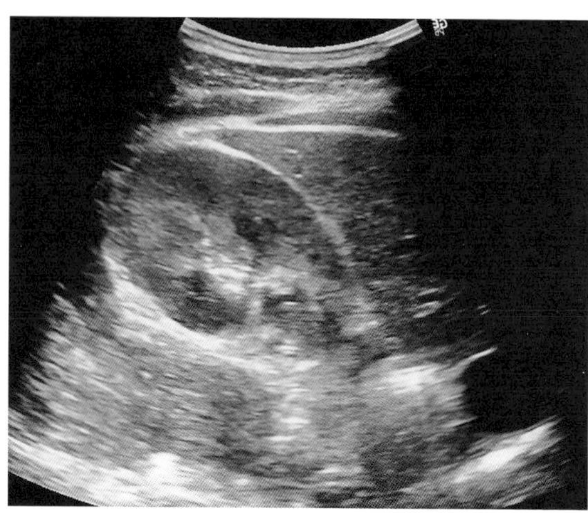

▶ **181** Kidney, liver

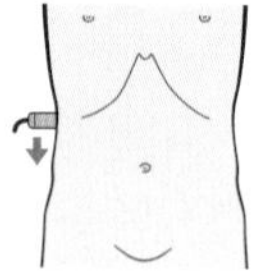

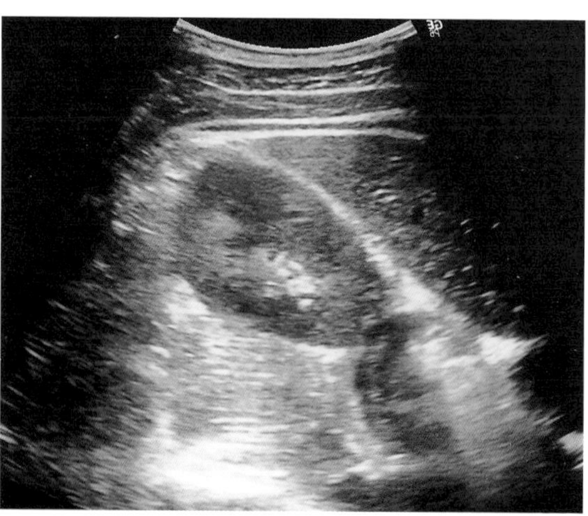

▶ **182** Kidney, liver

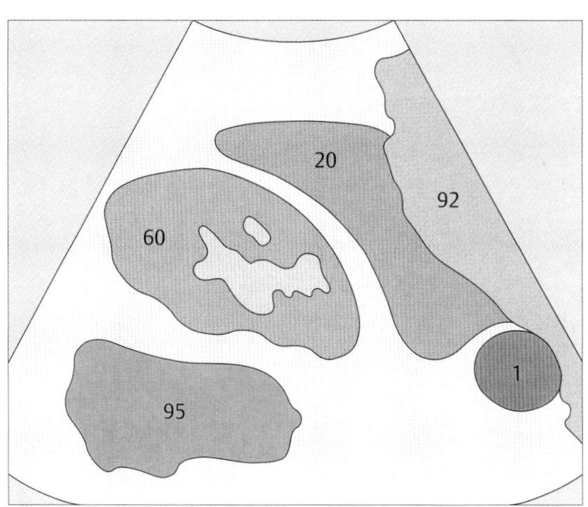

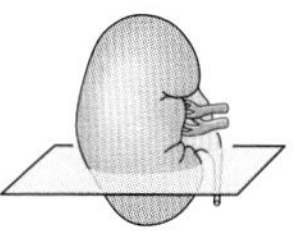

The psoas muscle is located medial to the kidney.

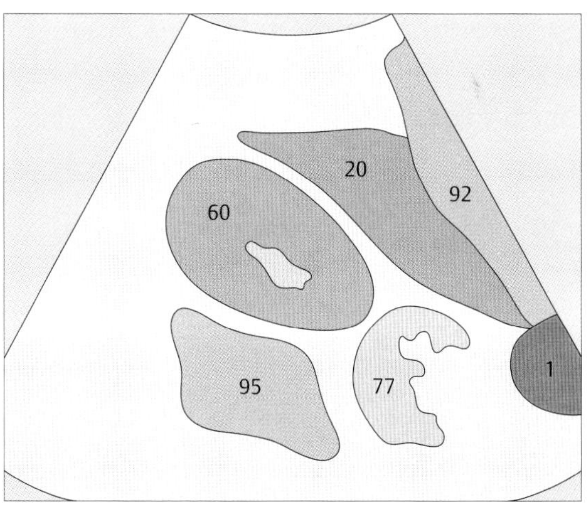

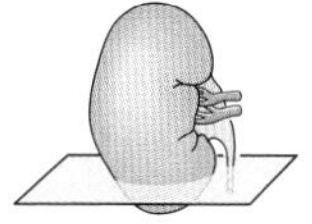

In most cases the right kidney can be clearly visualized as far as its upper pole when scanned from the lateral side.

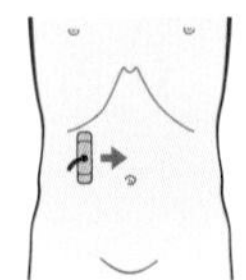

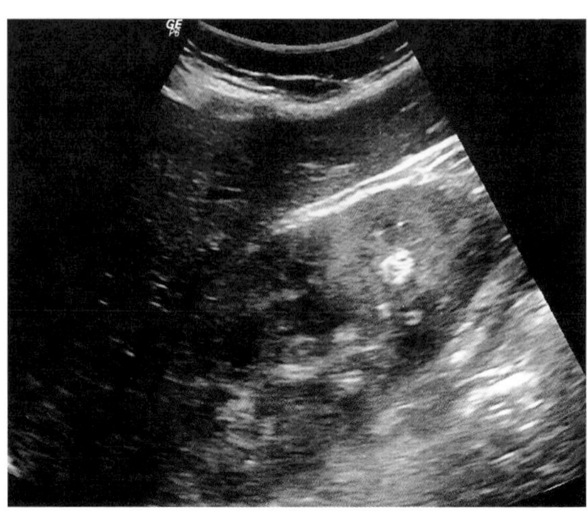

▶ **183** Kidney, liver

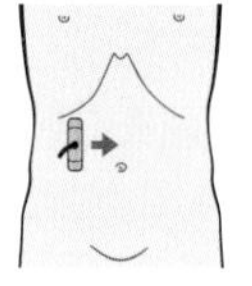

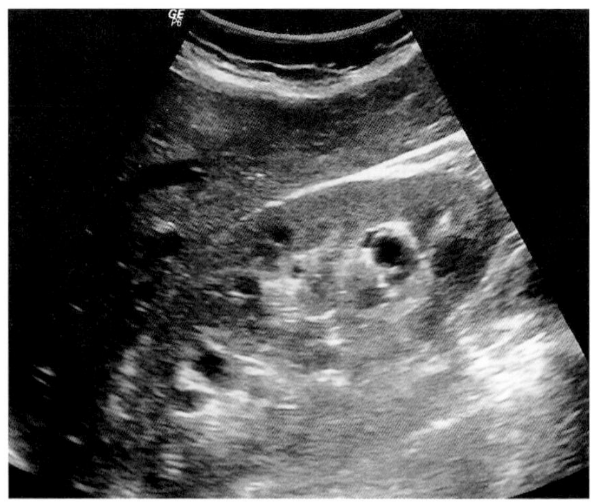

▶ **184** Kidney, liver

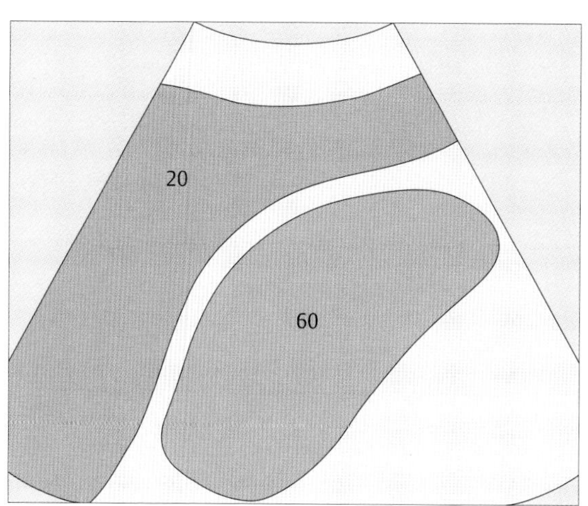

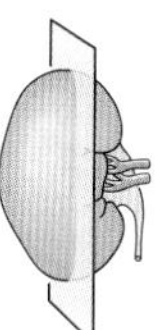

Unlike the left kidney, the right kidney can be clearly visualized from the anterior side using the liver as an acoustic window.

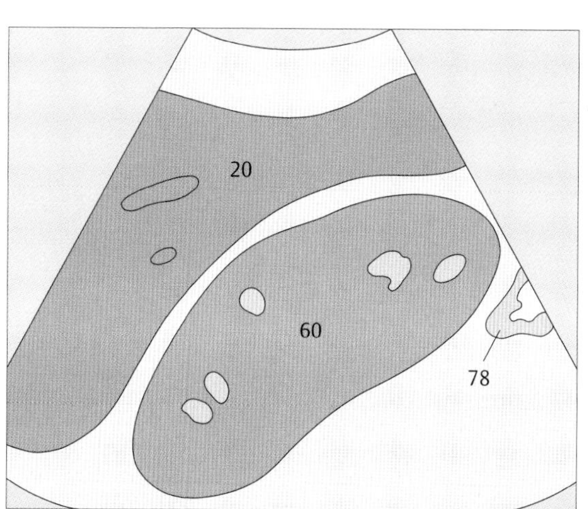

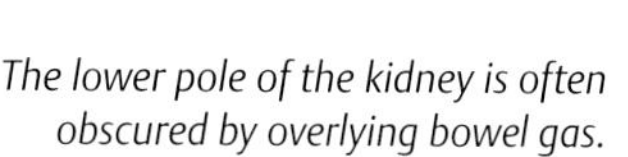

The lower pole of the kidney is often obscured by overlying bowel gas.

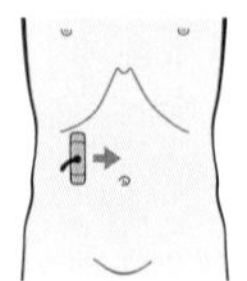

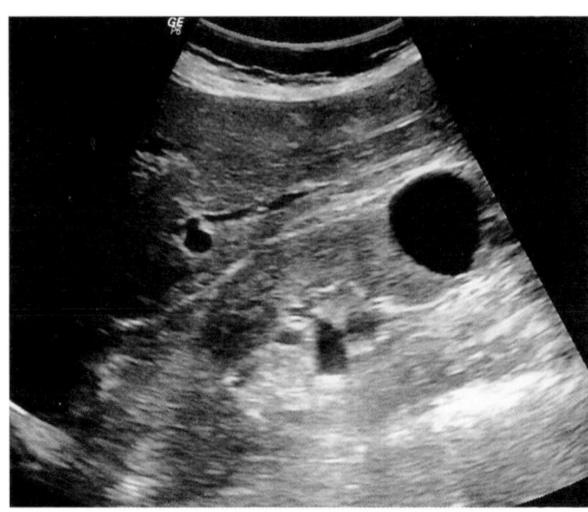

▶ **185** Kidney, liver, *renal cyst

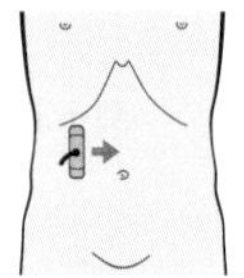

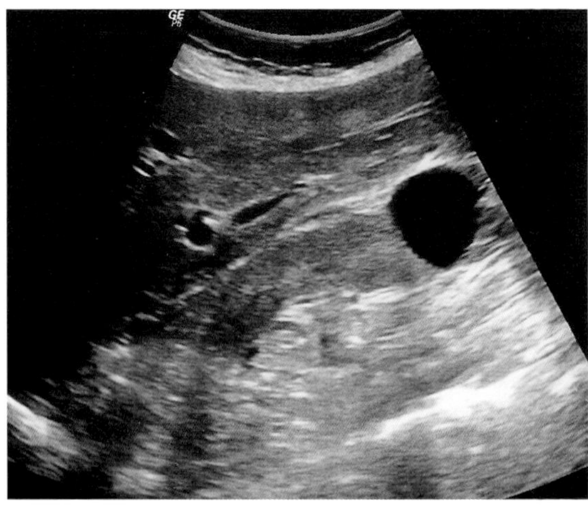

▶ **186** Kidney, liver, *renal cyst

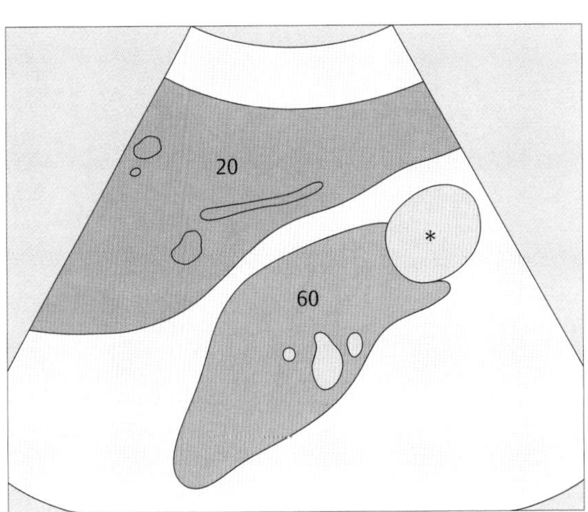

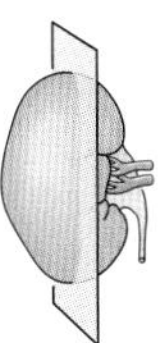

Renal cysts are common, irrelevant incidental findings.

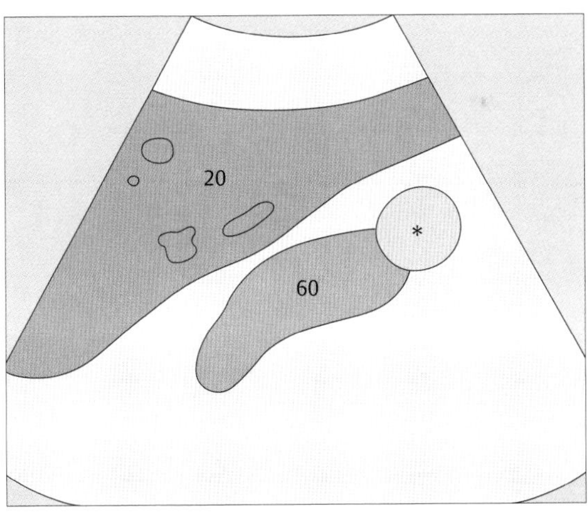

An anterior scan will often display the entire right kidney in thin patients.

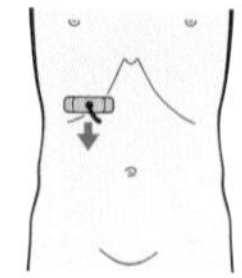

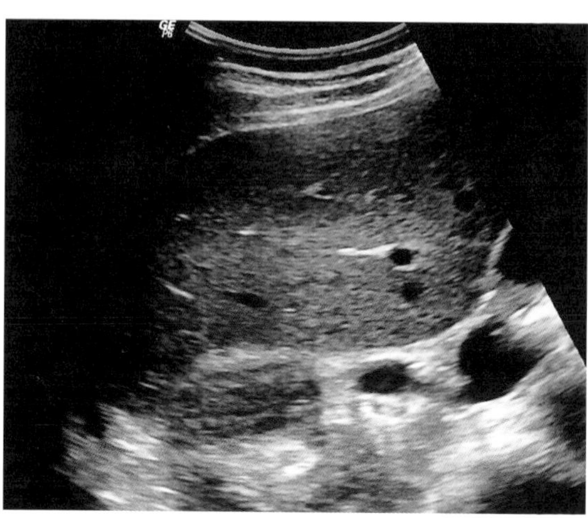

▶ **187** Kidney, right renal vein, vena cava

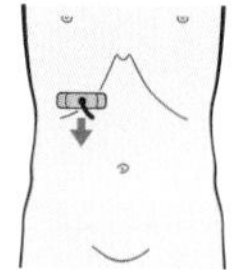

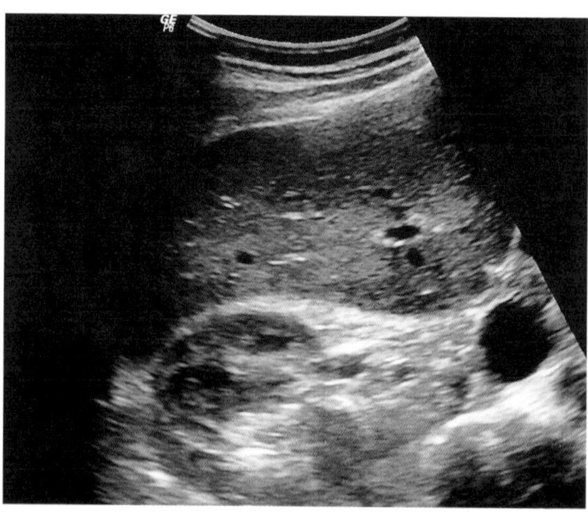

▶ **188** Kidney, right renal vein, vena cava, right renal artery

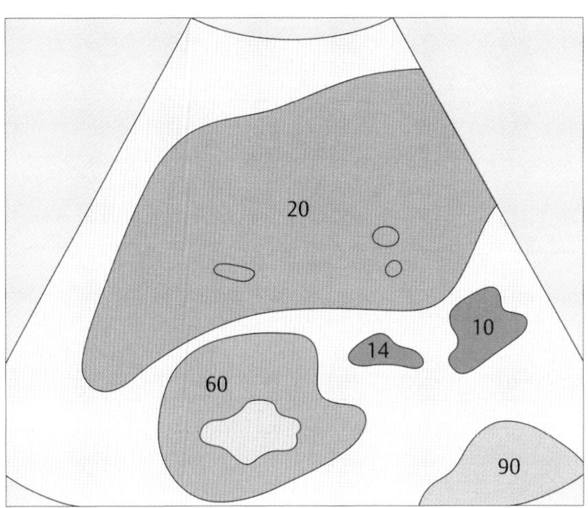

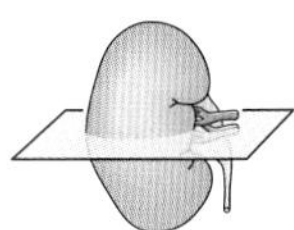

The renal vein enters the vena cava at the level of the renal upper pole.

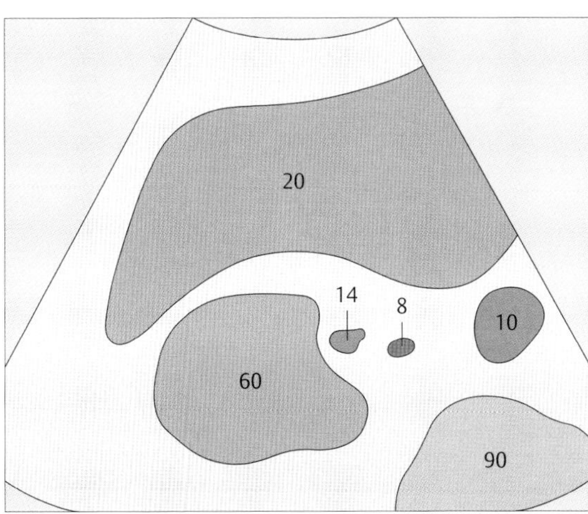

The renal artery is located posterior and superior to the renal vein, which is noticeably larger than the artery in most patients.

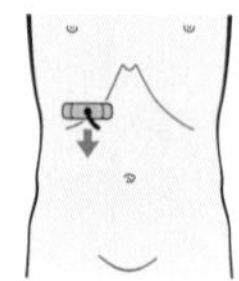

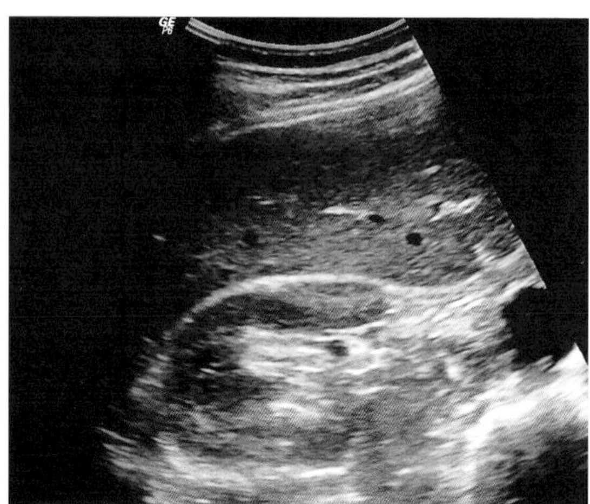

▶ **189** Kidneys, right renal artery

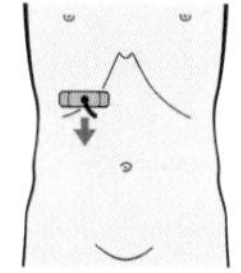

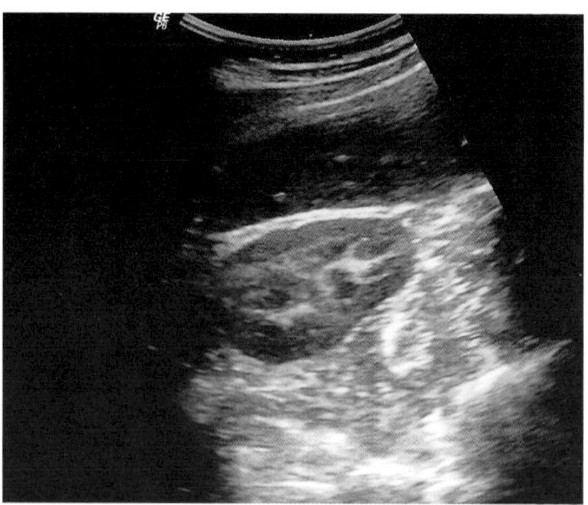

▶ **190** Kidney, spleen, psoas muscle

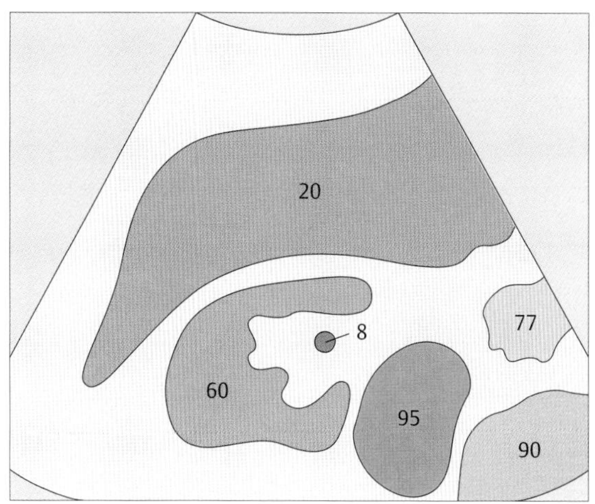

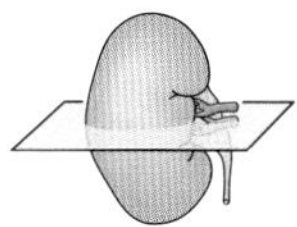

The kidney slides downward on the psoas muscle during inspiration.

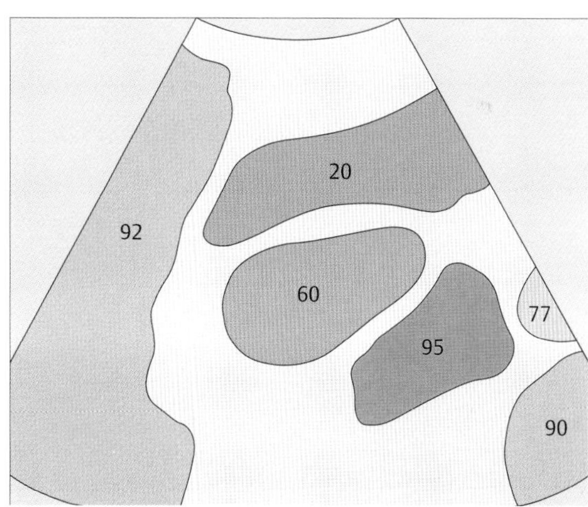

The right lobe of the liver extends a variable distance over the right kidney.

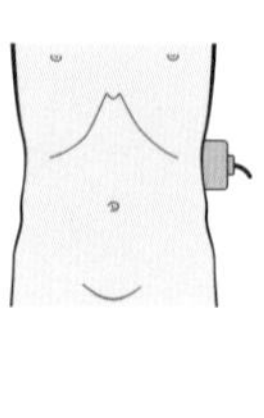

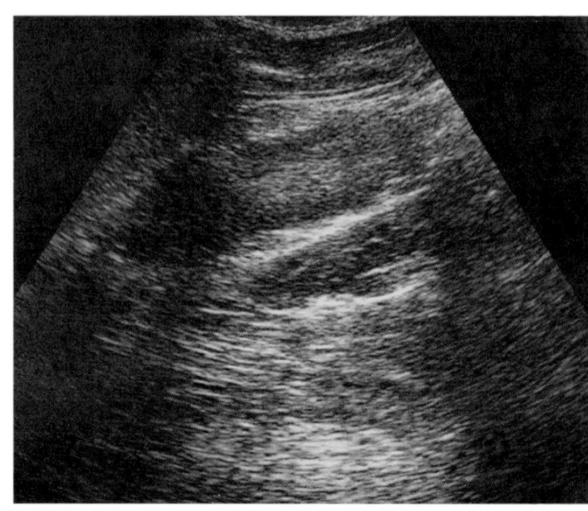

▶ **191** Kidney, spleen, psoas muscle

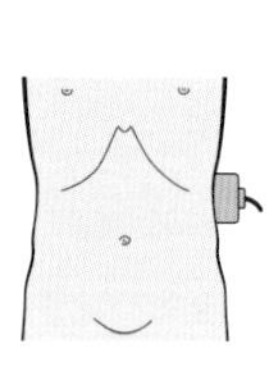

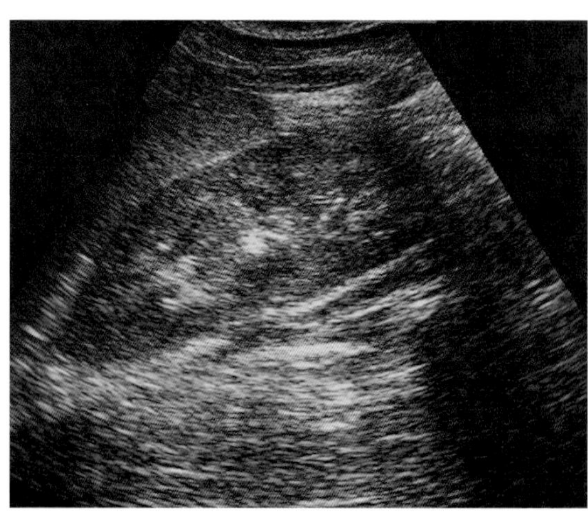

▶ **192** Kidney, spleen, psoas muscle

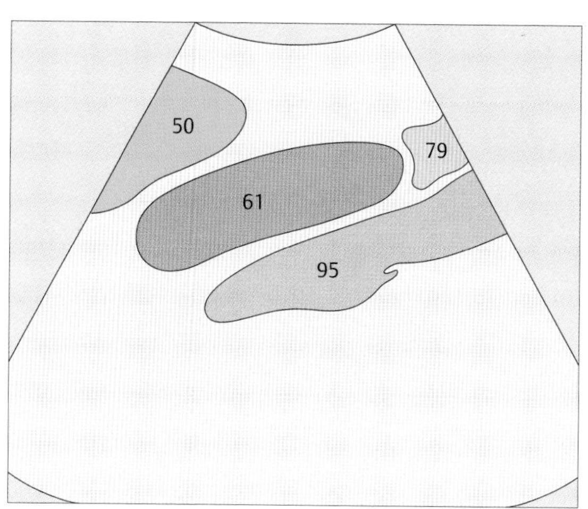

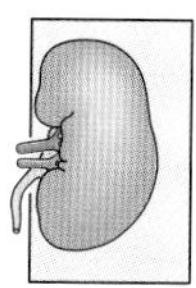

A good acoustic window is not available for scanning the left kidney.

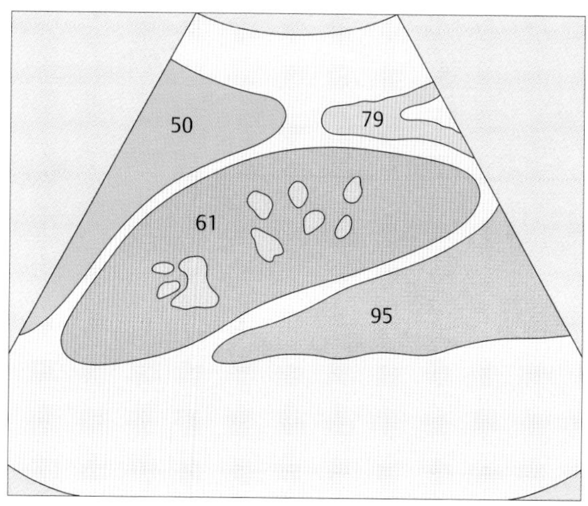

The spleen extends laterally to the approximate center of the left kidney.

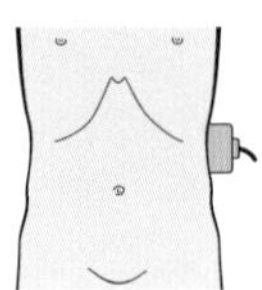

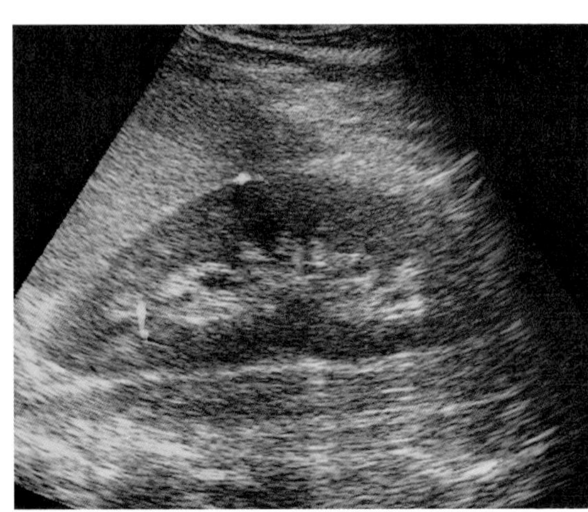

▶ **193** Kidney, spleen, psoas muscle

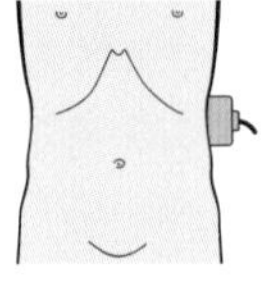

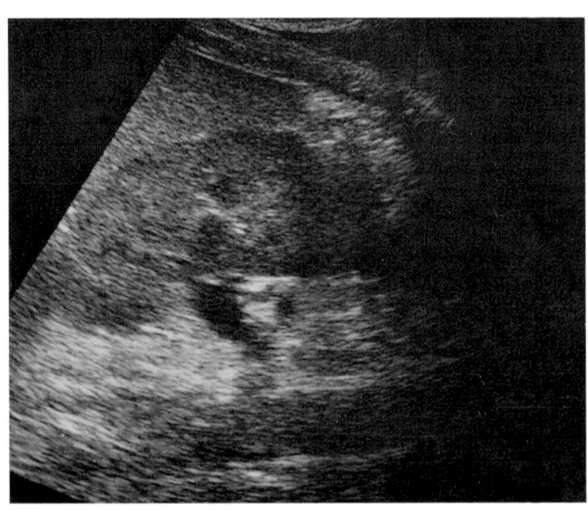

▶ **194** Kidney, renal vein, spleen, aorta

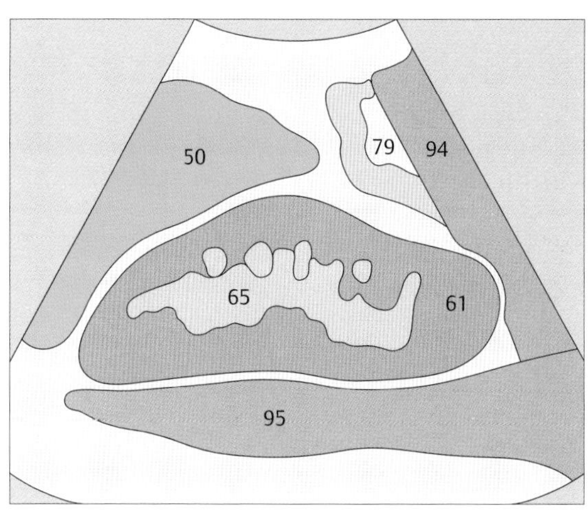

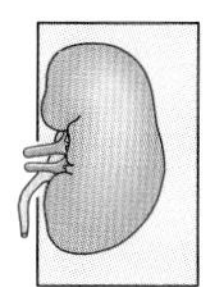

The lower half of the left kidney is covered laterally by the descending colon and left colic flexure.

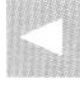

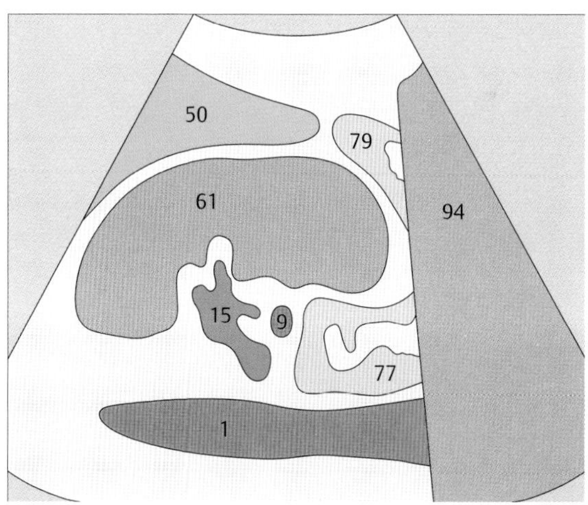

The aorta appears farthest from the transducer in a longitudinal scan from the left flank.

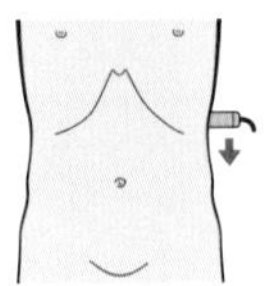

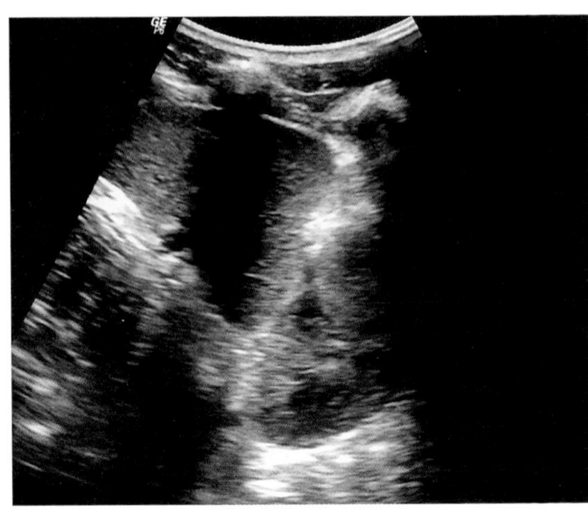

▶ **195** Kidney, spleen, stomach

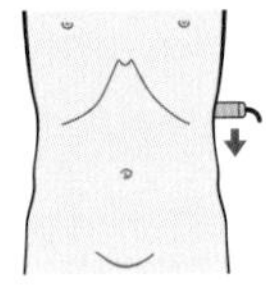

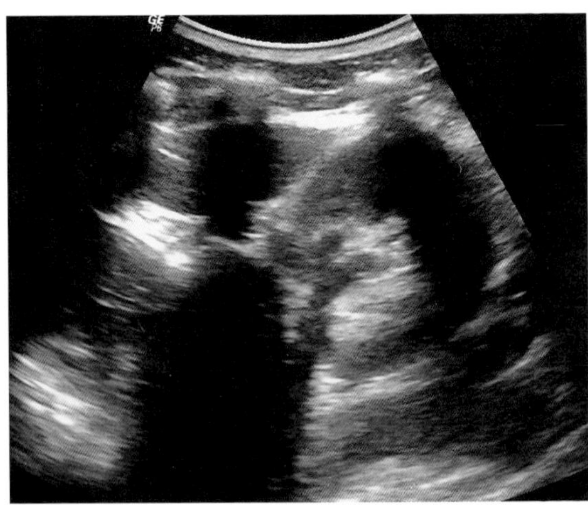

▶ **196** Kidney, left renal artery, spleen, stomach

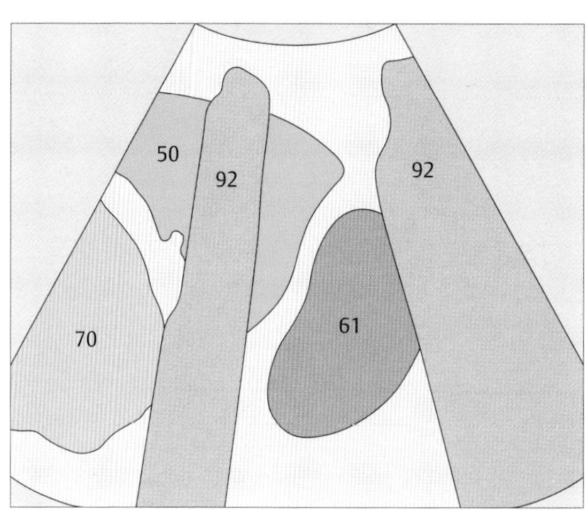

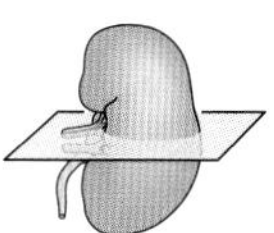

The ribs are an obstacle to scanning the left kidney through the spleen.

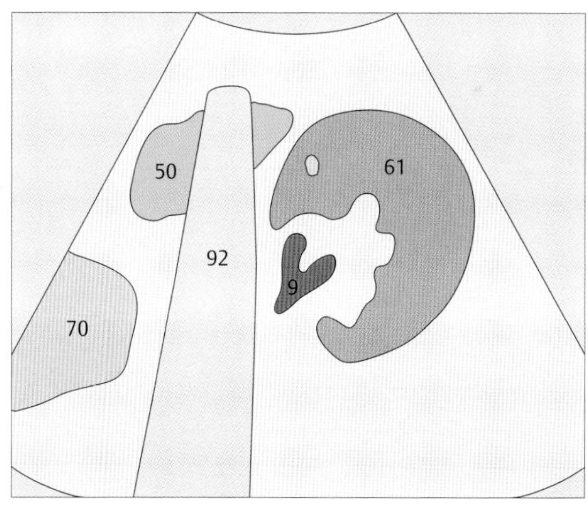

The renal vessels are often clearly visualized on the left side.

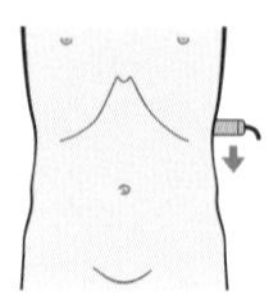

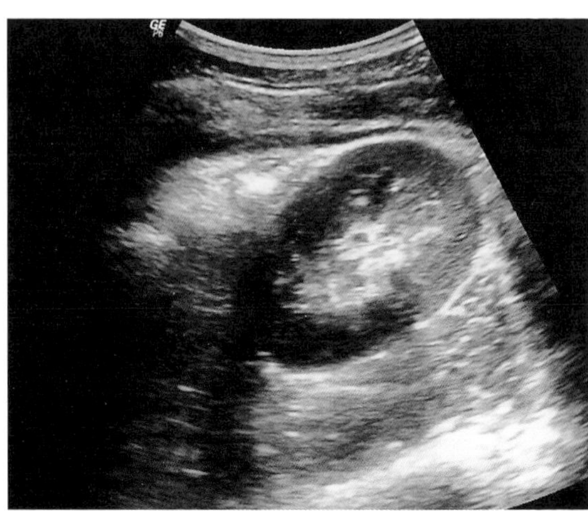

▶ **197** Kidney, right colic flexure

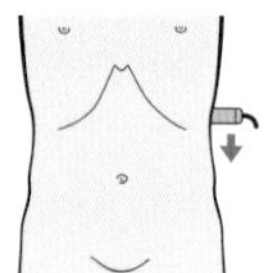

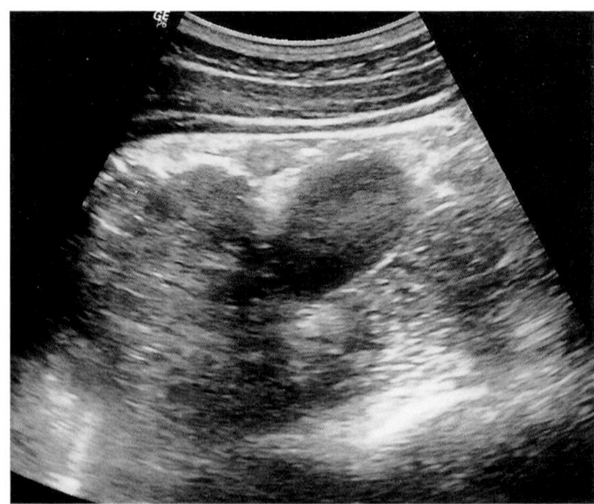

▶ **198** Kidney, right colic flexure

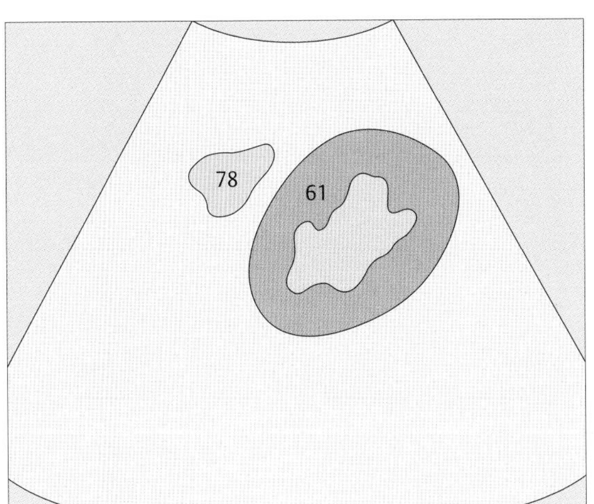

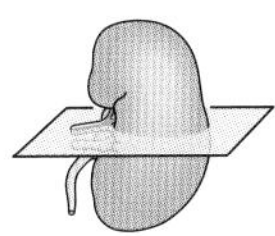

The lower pole of the left kidney is often difficult to define.

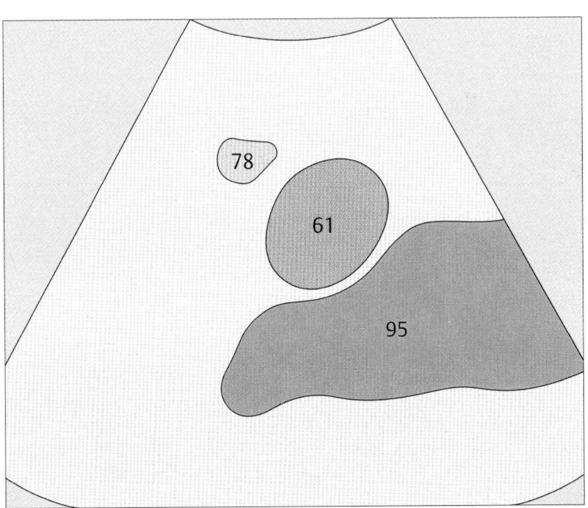

Because the kidney moves with respiratory excursions, it can be fully visualized in most cases despite being partially obscured by bowel gas and ribs.

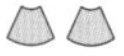

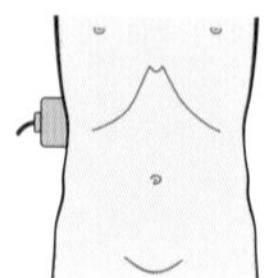

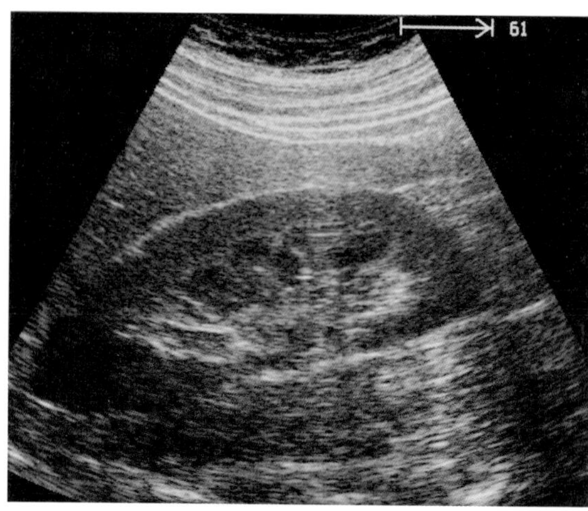

▶ **199** Medullary pyramids

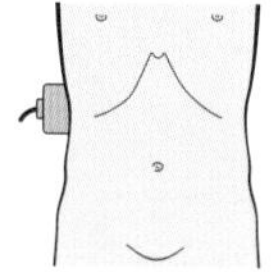

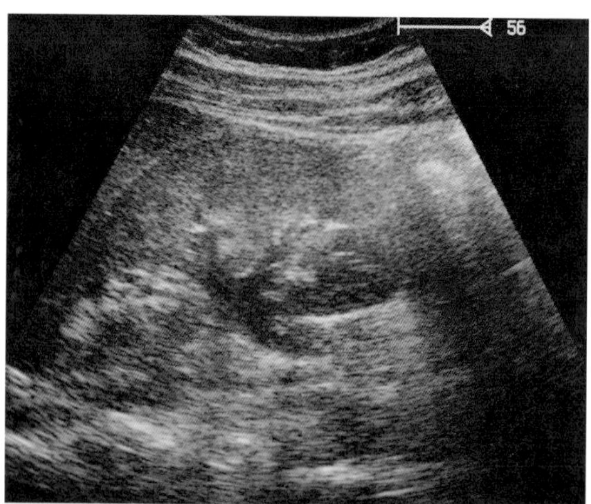

▶ **200** Collecting system

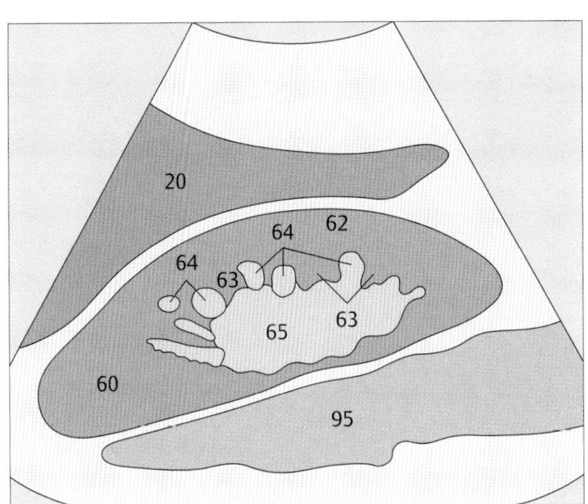

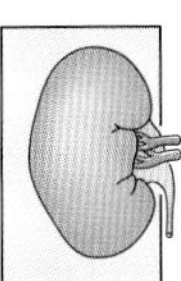

An imaginary line joining the bases of the hypoechoic medullary pyramids forms a dividing line between the cortical and medullary tissue in the ultrasound image.

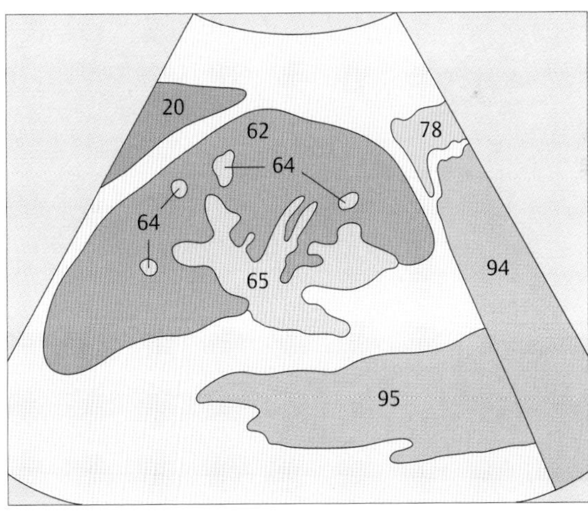

Intense diuresis has caused a bandlike or stellate fluid collection to appear in the renal pelvis.

7 Adrenal Glands

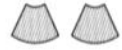
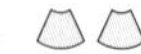

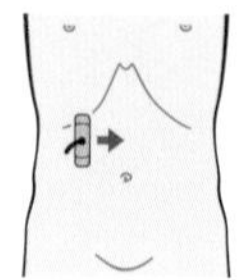

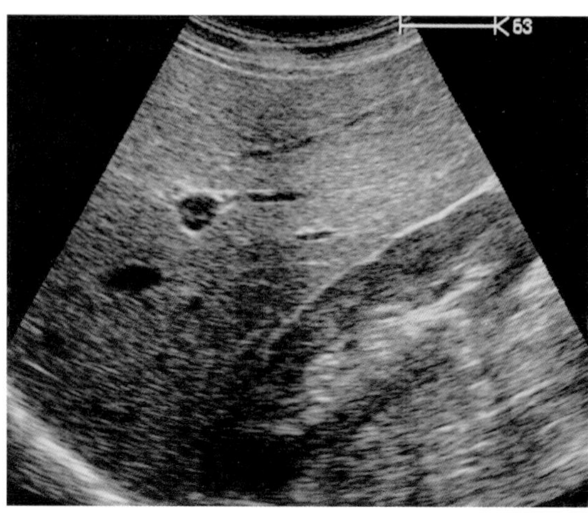

▶ **201** Kidney, liver

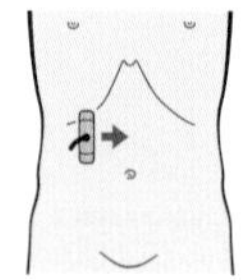

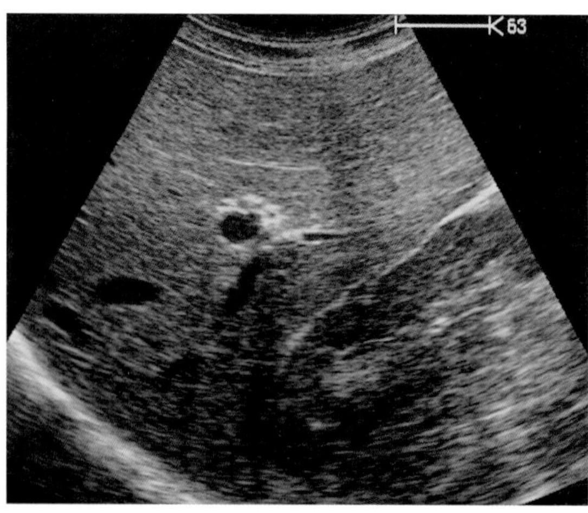

▶ **202** Kidney, liver

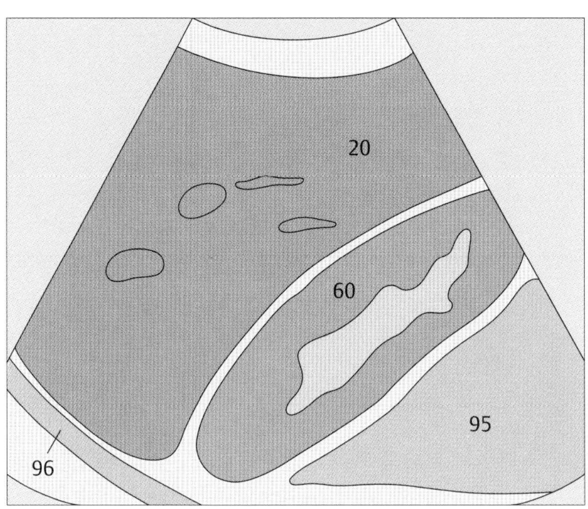

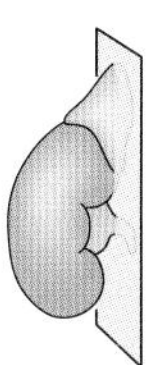

The right adrenal gland is located at the level of the upper renal pole, medial and anterior to the right kidney.

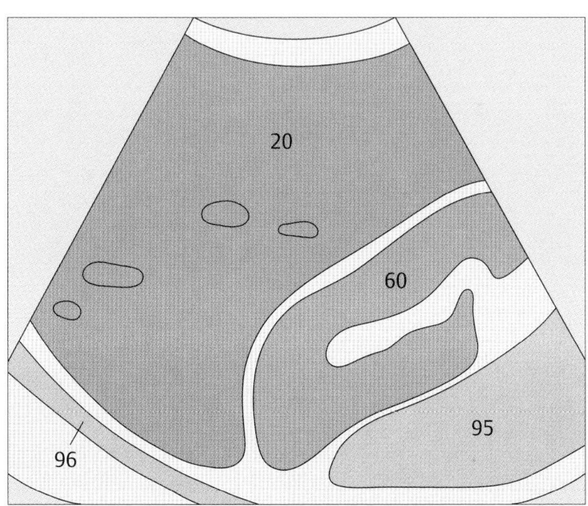

In an upper abdominal longitudinal scan from the anterior aspect, the kidney is used as a landmark for locating the right adrenal gland.

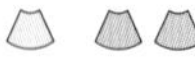

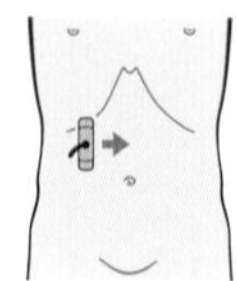

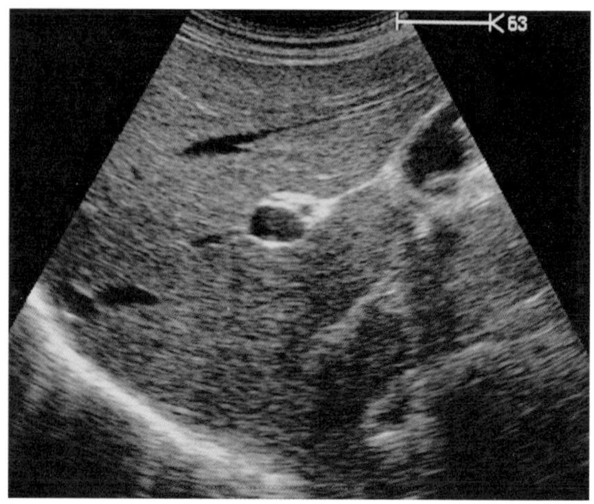

▶ **203** Adrenal gland, liver

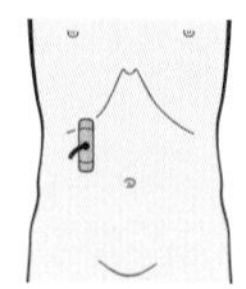

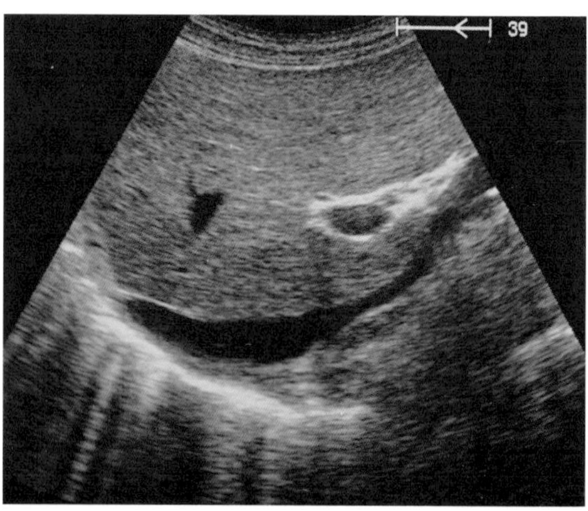

▶ **204** Adrenal gland, vena cava, renal artery

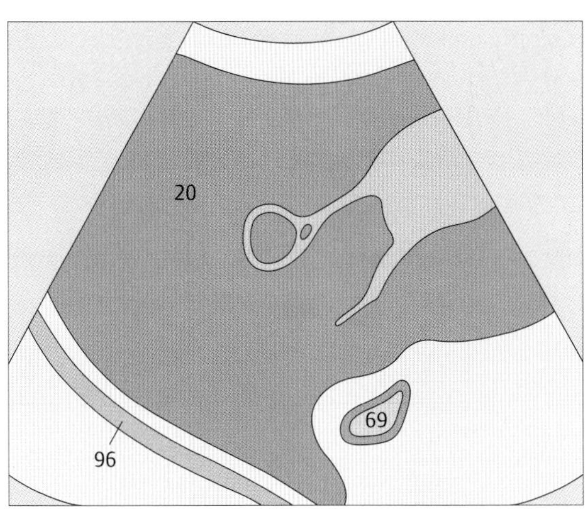

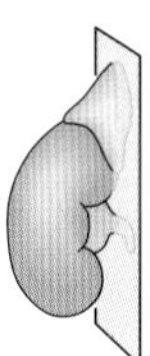

In a scan across the kidney from right to left, when the upper renal pole is just disappearing from the image the region of the right adrenal gland has been located.

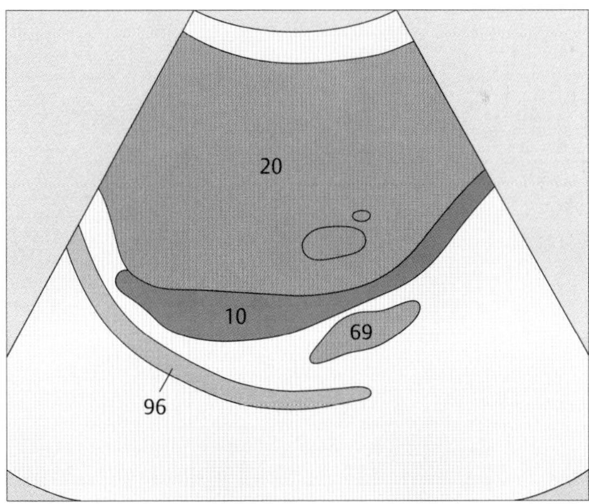

The right adrenal gland extends behind the vena cava, above the renal vessels.

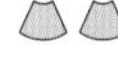

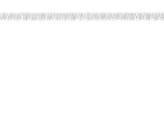

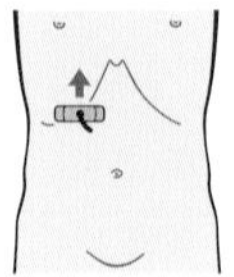

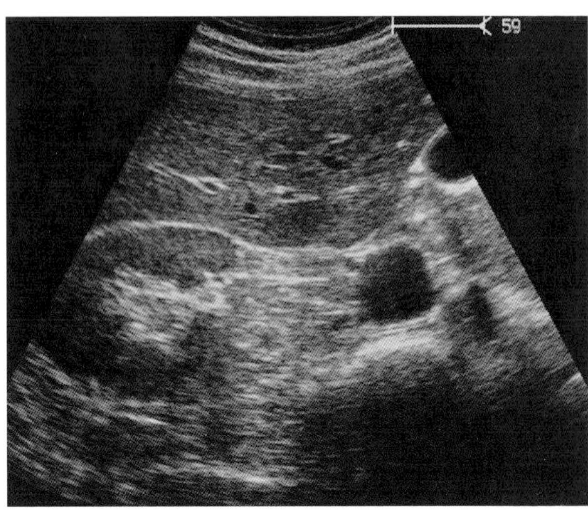

▶ **205** Kidney, vena cava

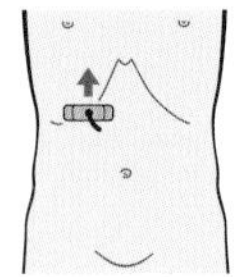

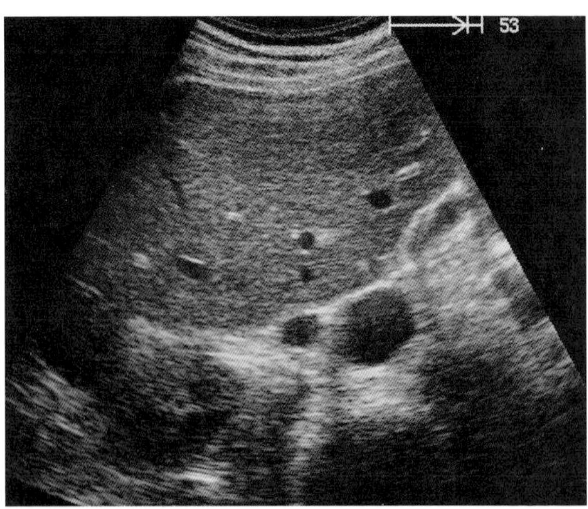

▶ **206** Kidney, renal vein, vena cava

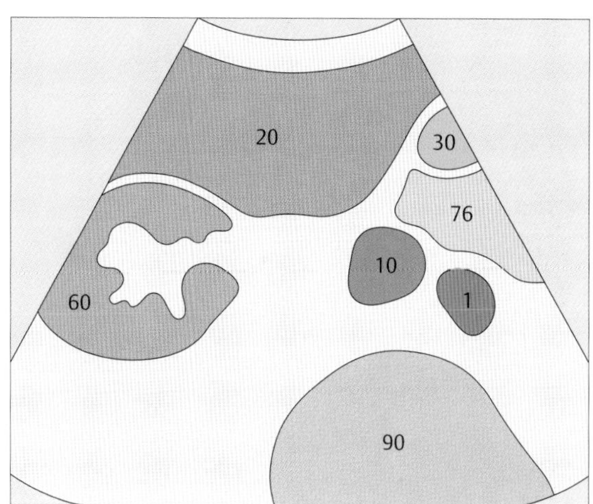

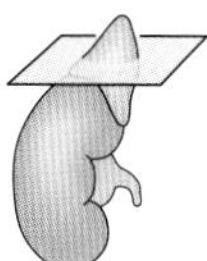

The landmarks for identifying the right adrenal gland region in transverse section are the kidney, the inferior surface of the liver, and the vena cava.

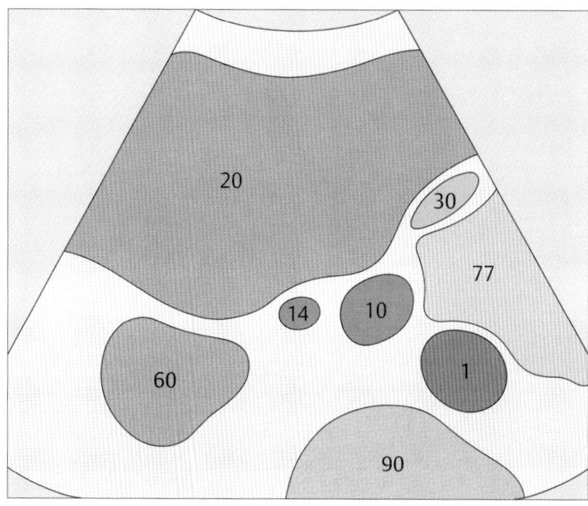

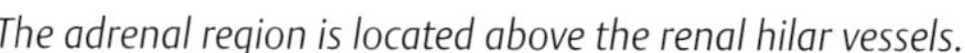

The adrenal region is located above the renal hilar vessels.

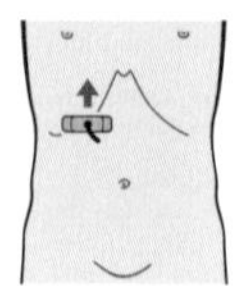

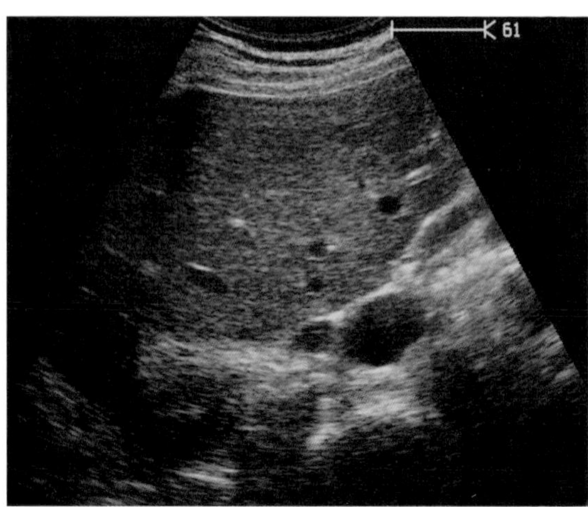

▶ **207** Renal vein, vena cava

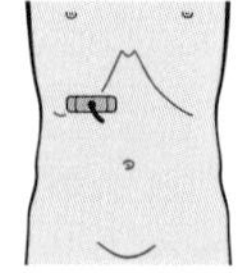

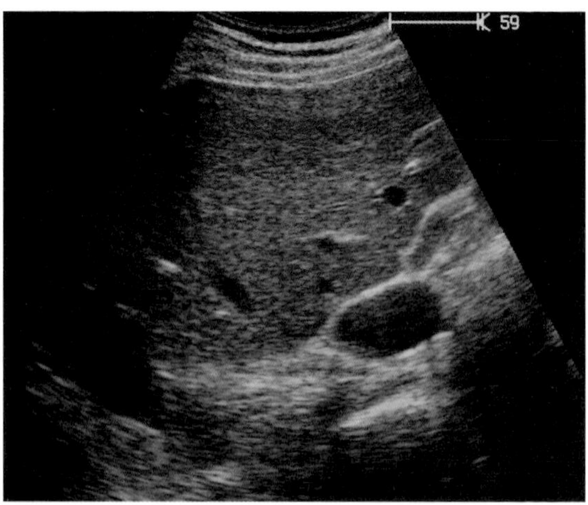

▶ **208** Adrenal gland, vena cava

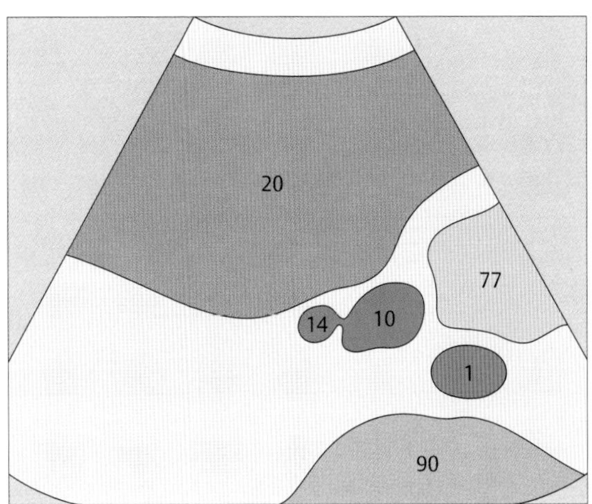

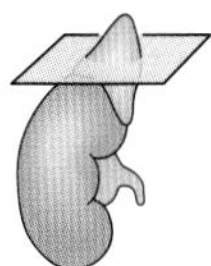

The right adrenal gland is identified just above the renal pole, lateral and posterior to the vena cava.

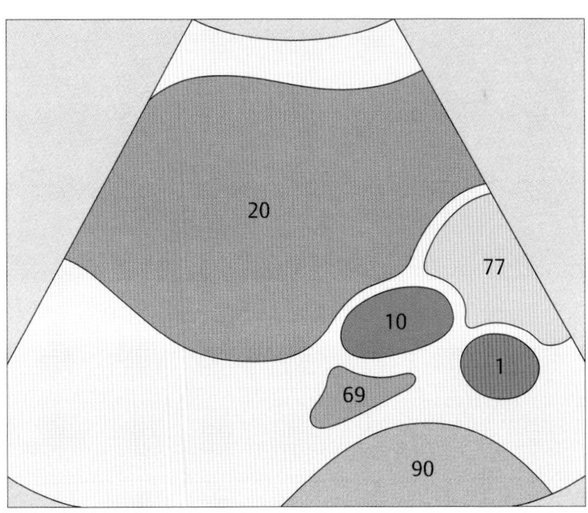

The right adrenal gland appears as a narrow, triangular, hypoechoic structure with an echodense rim.

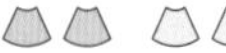

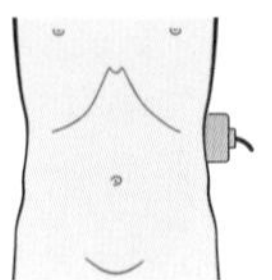

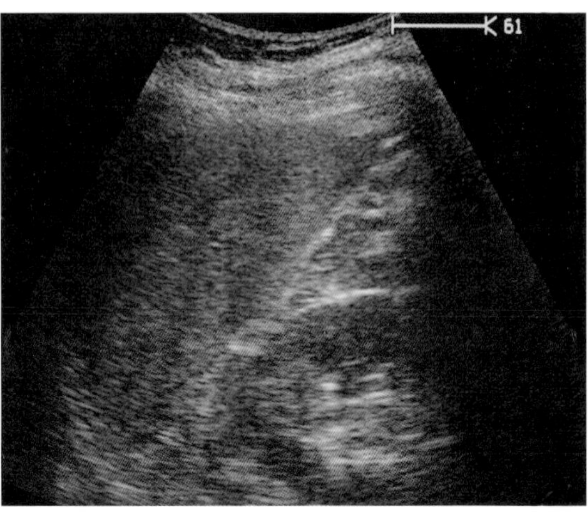

▶ **209** Kidney, spleen

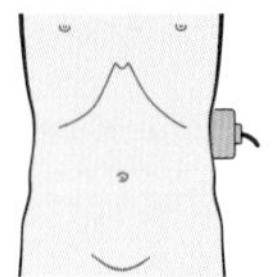

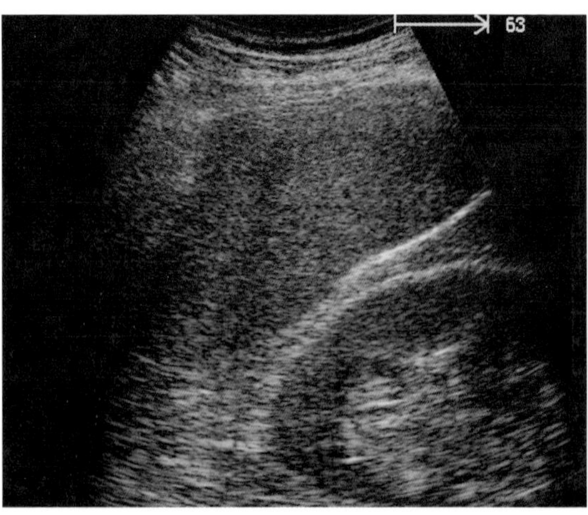

▶ **210** Adrenal gland, kidney, spleen

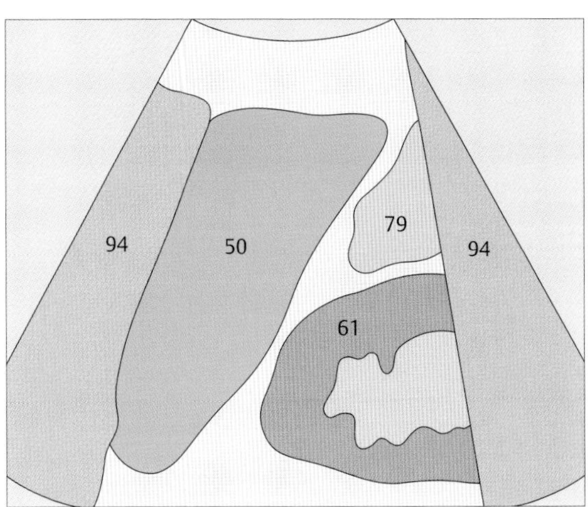

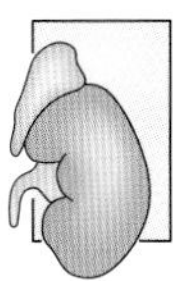

The left adrenal gland is usually more difficult to locate than the right adrenal gland.

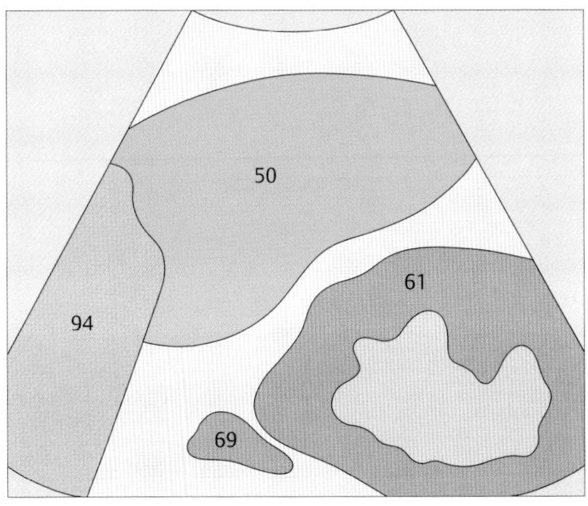

The left adrenal gland is identified between the upper renal pole, spleen, and aorta.

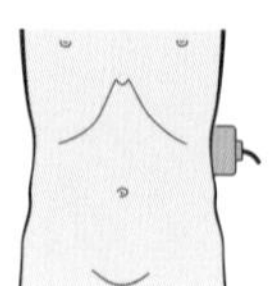

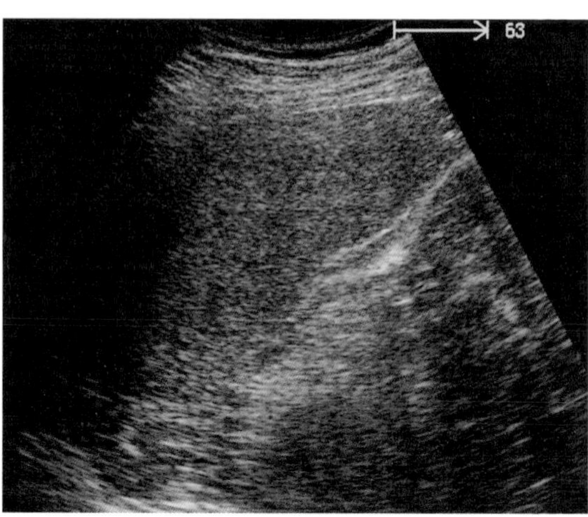

▶ **211** Adrenal gland, kidney, spleen

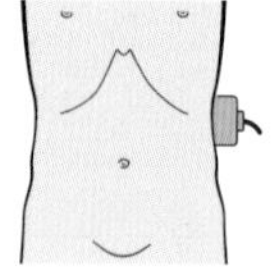

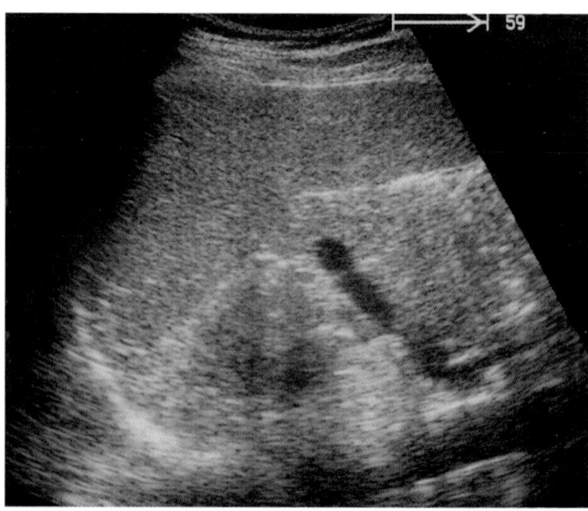

▶ **212** Spleen, tail of pancreas

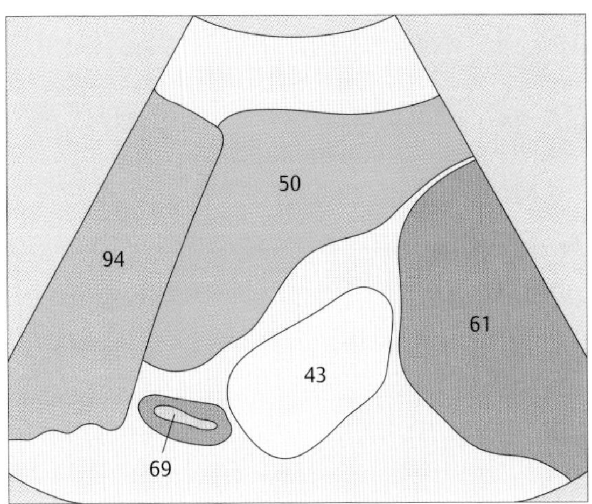

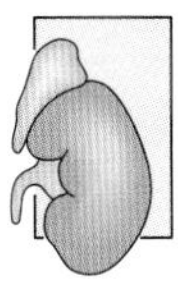

The left adrenal gland is frequently crescent-shaped.

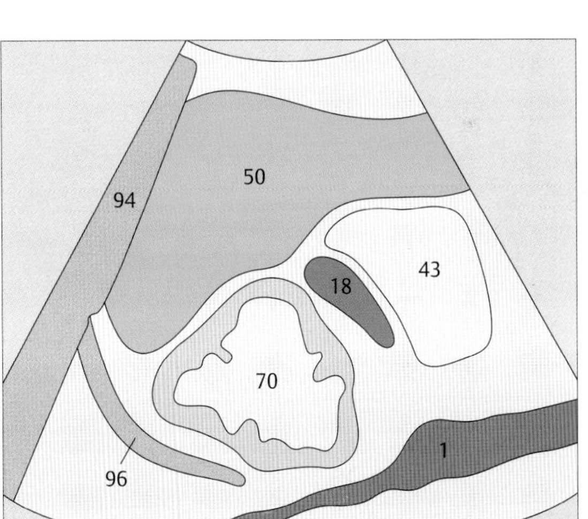

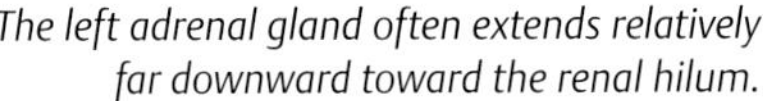

The left adrenal gland often extends relatively far downward toward the renal hilum.

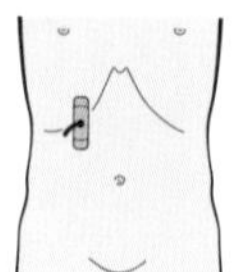

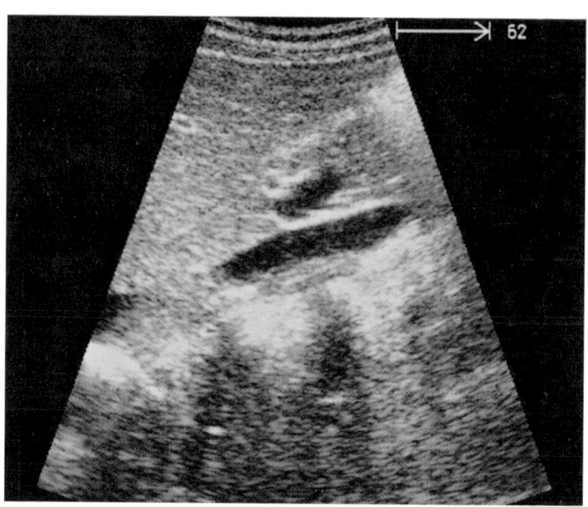

▶ **213** Layers of adrenal gland

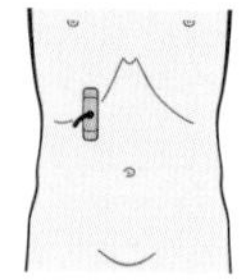

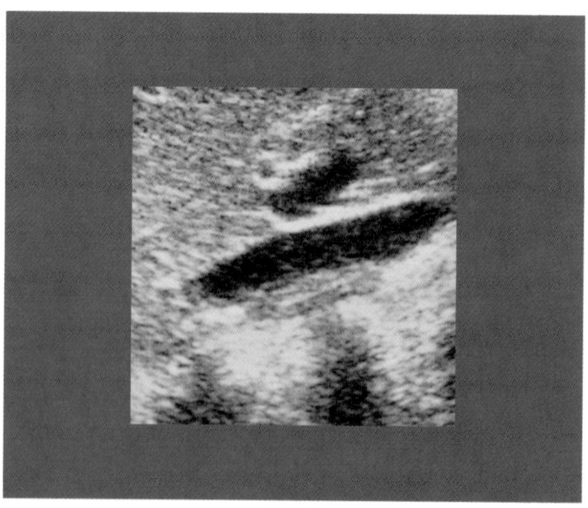

▶ **214** Layers of adrenal gland

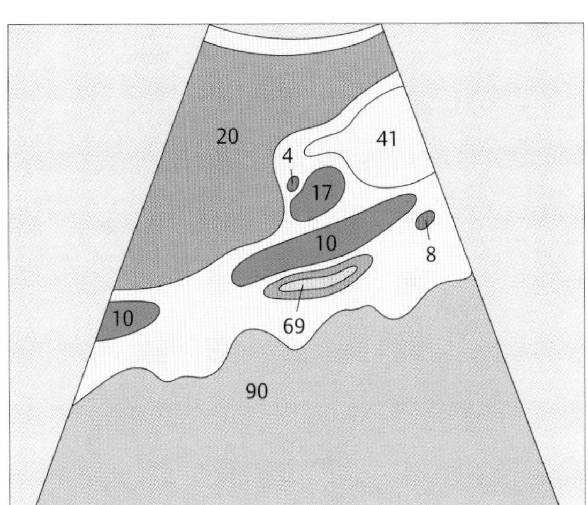

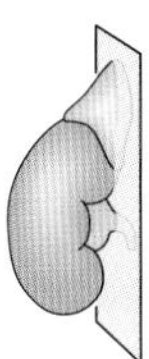

The adrenal gland is seen to consist of three layers:
two echodense outer layers and a hypoechoic middle layer.

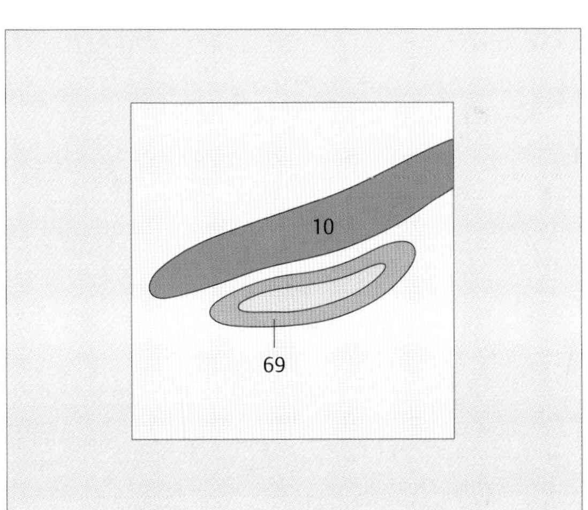

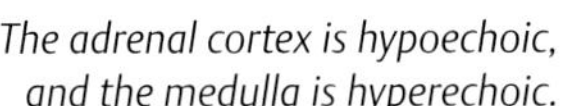

The adrenal cortex is hypoechoic,
and the medulla is hyperechoic.

8 Stomach

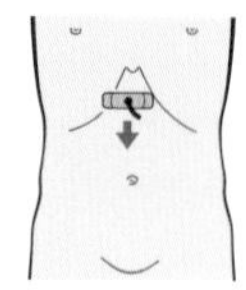

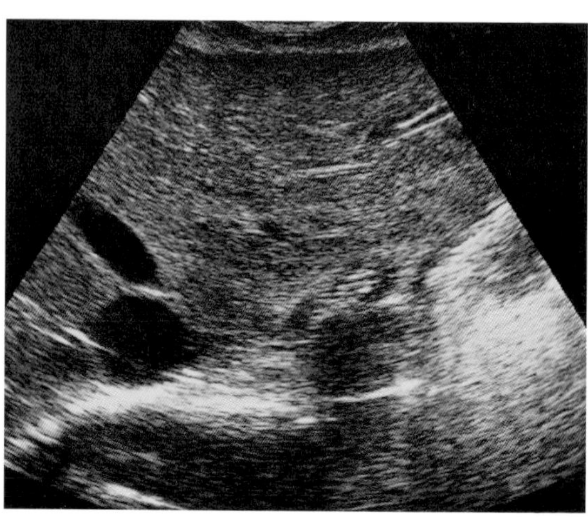

▶ **215** Esophagus, aorta, liver

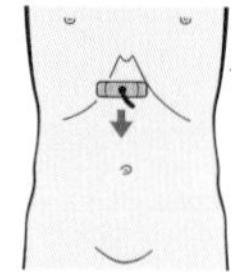

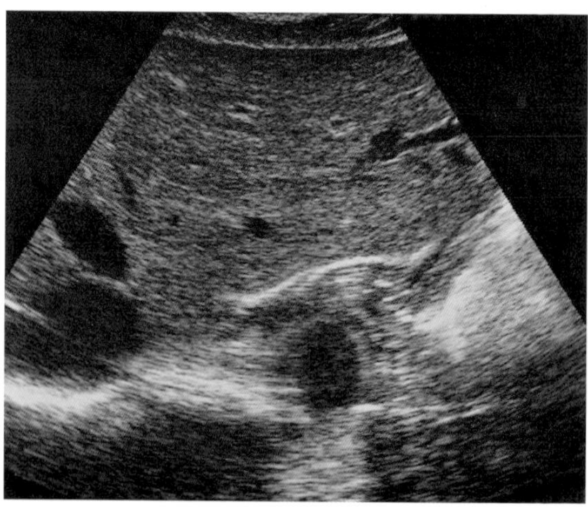

▶ **216** Cardia, aorta, liver

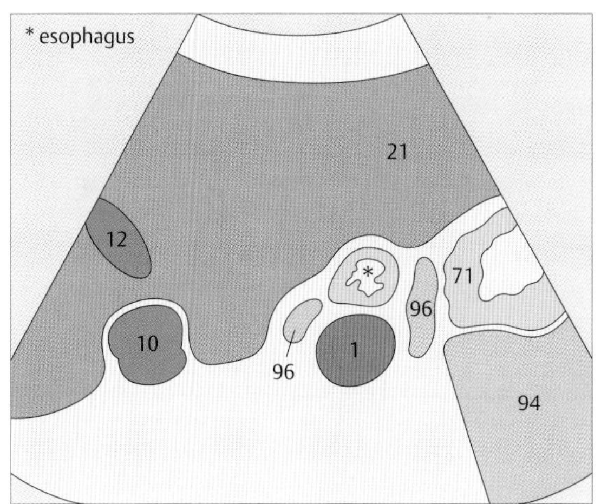

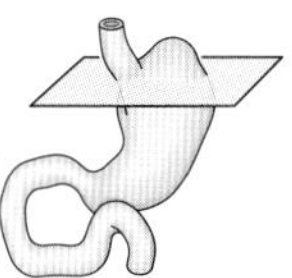

The gastroesophageal junction is identified between the liver, aorta, and crura of the diaphragm.

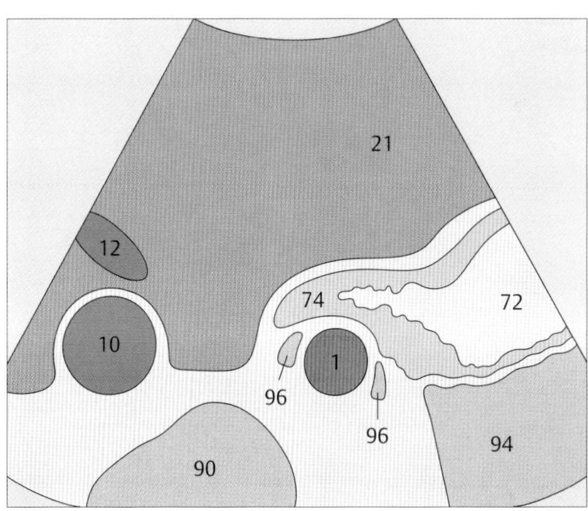

The cardia opens into a sharply tapered triangular structure when viewed in transverse section.

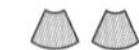

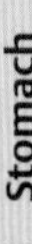

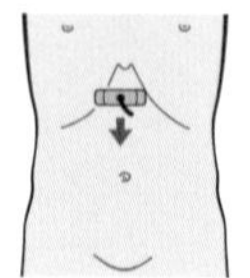

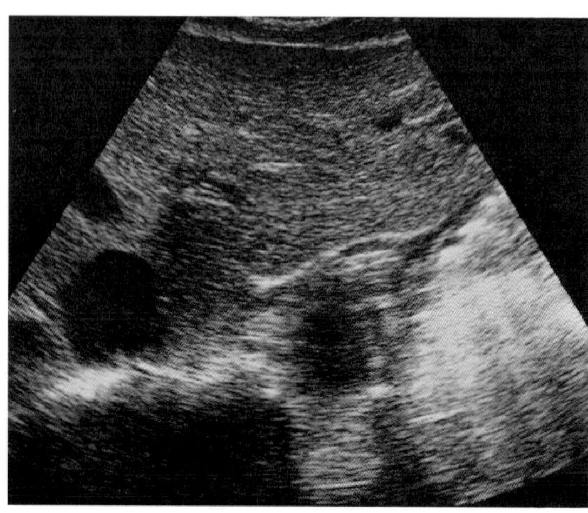

▶ **217** Cardia, gastric body, aorta, liver

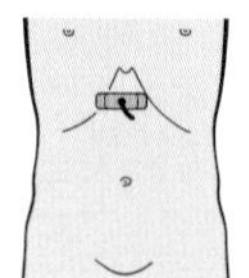

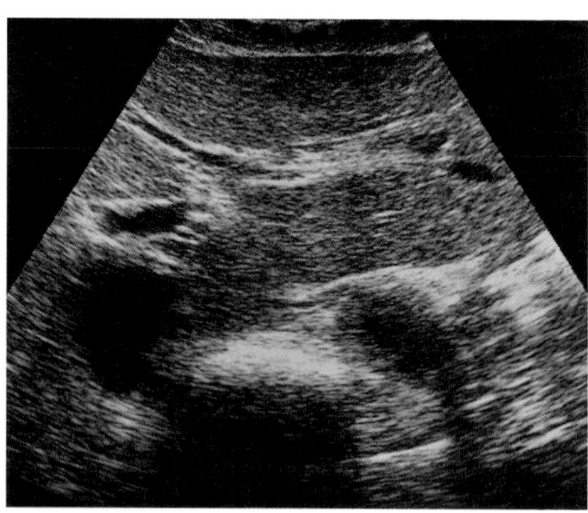

▶ **218** Gastric body, aorta, liver

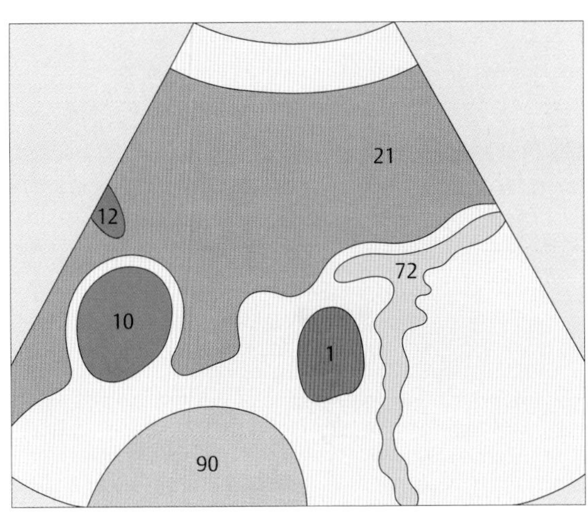

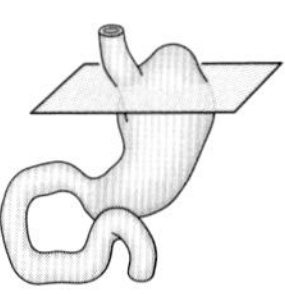

Next to the cardia, the gastric body presents a seemingly chaotic pattern of solid, liquid and gaseous material.

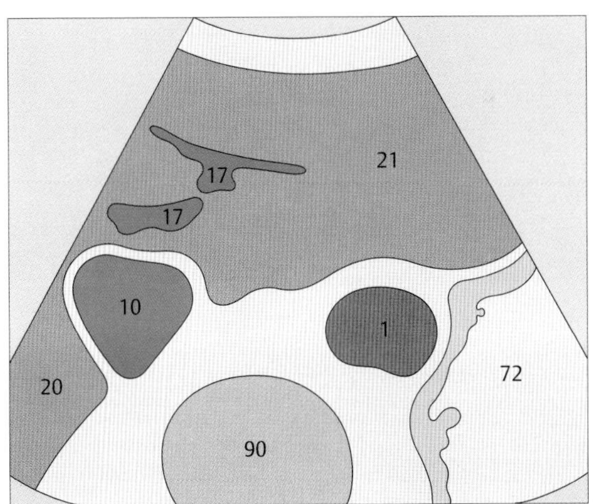

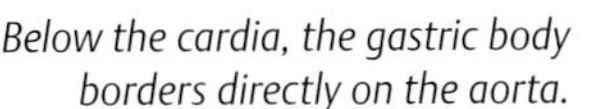

Below the cardia, the gastric body borders directly on the aorta.

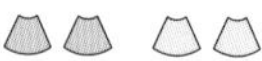

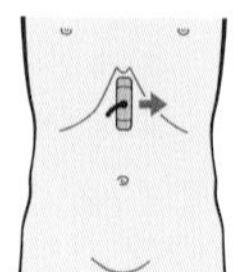

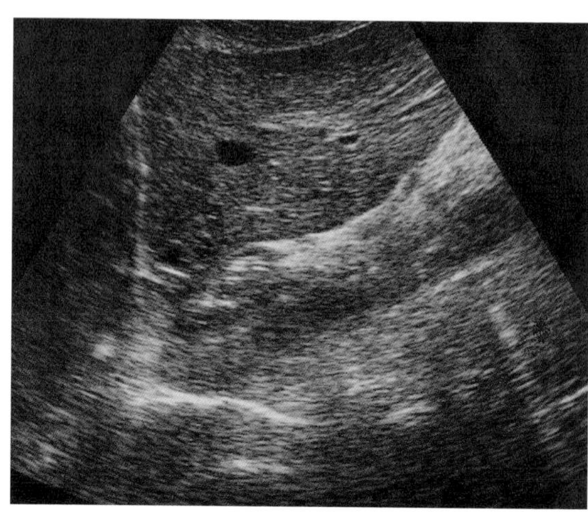

▶ **219** Esophagus, aorta, liver

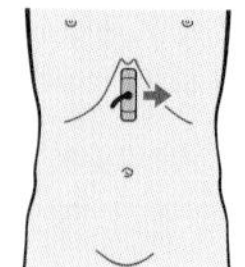

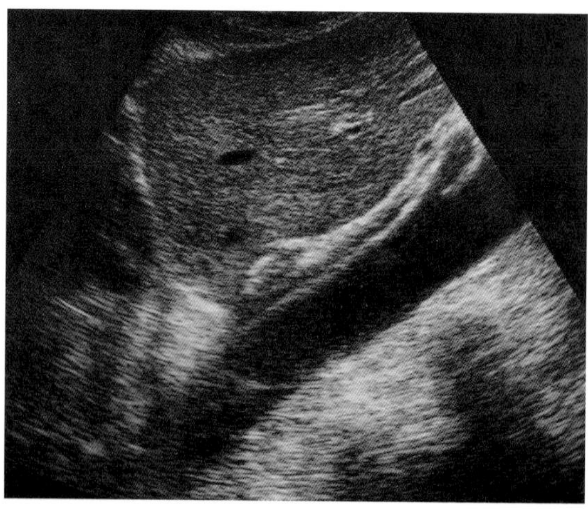

▶ **220** Esophagus, aorta, liver

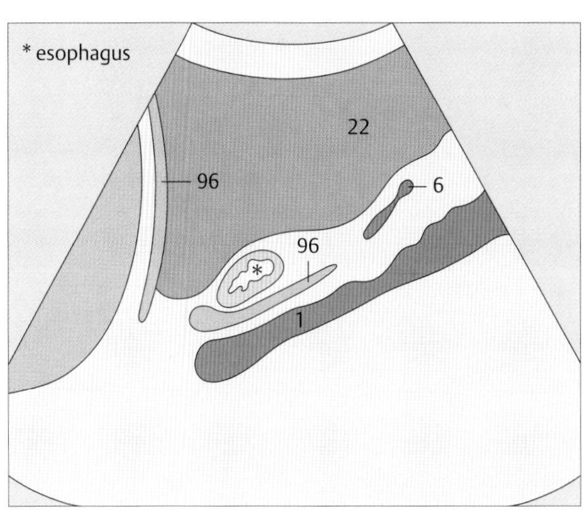

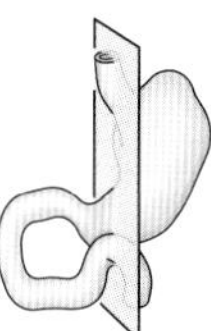

The abdominal esophagus is identified just to the right of, and anterior to, the aorta.

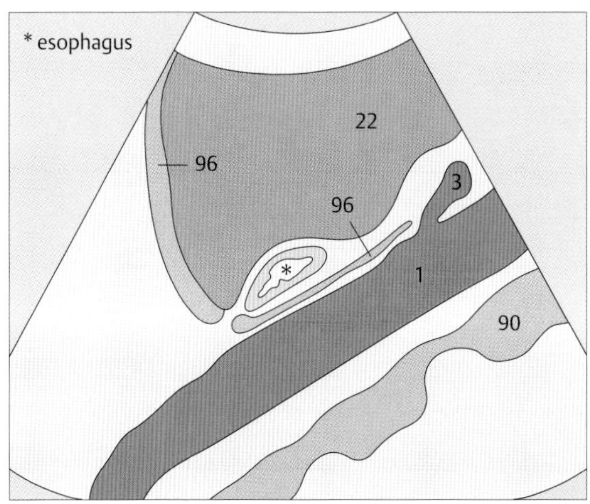

The esophagus and cardia are located between the liver and aorta in an upper abdominal longitudinal scan.

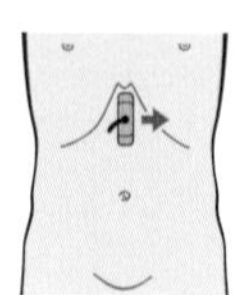

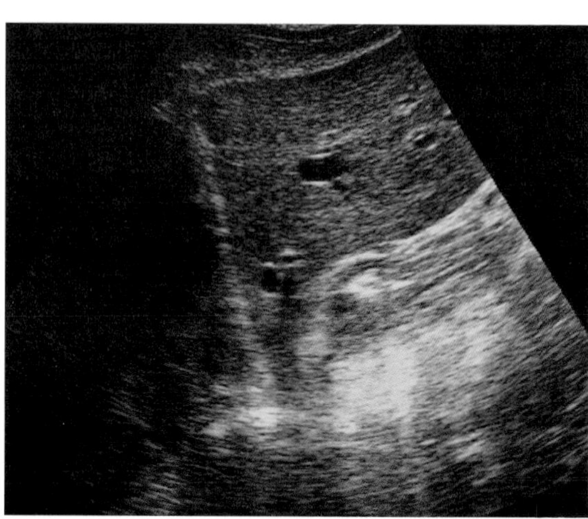

▶ **221** Cardia, liver

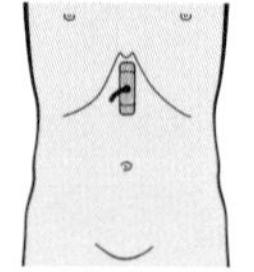

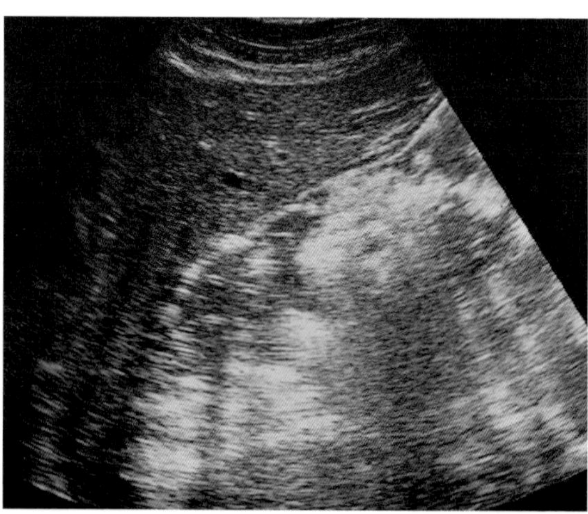

▶ **222** Gastric body, liver

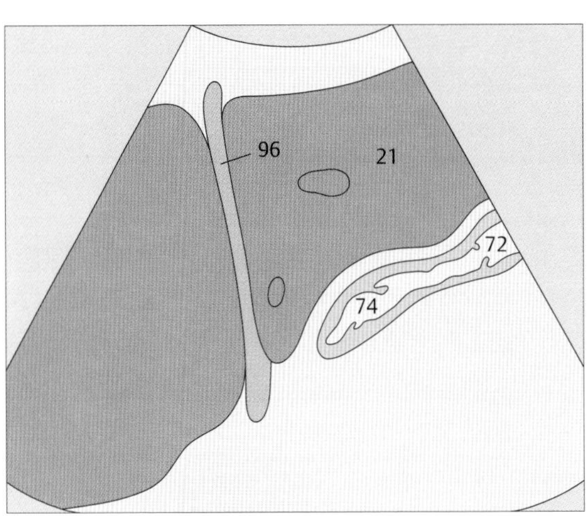

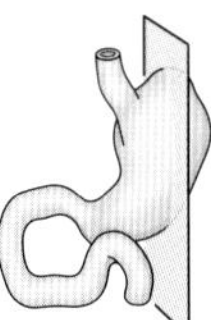

The cardia and body of the stomach are located and identified by first defining the gastroesophageal junction.

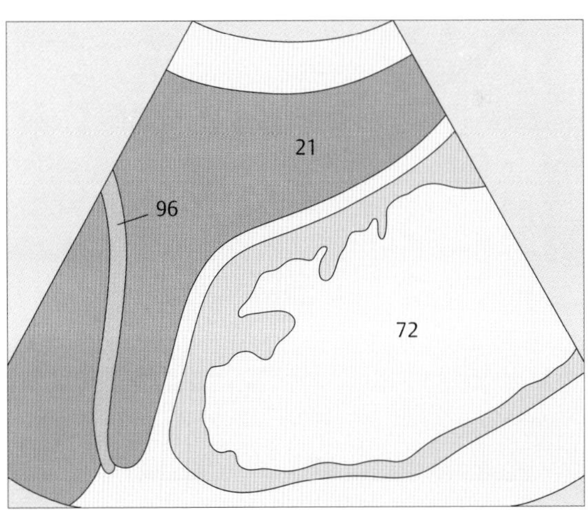

In subjects who have not been specially prepared, the gastric body presents a heterogeneous echo pattern located behind the left lobe of the liver.

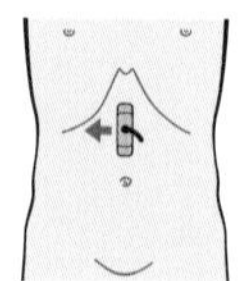

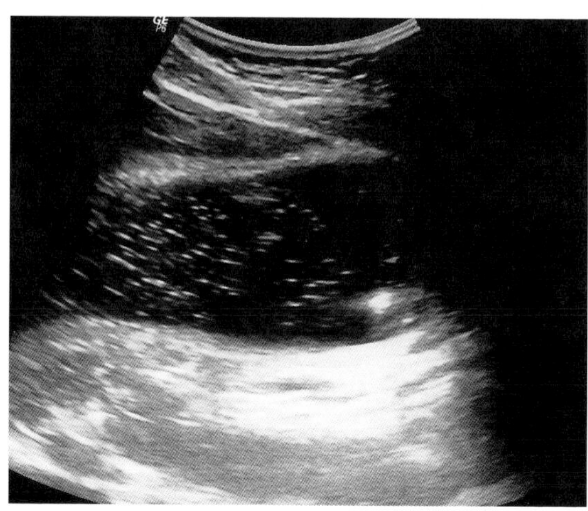

▶ **223** Gastric body, liver

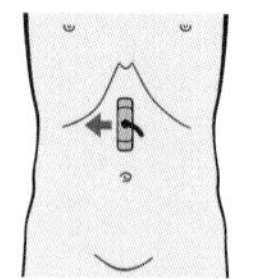

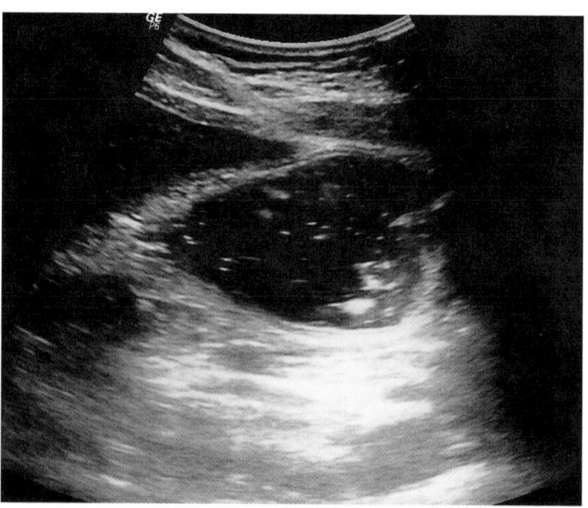

▶ **224** Antrum, liver, pancreas

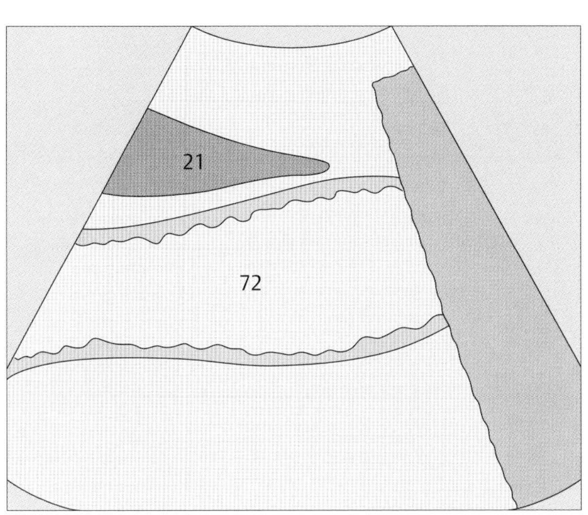

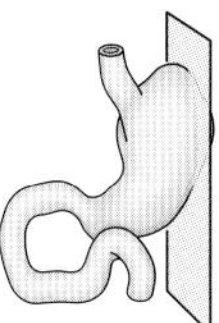

The gastric body is consistently located behind the left lobe of the liver.

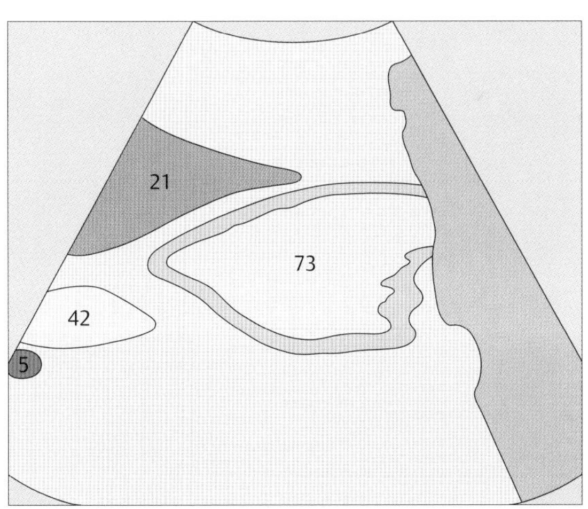

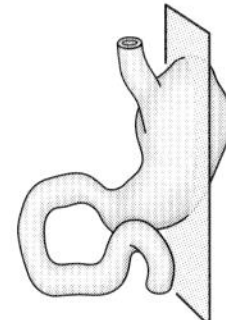

The appearance of the stomach depends on its degree of distention.

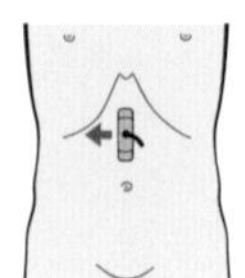

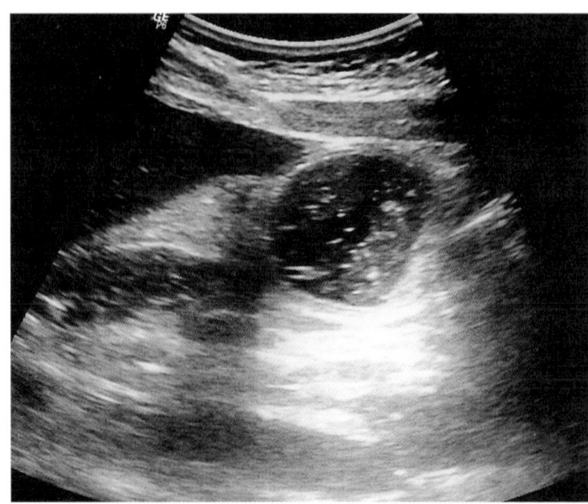

▶ **225** Antrum, liver, pancreas

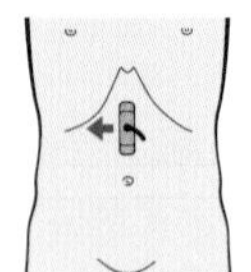

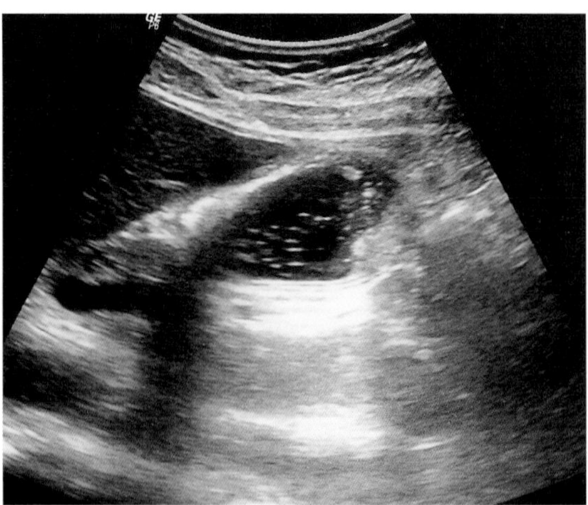

▶ **226** Antrum, liver, pancreas

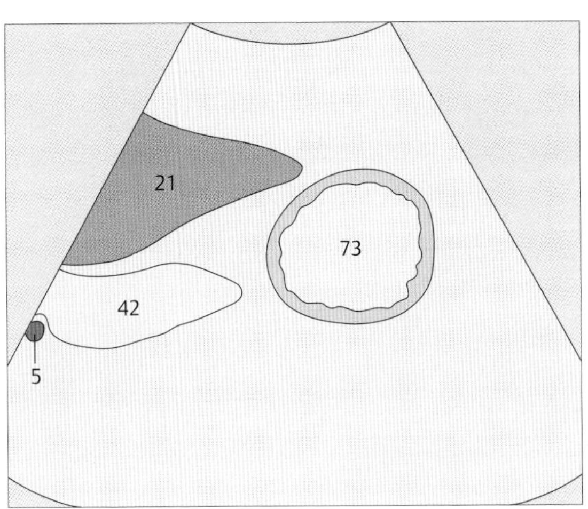

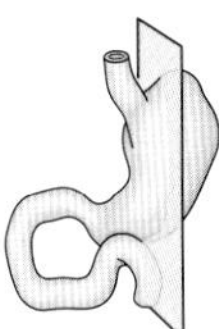

Generally the fluid-filled stomach can be clearly visualized with ultrasound.

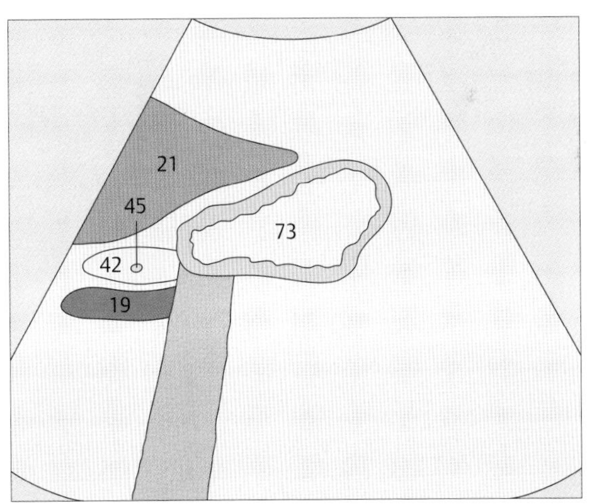

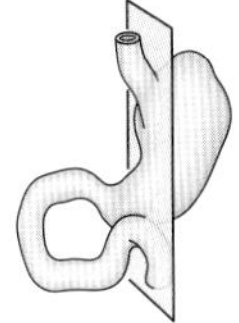

A longitudinal scan at the center of the upper abdomen displays the triad of the stomach, liver, and pancreas.

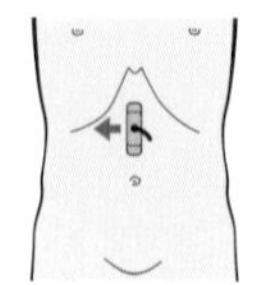

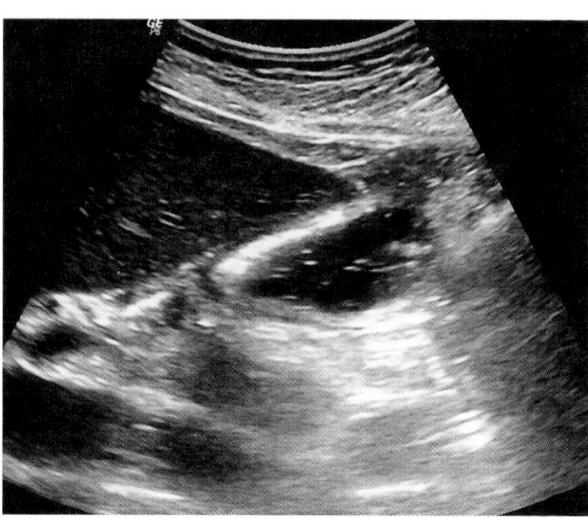

▶ **227** Antrum, liver, duodenum

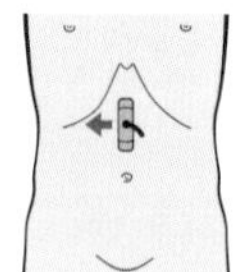

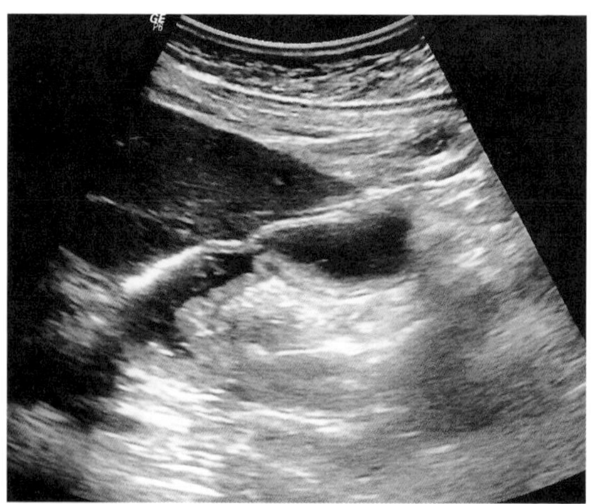

▶ **228** Antrum, duodenal bulb, *pylorus

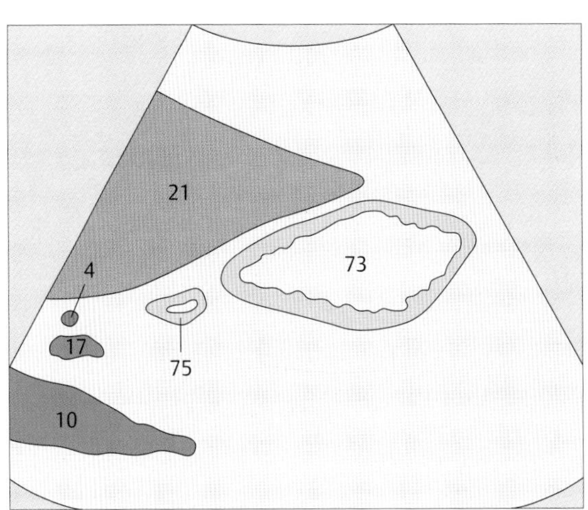

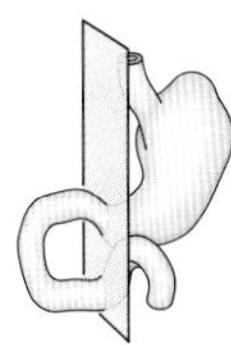

The typical target pattern of the gastric antrum is seen most clearly in a longitudinal scan at the inferior border of the liver.

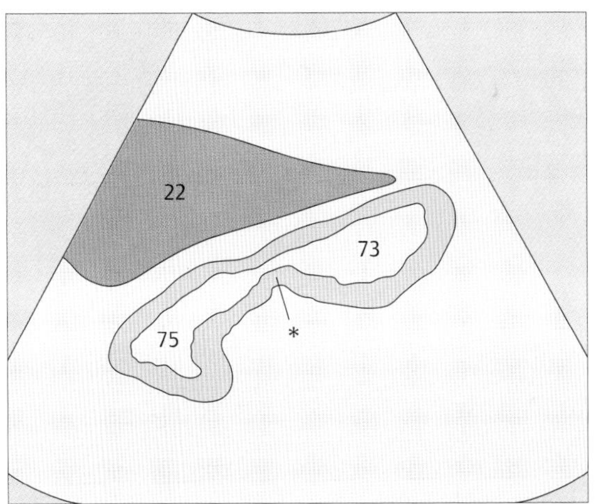

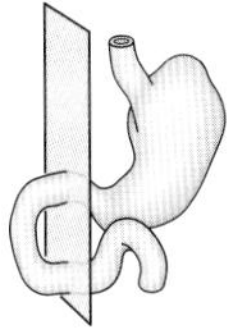

A definite thickening of the muscularis marks the location of the pylorus.

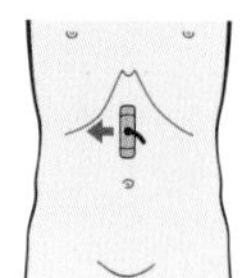

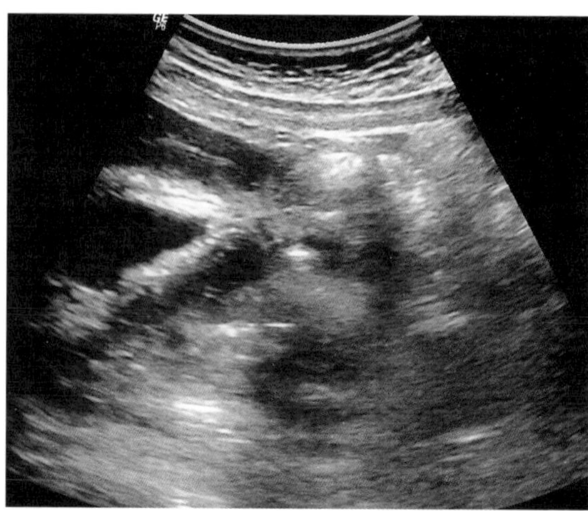

► **229** Duodenum, gallbladder, liver

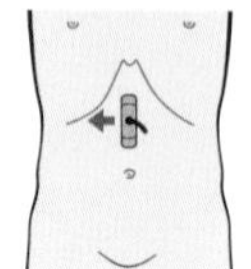

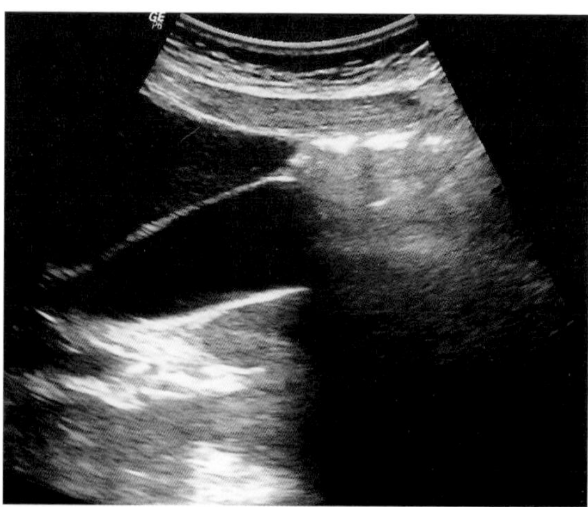

► **230** Gallbladder, liver

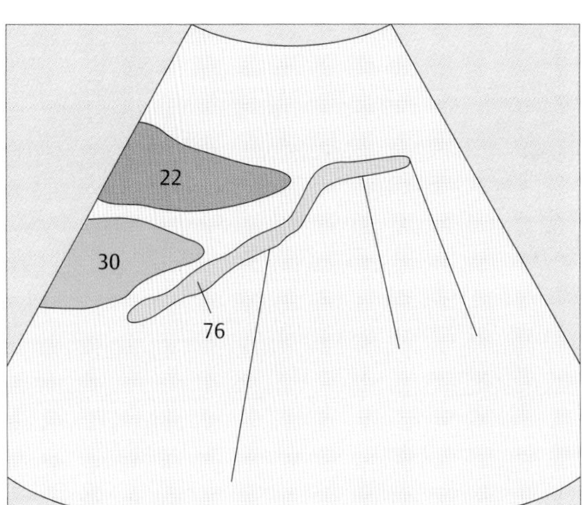

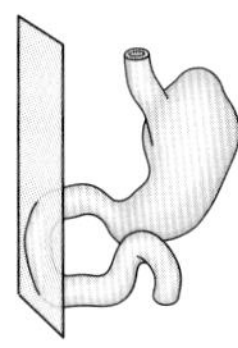

The descending duodenum is imaged posterior to the gallbladder.

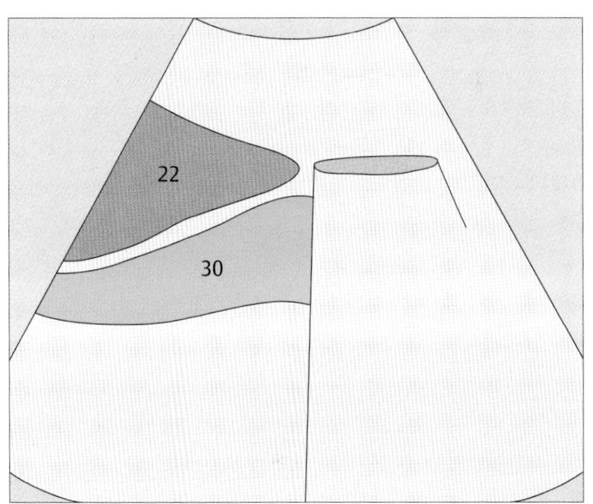

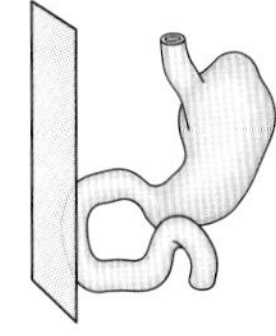

Bowel gas often produces artifacts in the gallbladder region.

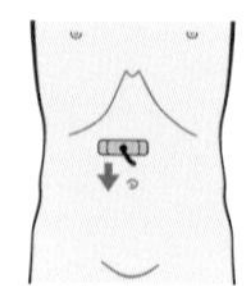

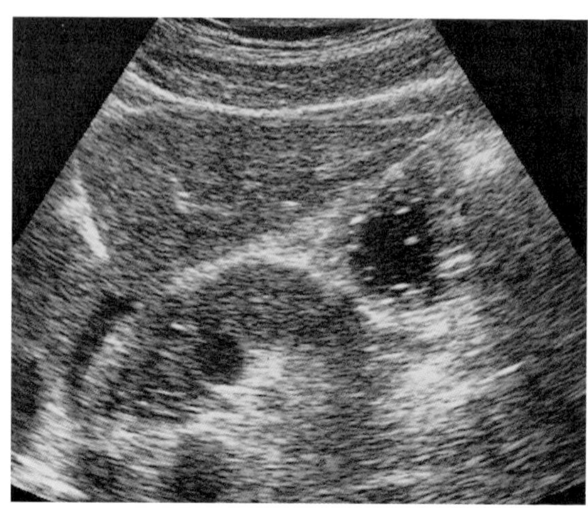

▶ **231** Antrum, liver, pancreas

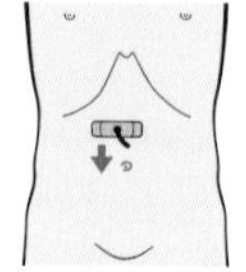

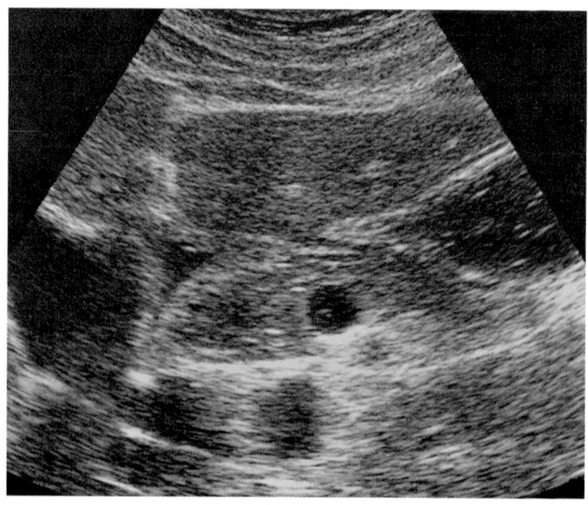

▶ **232** Antrum, duodenum, liver, pancreas, gallbladder

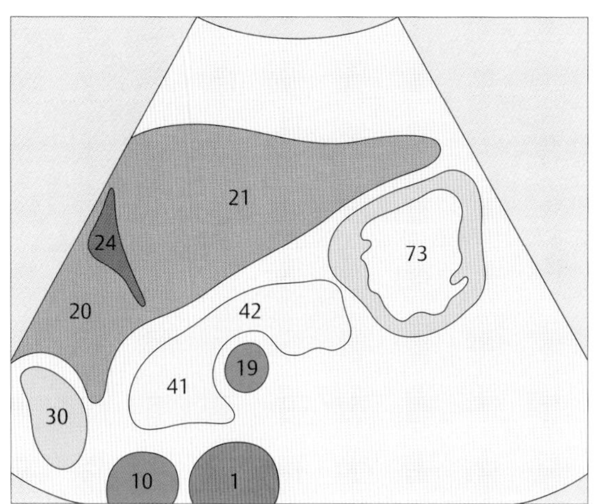

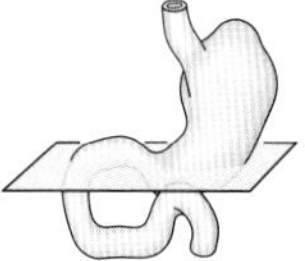

The pancreas lies against the posterior surface of the stomach.

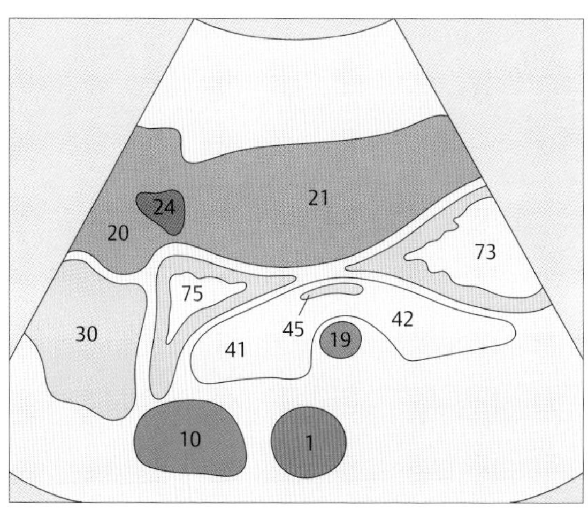

The antrum extends to the right, coming between the pancreas and liver. It is difficult to visualize at that location.

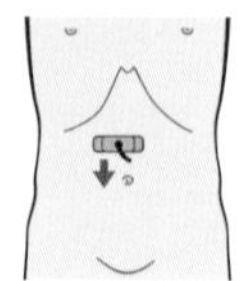

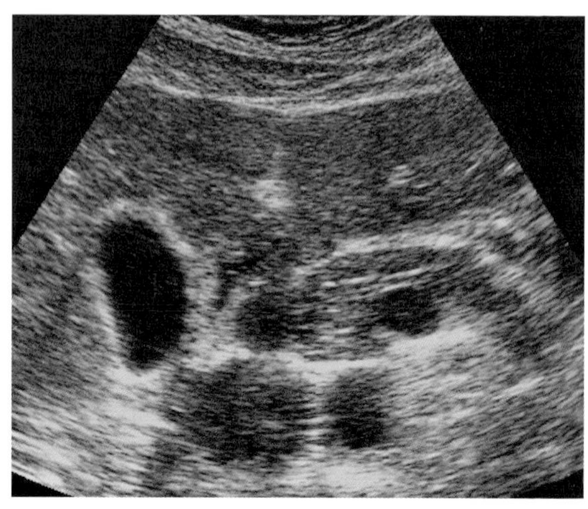

▶ **233** Antrum, duodenum, liver, pancreas, gallbladder

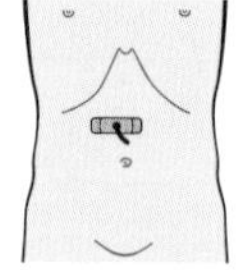

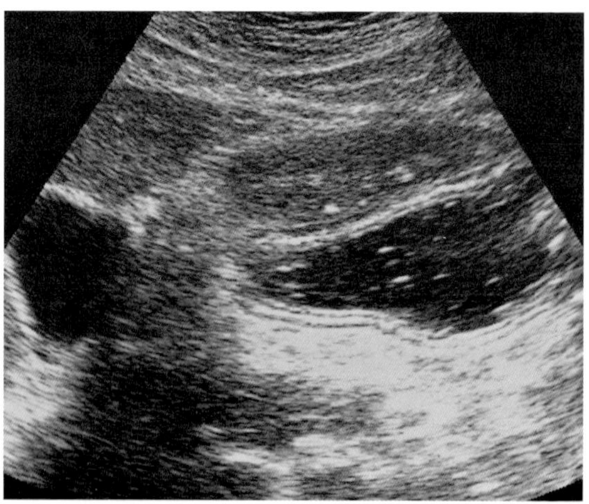

▶ **234** Antrum, gallbladder

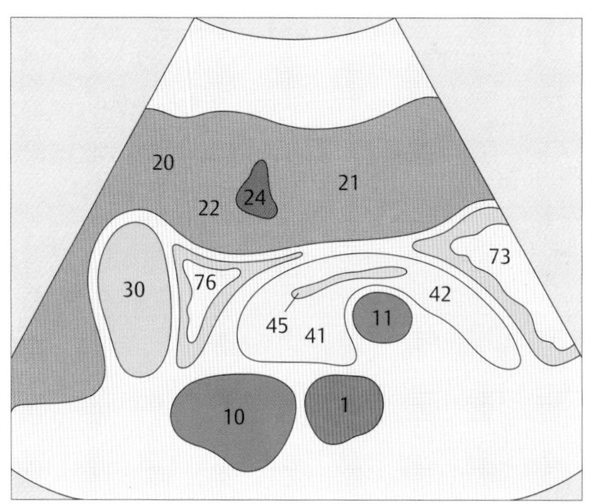

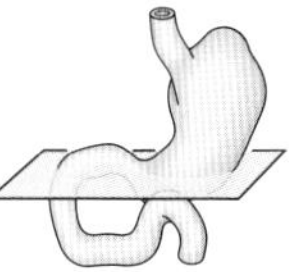

The second part of the duodenum lies between the liver, gallbladder, vena cava, and head of pancreas.

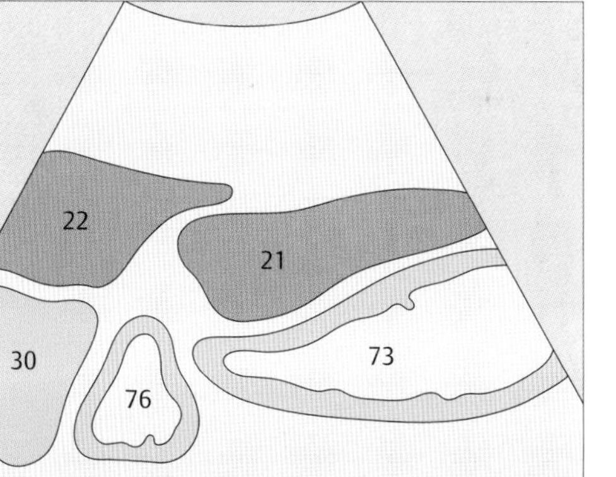

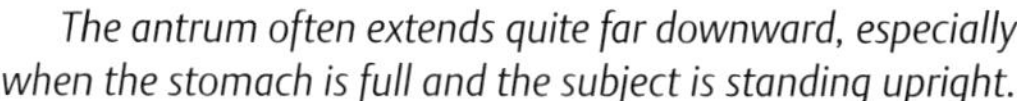

The antrum often extends quite far downward, especially when the stomach is full and the subject is standing upright.

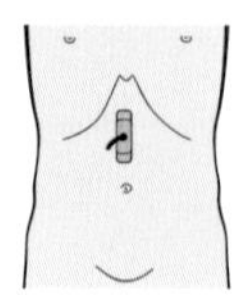

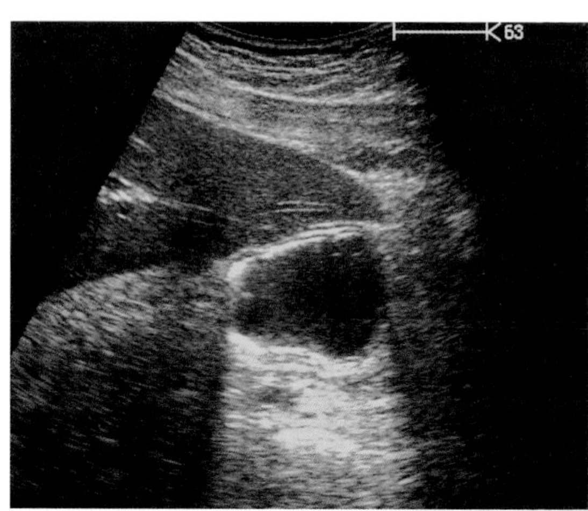

▶ **235** Layers of gastric wall

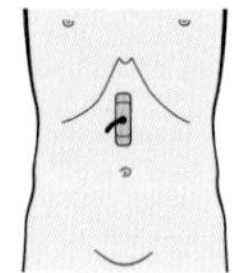

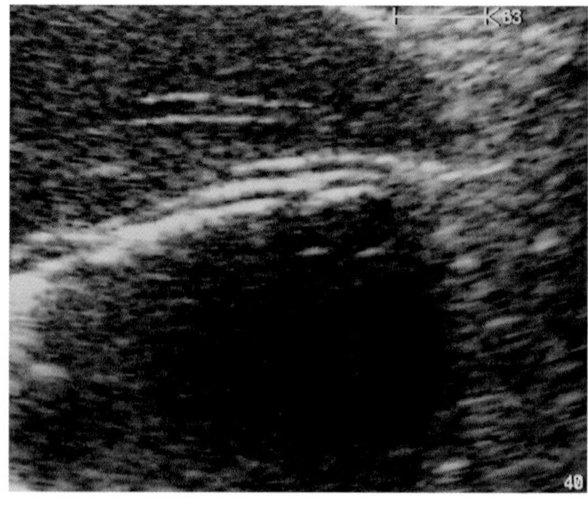

▶ **236** Layers of gastric wall

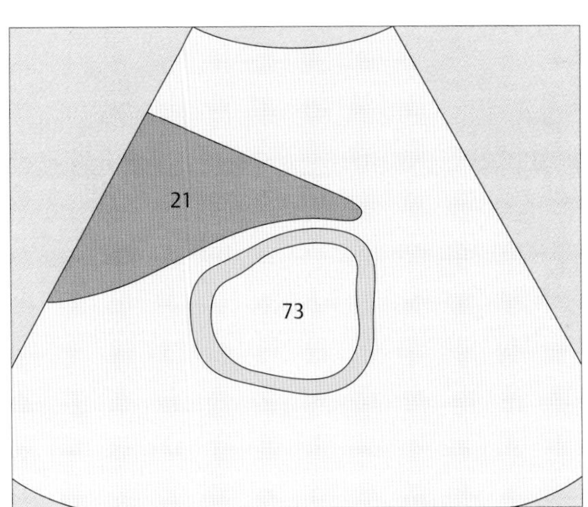

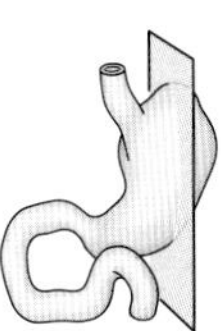

With a high-resolution device and favorable scanning conditions, five layers can be distinguished in the gastric wall.

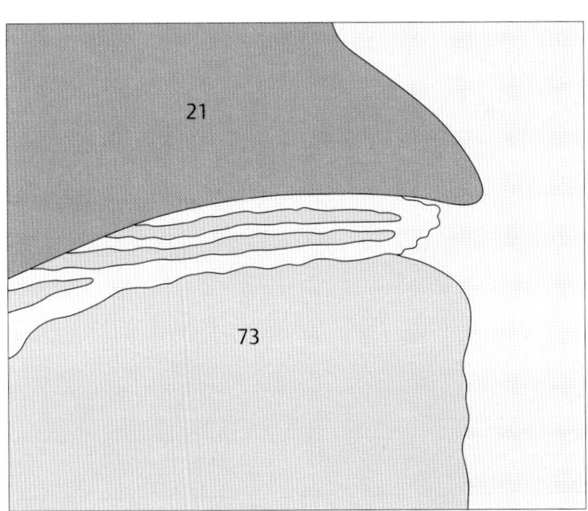

A scan through the antrum is best for differentiating the layers of the gastric wall.

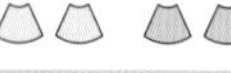

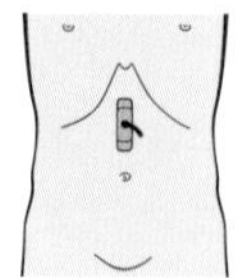

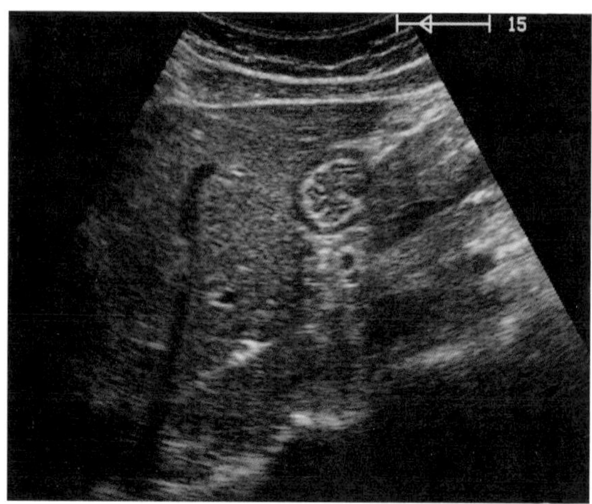

▶ **237** Gastric folds

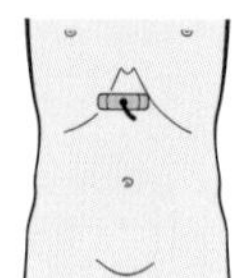

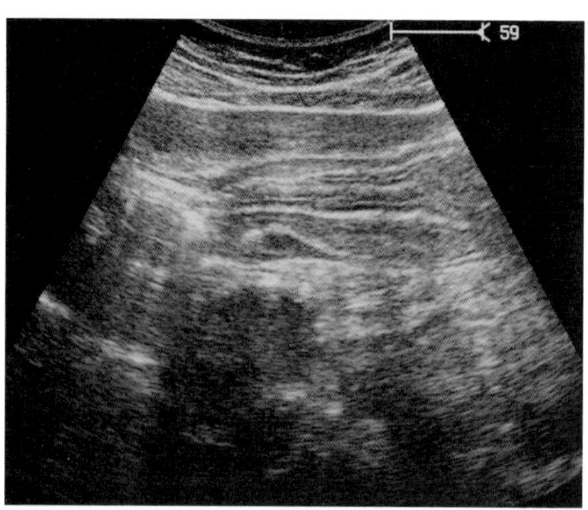

▶ **238** Gastric folds

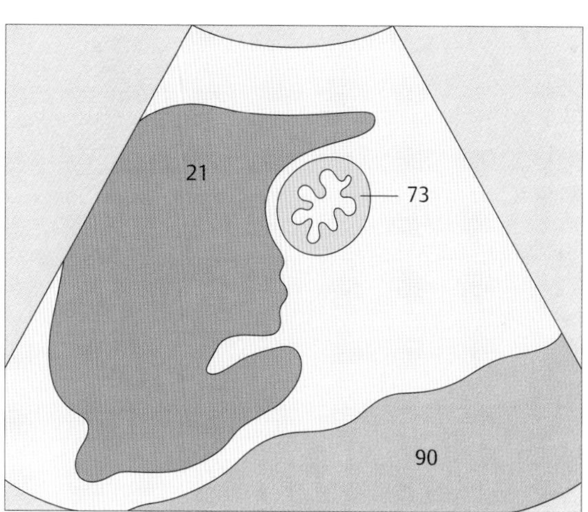

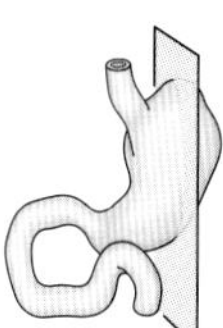

The rugal folds of the stomach are demonstrated most clearly in the fasted state.

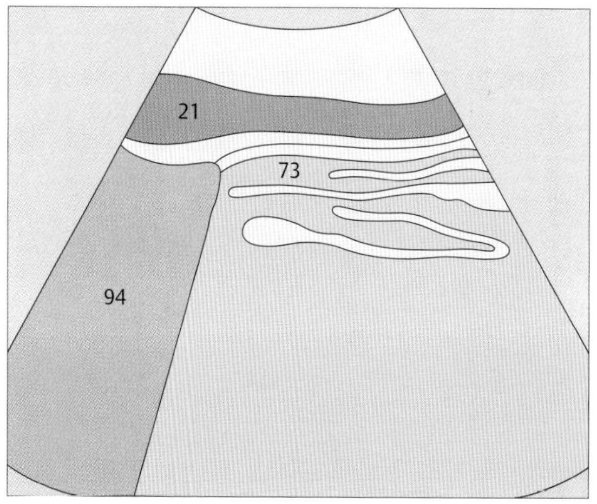

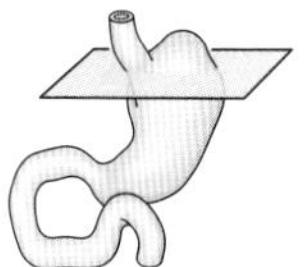

In an upper abdominal transverse scan, the gastric folds produce a confusing pattern in which numerous wall layers are seen.

9 Bladder

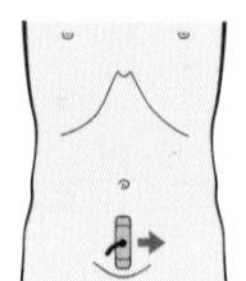

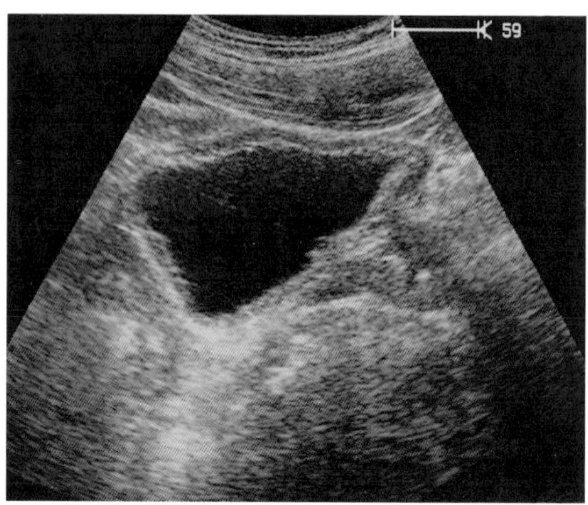

▶ **239** Bladder, prostate, rectum

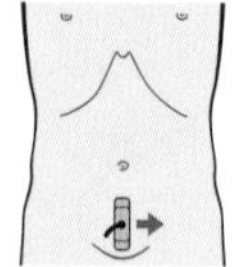

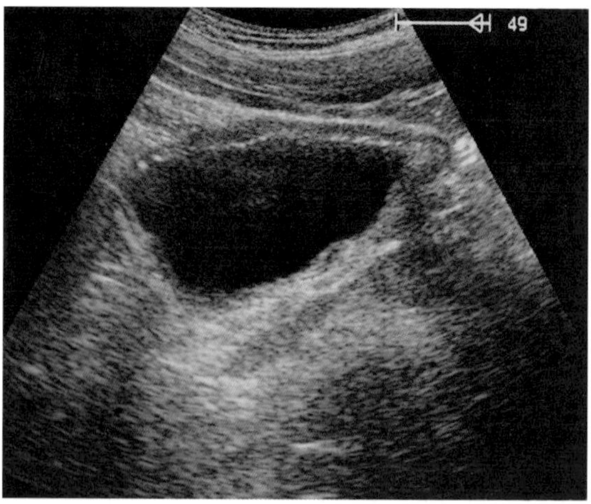

▶ **240** Bladder, ureteral orifice, prostate, rectum

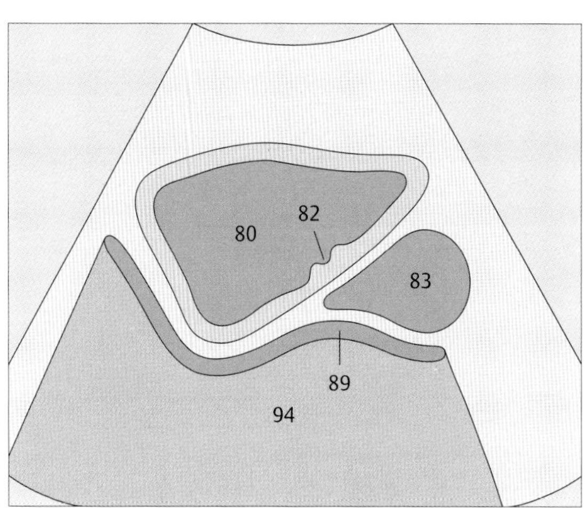

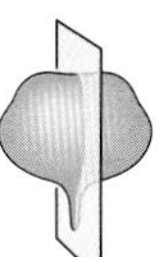

The full bladder appears in longitudinal section as a triangular structure devoid of internal echoes.

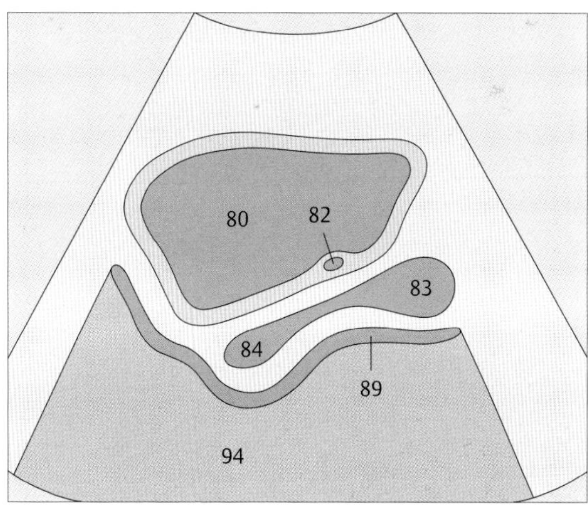

The internal genitalia are seen posterior to the bladder in the midsagittal scan.

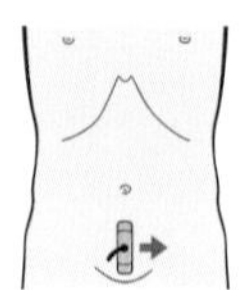

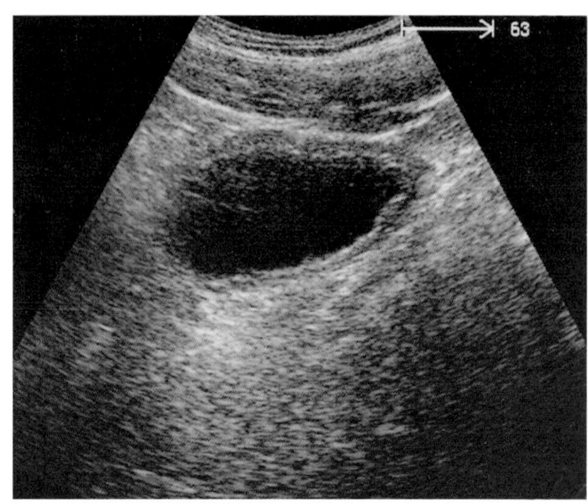

▶ **241** Bladder, rectum

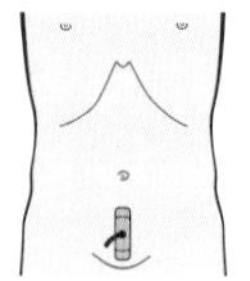

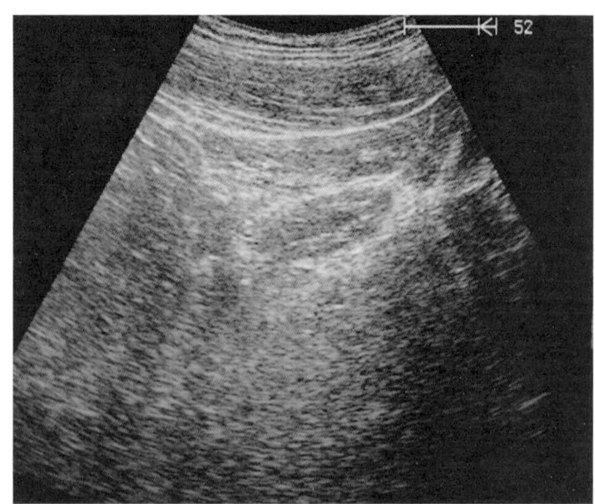

▶ **242** Bladder, bowel

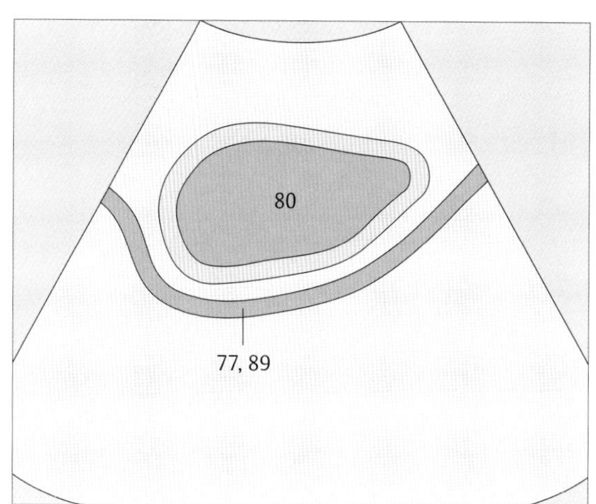

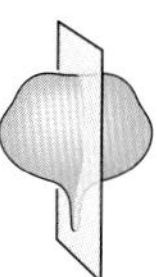

The anterior wall of the bladder is loosely attached to the anterior abdominal wall by the vesicoumbilical fascia. This keeps gas-containing bowel loops from coming between the abdominal wall and the anterior surface of the full bladder.

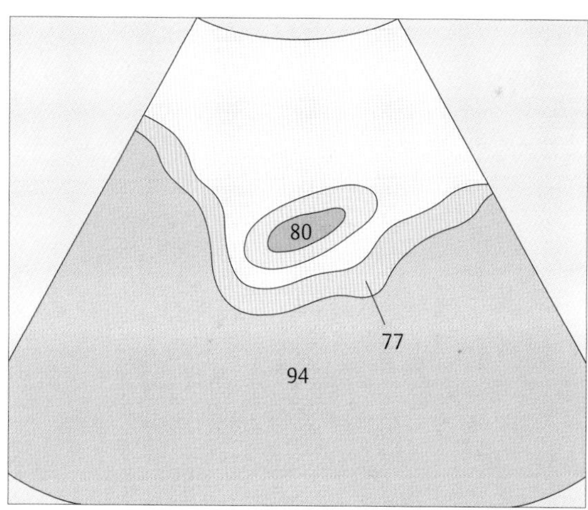

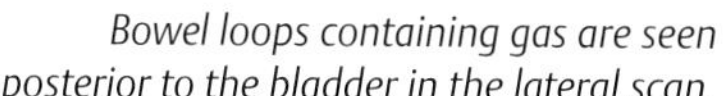

Bowel loops containing gas are seen posterior to the bladder in the lateral scan.

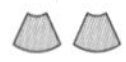

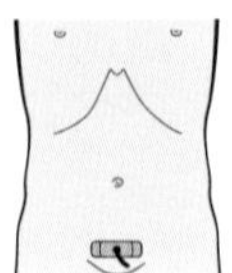

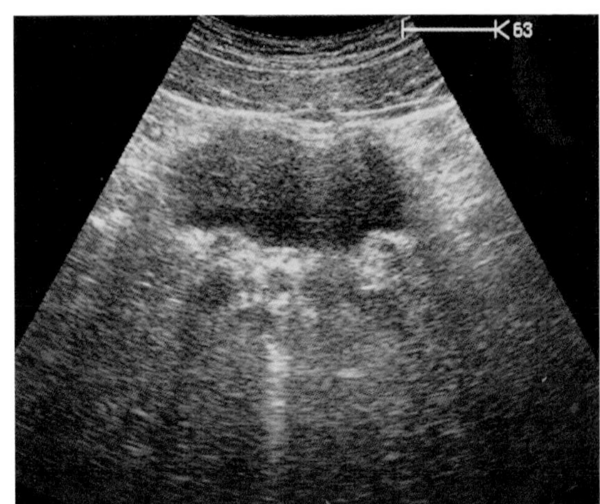

▶ **243** Bladder, ureteral orifices

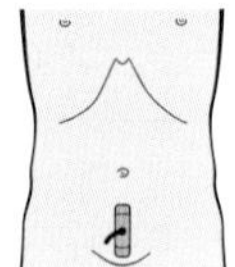

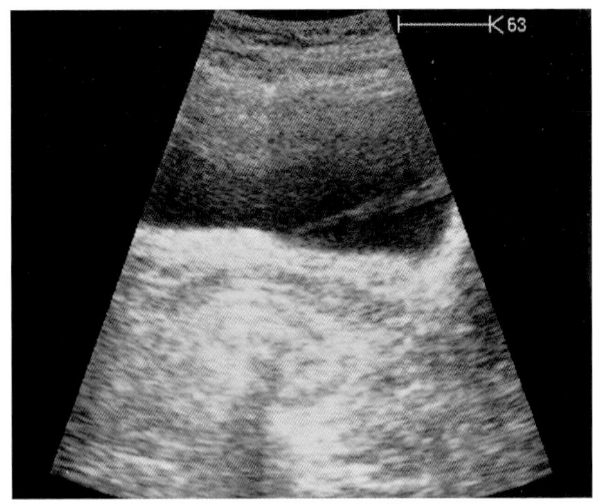

▶ **244** Bladder, inflow of urine

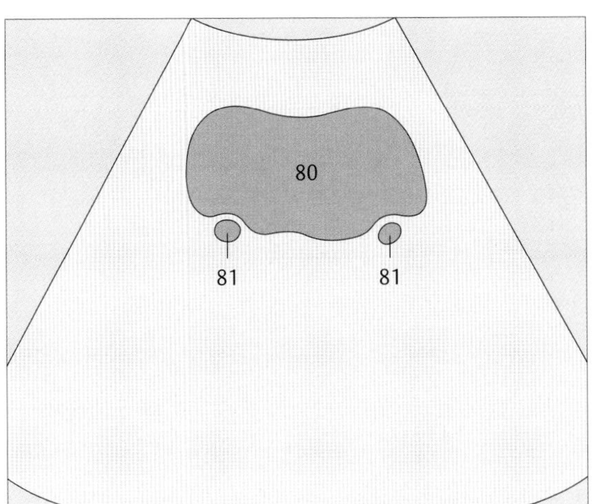

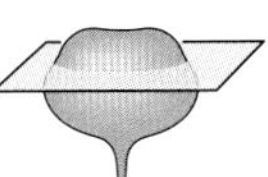

The ureters appear as fine tubular structures in the posterior bladder wall.

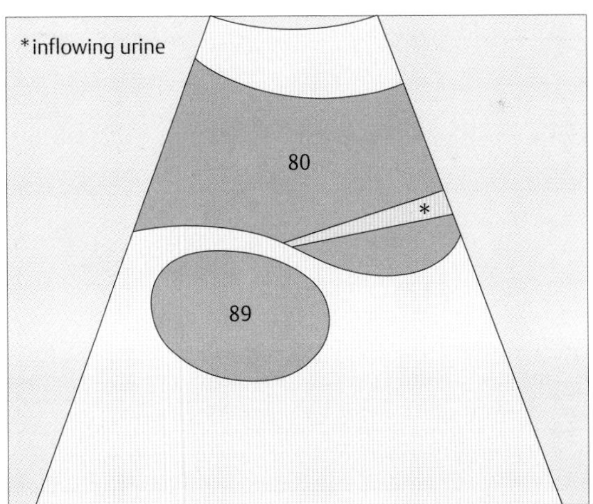

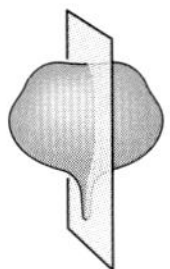

Ultrasound can often demonstrate urine flowing into the bladder from a ureteral orifice.

10 Prostate

Prostate in Longitudinal Sections ... p. 278

Prostate in Transverse Scans from Below Upward ... p. 282

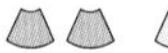
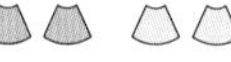

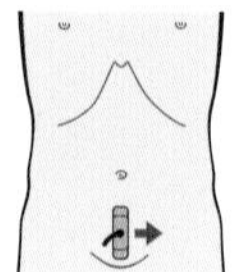

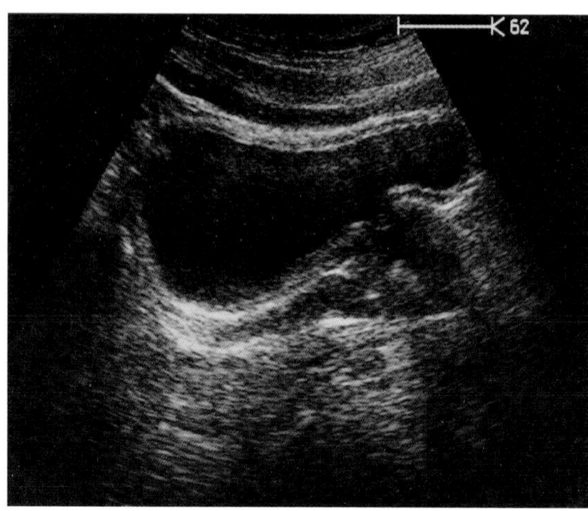

▶ **245** Prostate, rectum, bladder

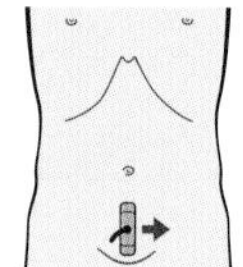

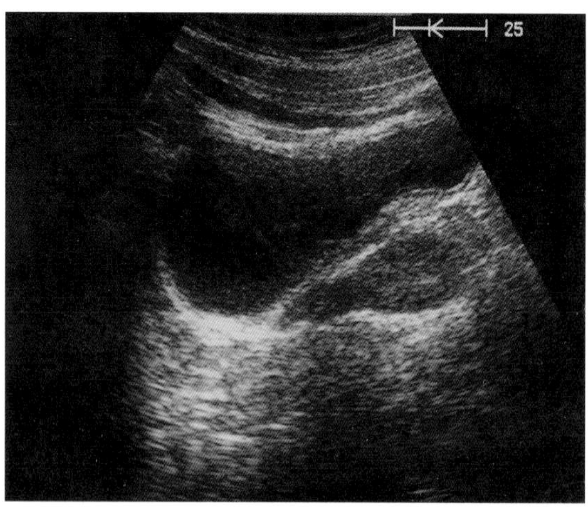

▶ **246** Prostate, rectum, bladder

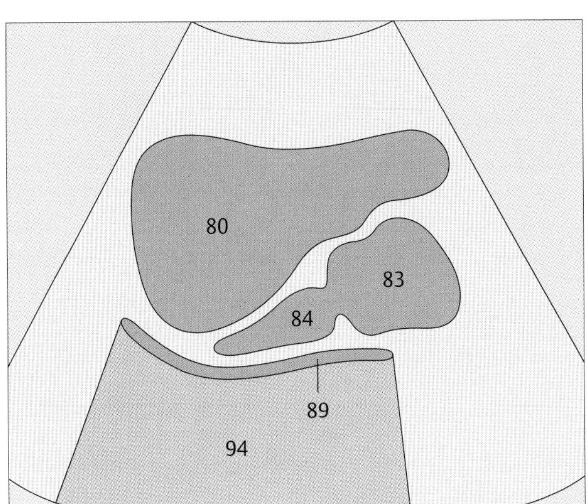

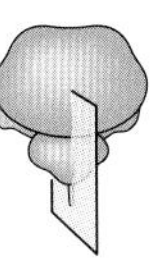

The prostate displays a bulbous shape in longitudinal section.

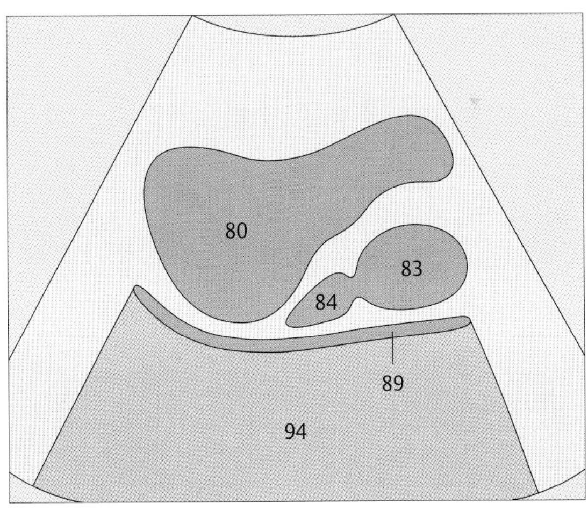

The rectum usually appears as an air-filled structure posterior to the prostate.

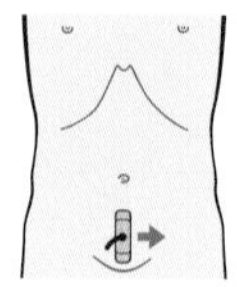

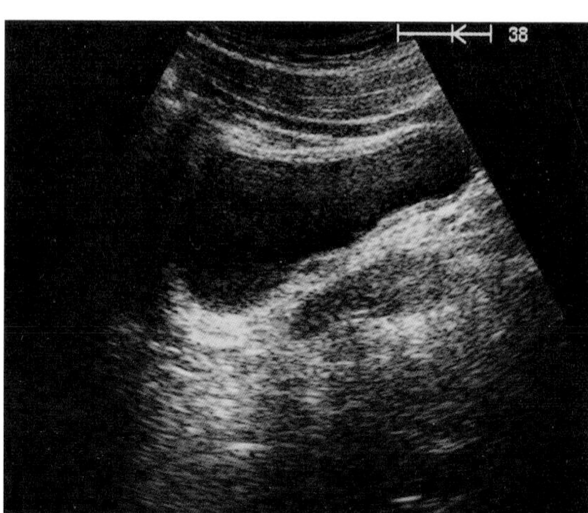

▶ **247** Prostate, seminal vesicles

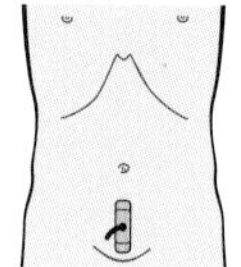

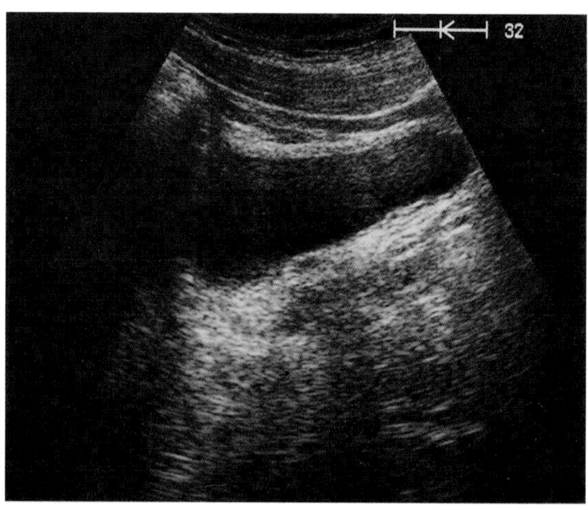

▶ **248** Prostate, seminal vesicles

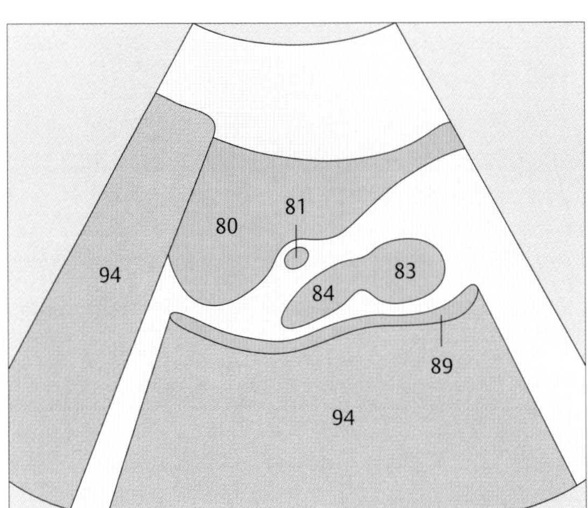

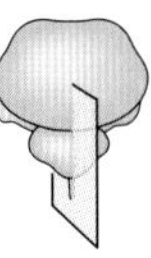

The seminal vesicles are in contact with the bladder over their full length.

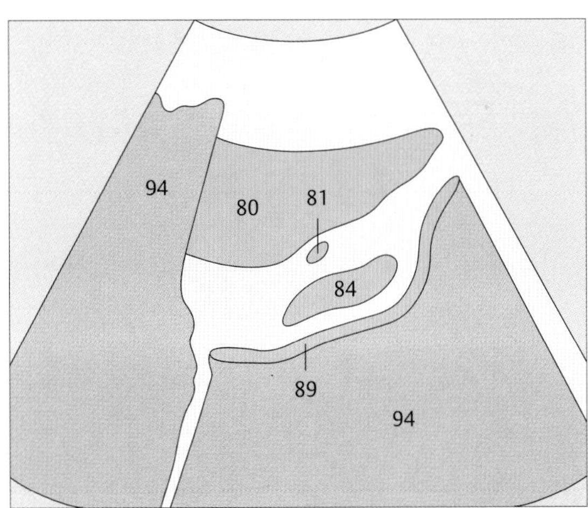

The seminal vesicles are located lateral and superior to the prostate.

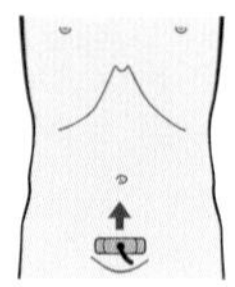

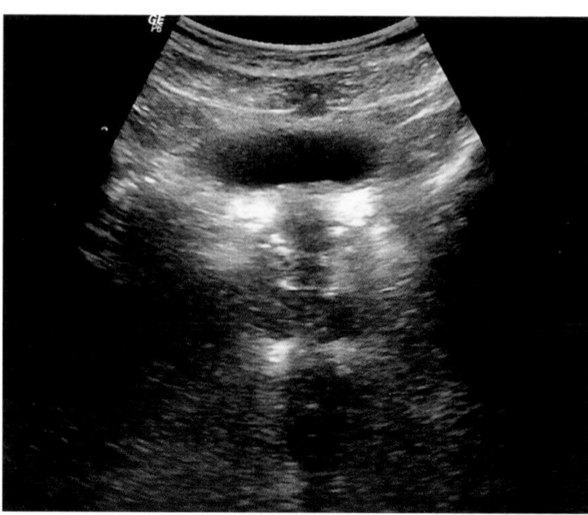

▶ **249** Prostate, urethra, bladder

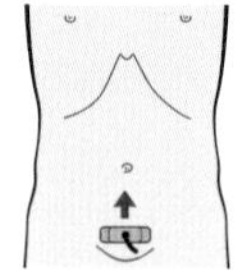

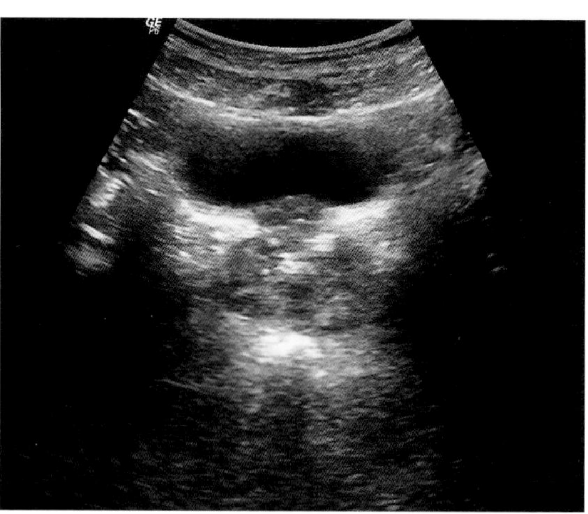

▶ **250** Prostate, urethra, bladder

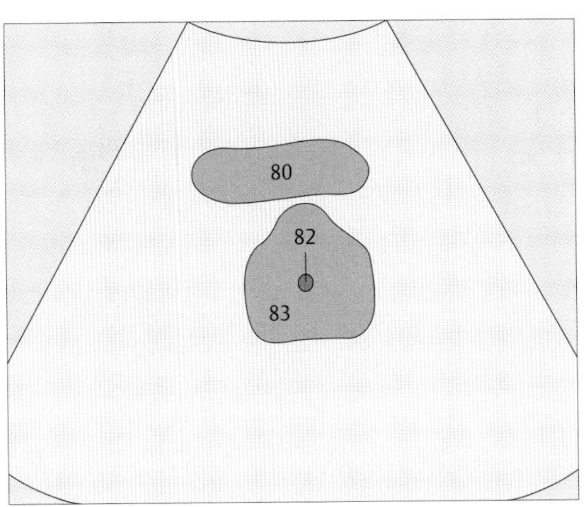

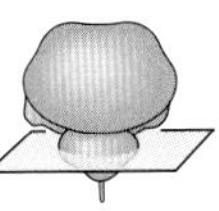

The prostate presents an elliptical "chestnut" shape when viewed in transverse section.

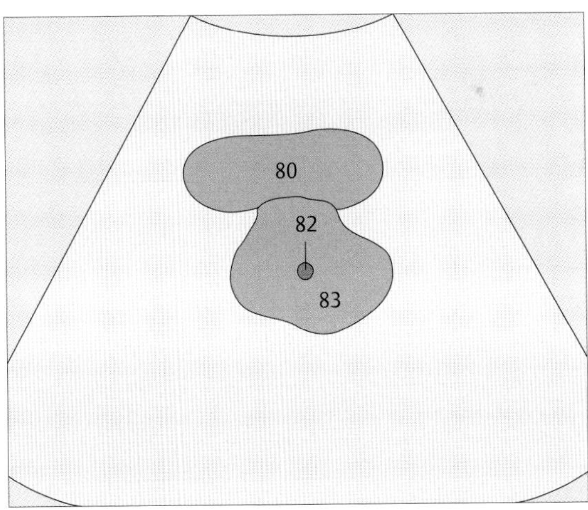

The middle lobe of the prostate sometimes bulges a short distance into the bladder lumen.

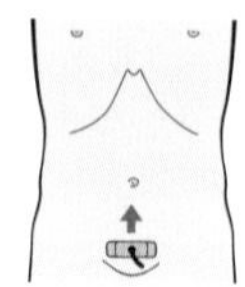

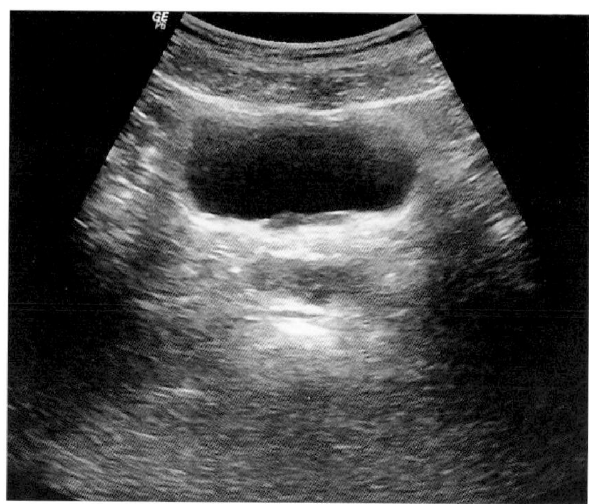

▶ **251** Prostate, urethra, bladder, rectum

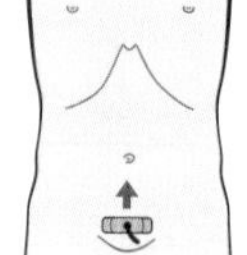

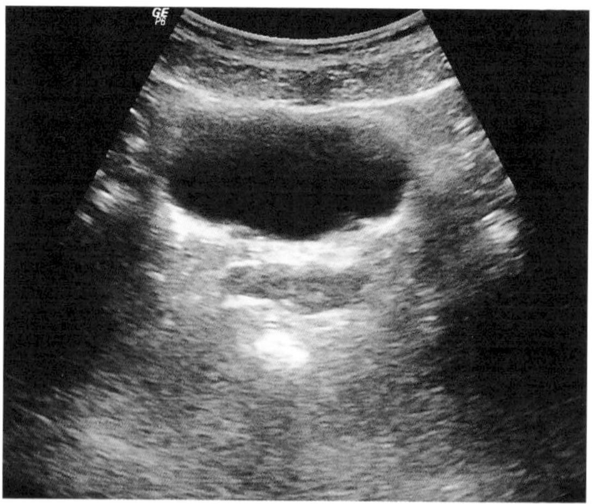

▶ **252** Seminal vesicles, rectum, bladder, *ampulla of vas deferens

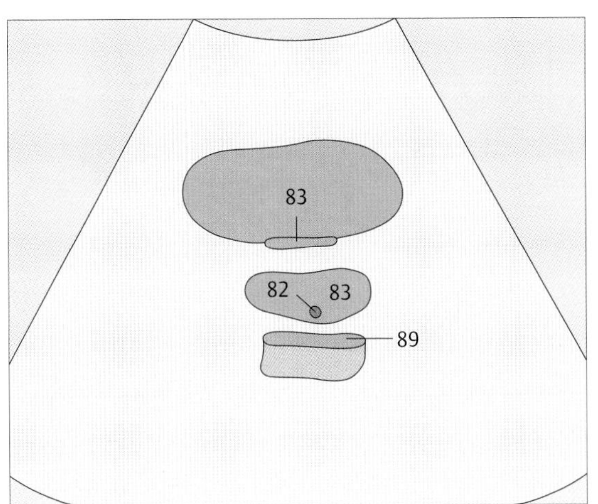

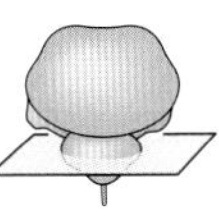

The urethra appears as a round, hypoechoic structure within the prostate.

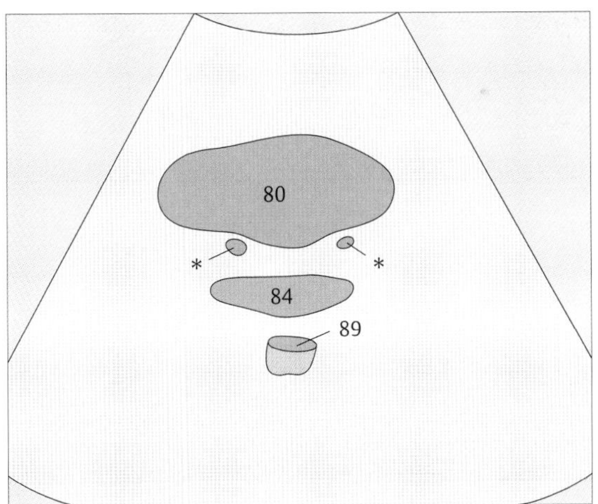

The rectum is consistently visualized posterior to the prostate.

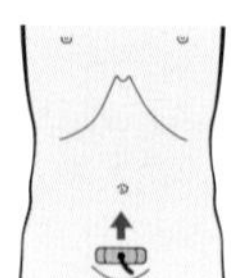

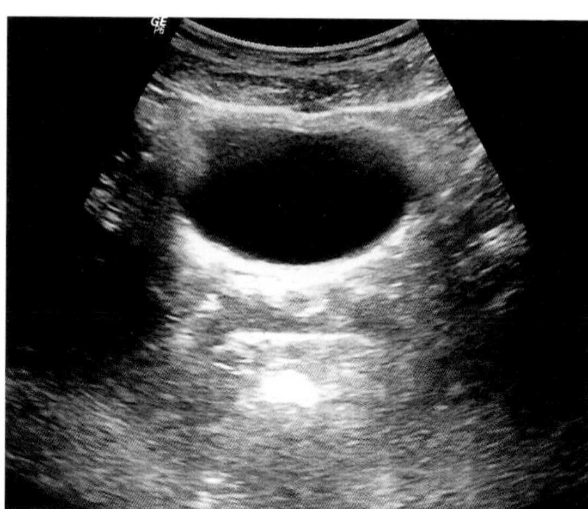

▶ **253** Seminal vesicles, rectum, bladder, *ampulla of vas deferens

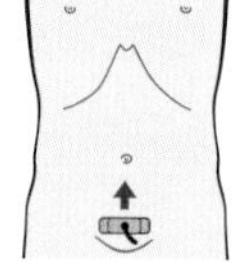

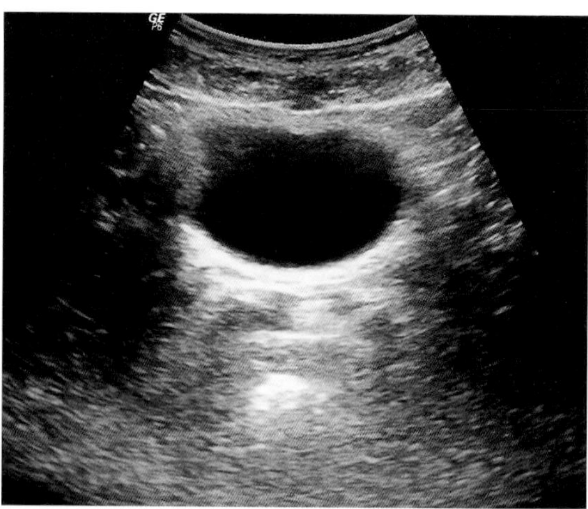

▶ **254** Seminal vesicles, rectum, bladder, *ampulla of vas deferens

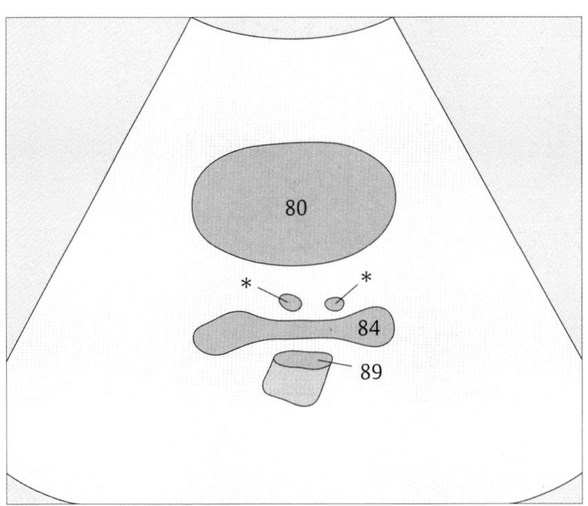

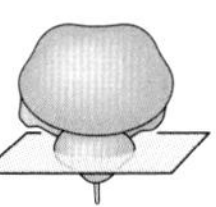

The seminal vesicles are approximately 5 cm long and 1 cm in diameter and are located on the posterior bladder wall.

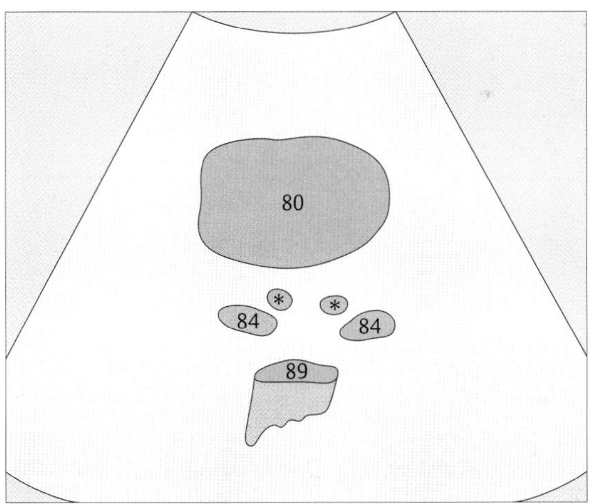

The vasa deferentia are located between the seminal vesicles and bladder.

11 Uterus

Uterus in Longitudinal Sections from Left to Right ... p. 290

Uterus in Transverse Sections from Below Upward ... p. 294

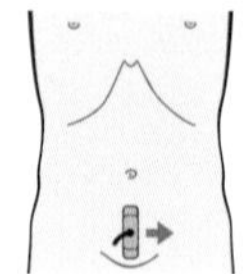

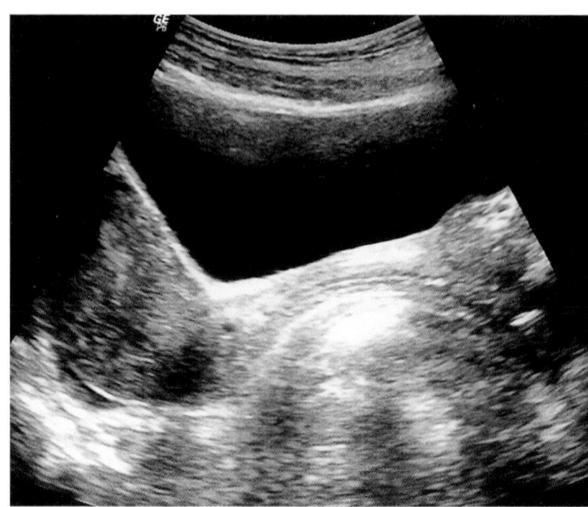

▶ **255** Uterus, vagina, bladder, rectum

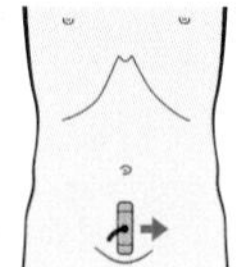

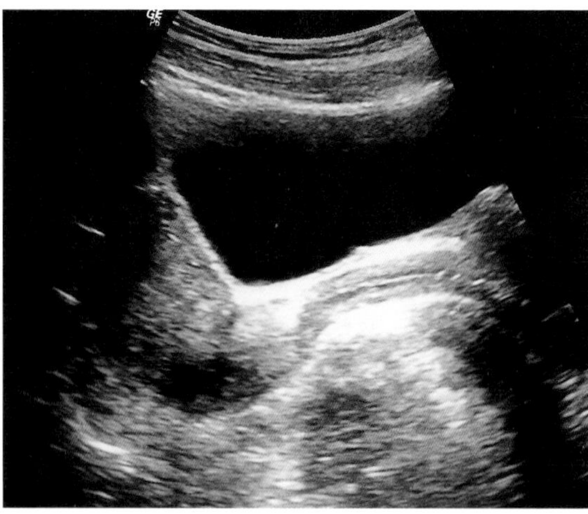

▶ **256** Uterus, vagina, bladder, rectum

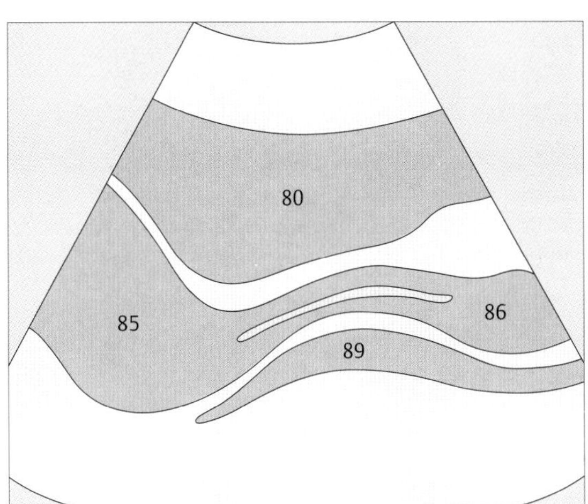

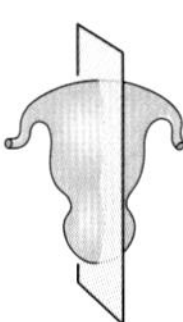

The vagina appears behind the bladder as an elongated, hypoechoic structure with a central band of higher-level echoes.

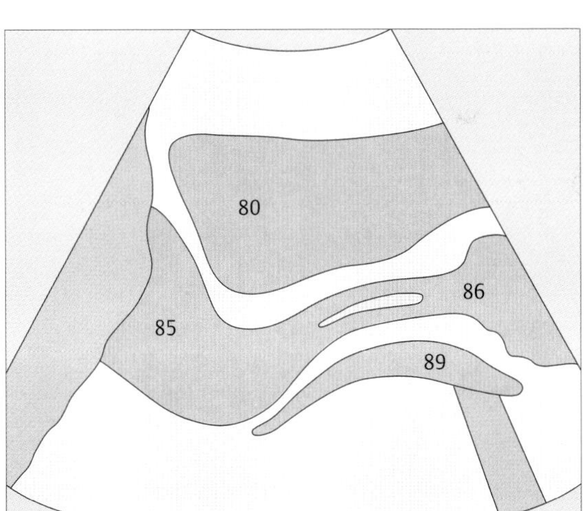

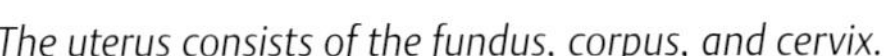

The uterus consists of the fundus, corpus, and cervix.

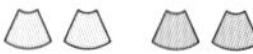

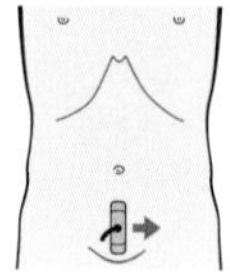

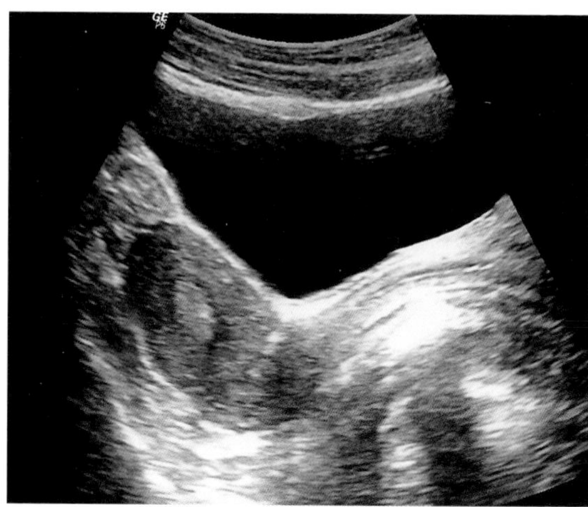

▶ **257** Uterus, vagina, bladder, rectum

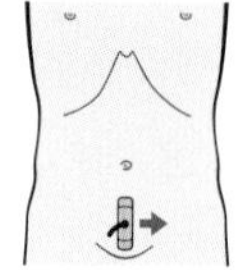

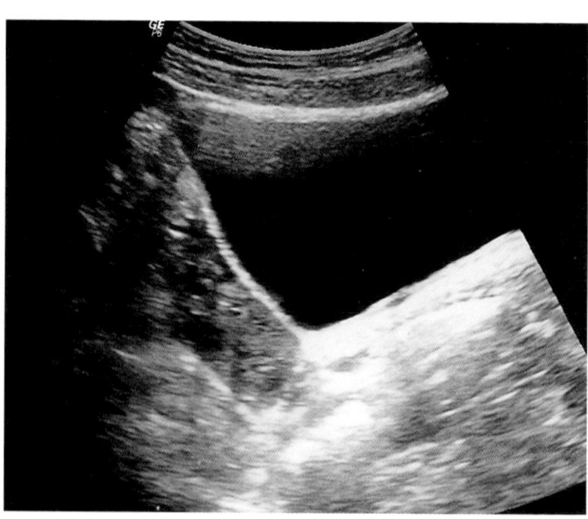

▶ **258** Ovary

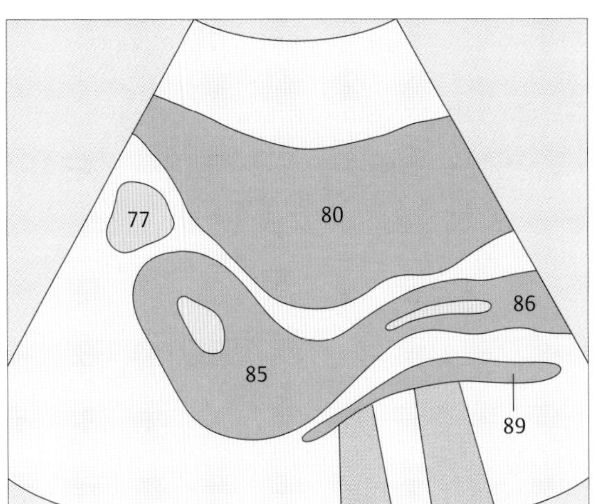

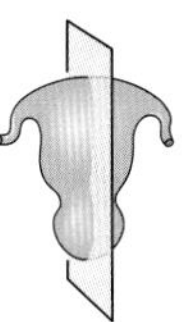

The uterine cavity is visible sonographically only during menstruation and pregnancy.

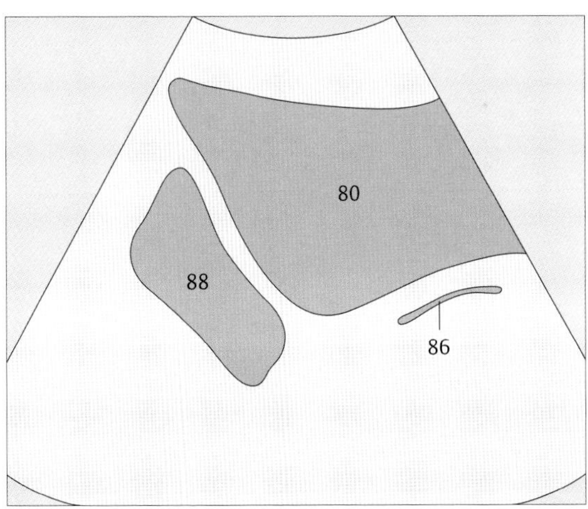

The ovaries flank the superior border of the full urinary bladder.

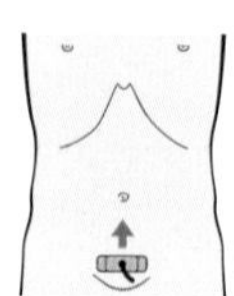

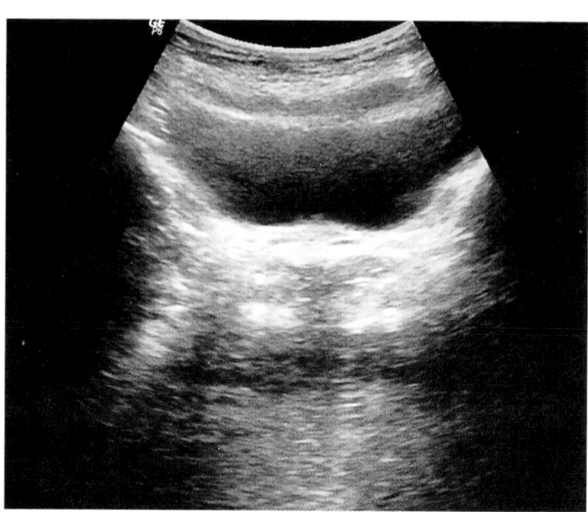

► **259** Vagina, bladder, rectum

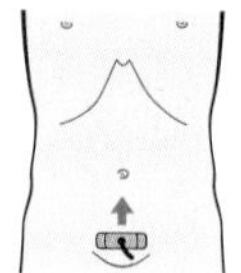

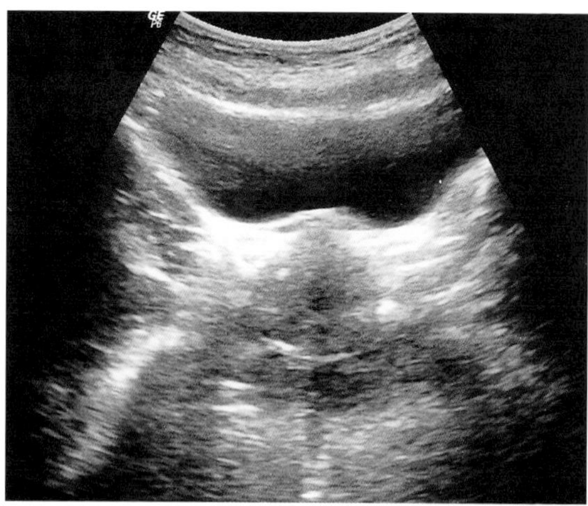

► **260** Vagina, bladder

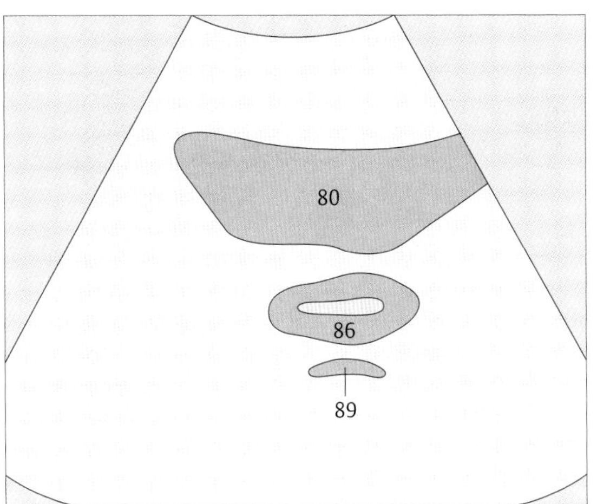

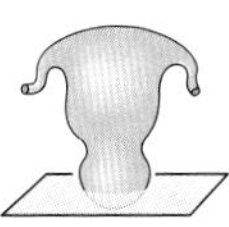

The vaginal lumen has a streaklike appearance in transverse section.

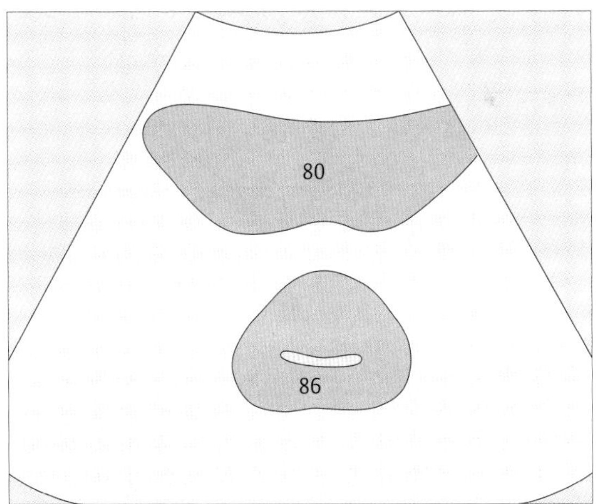

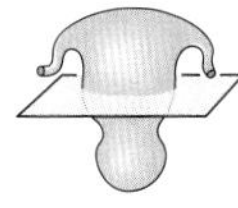

The uterus impresses on the posterior bladder wall.

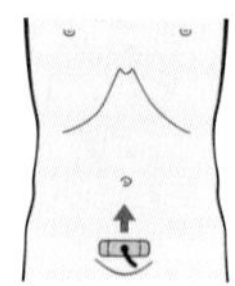

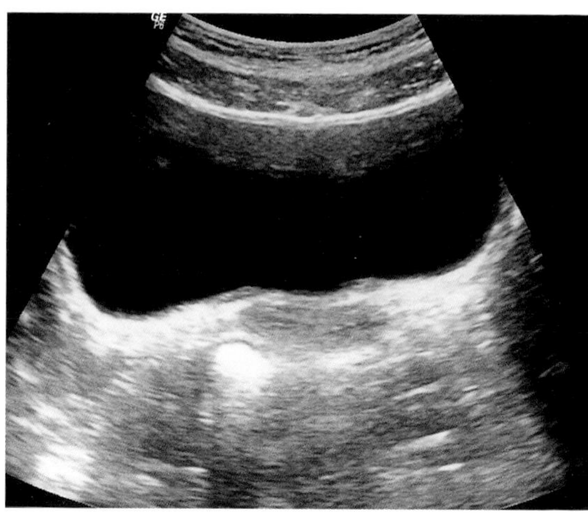

▶ **261** Vagina, bladder, rectum

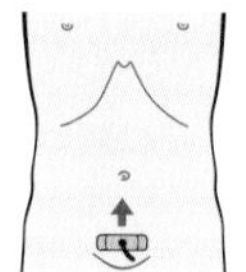

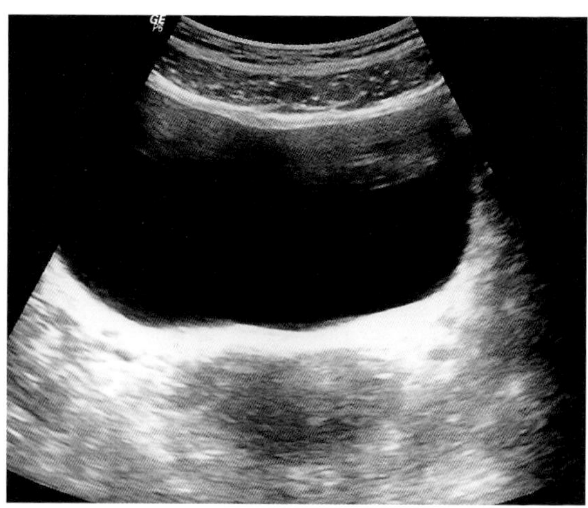

▶ **262** Uterus, bladder

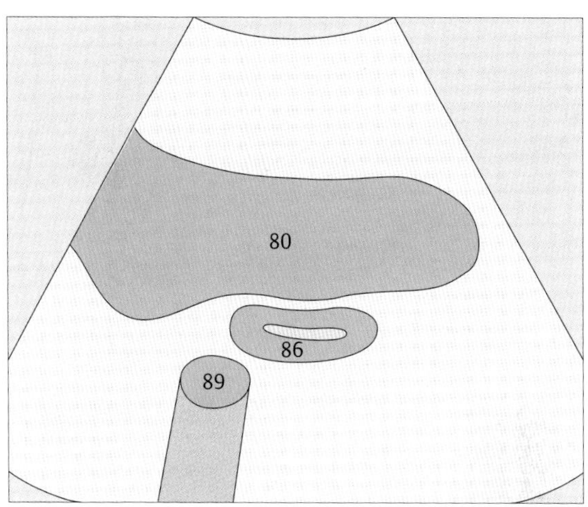

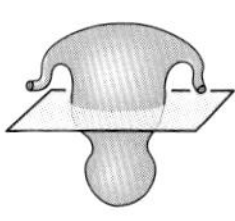

Transverse scan of the female pelvis displays, from anterior to posterior, the urinary bladder, vesicouterine pouch, uterus, and rectum.

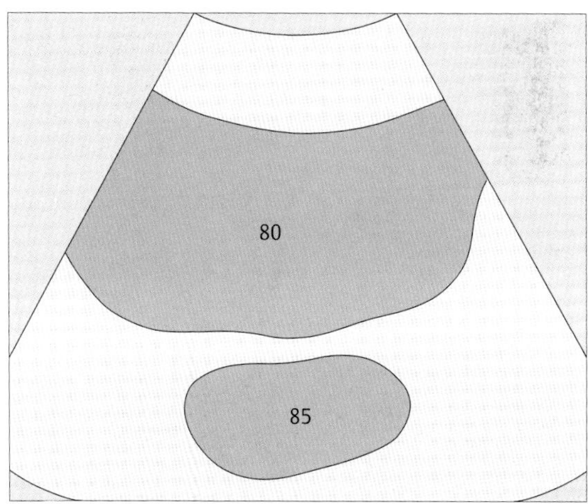

With the bladder distended, the uterus can be clearly visualized from the anterior side.

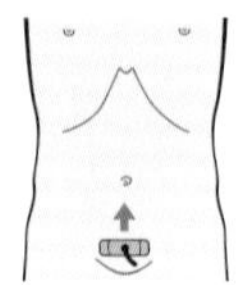

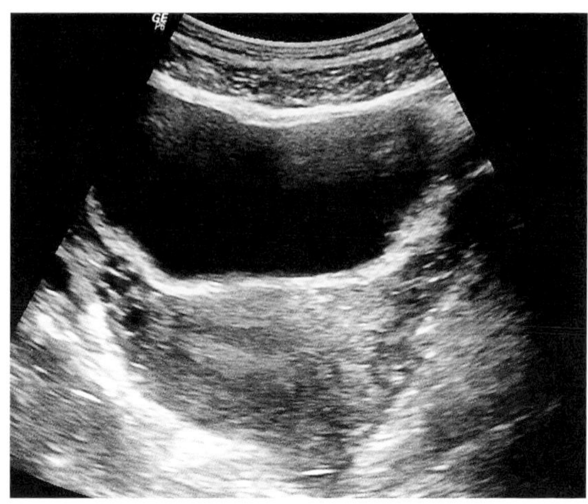

▶ **263** Uterus, bladder, ovaries

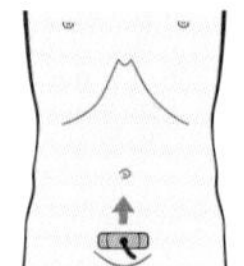

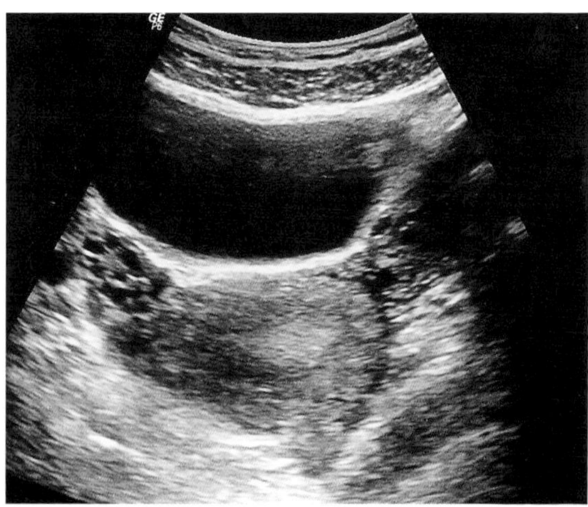

▶ **264** Uterus, bladder, ovaries

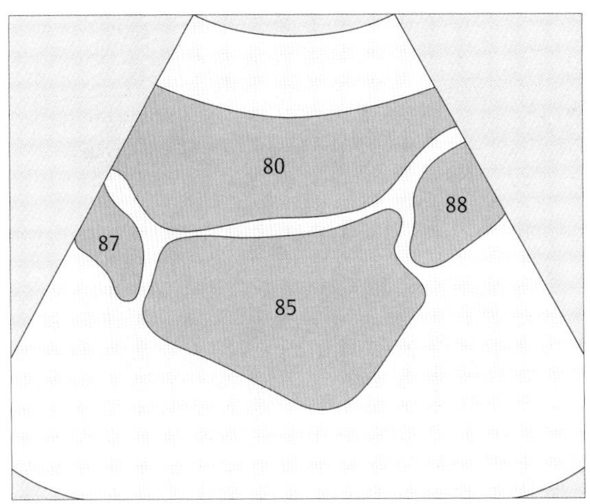

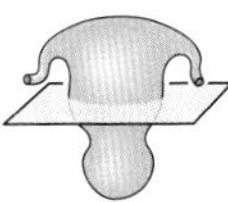

The ovaries are usually located lateral to the uterus at the level of the uterine corpus.

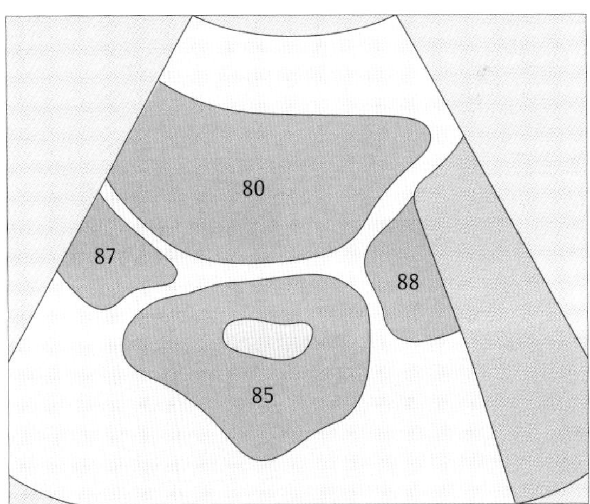

The ovaries appear as rounded structures approximately 3 cm long and are extremely variable in their location.

12 Thyroid Gland

Left Thyroid Lobe in Longitudinal Scans from Right to Left ... p. 302

265 Isthmus of thyroid gland
266 Isthmus of thyroid gland
267 Left lobe of thyroid gland, sternohyoid muscle, sternothyroid muscle
268 Left lobe of thyroid gland, sternohyoid muscle, sternothyroid muscle
269 Left lobe of thyroid gland, sternohyoid muscle, sternothyroid muscle
270 Left lobe of thyroid gland, common carotid artery
271 Internal jugular vein, sternocleidomastoid muscle
272 Internal jugular vein, sternocleidomastoid muscle

Left Thyroid Lobe in Transverse Scans from Below Upward ... p. 310

273 Left lobe of thyroid gland, common carotid artery, internal jugular vein
274 Left lobe of thyroid gland, common carotid artery, internal jugular vein
275 Left lobe of thyroid gland, common carotid artery, internal jugular vein
276 Left lobe of thyroid gland, common carotid artery, internal jugular vein
277 Left lobe of thyroid gland
278 Left lobe of thyroid gland

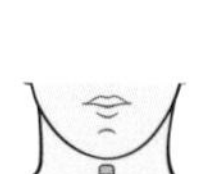

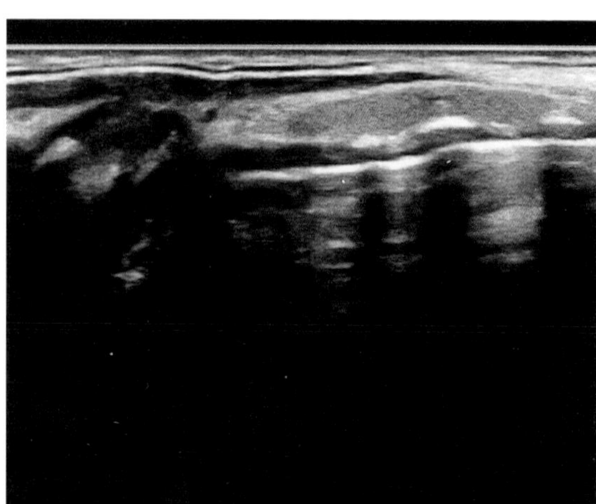

▶ **265** Isthmus of thyroid gland

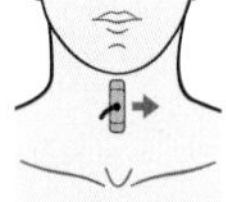

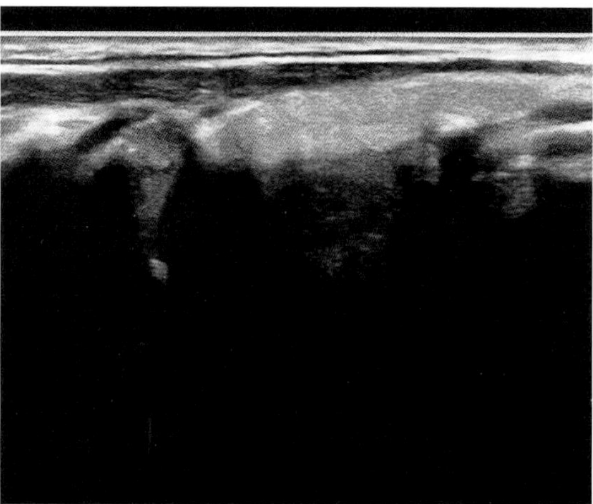

▶ **266** Isthmus of thyroid gland

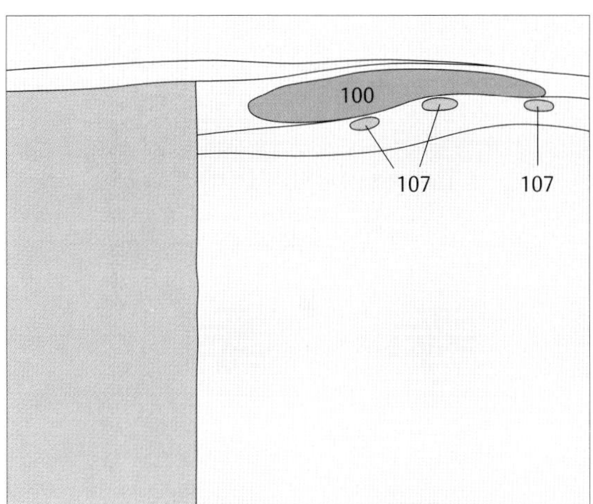

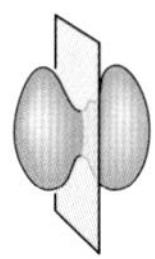

The trachea is located directly behind the isthmus of the thyroid gland.

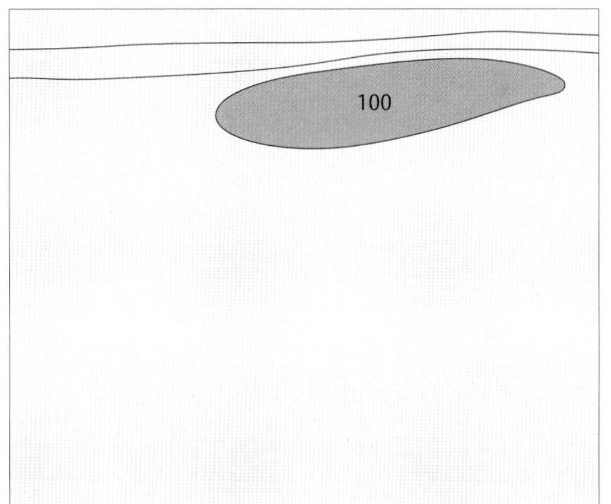

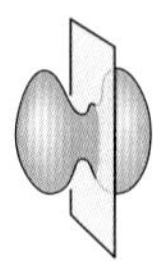

The thyroid gland is imaged with a high-resolution transducer.

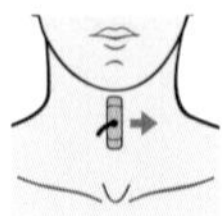

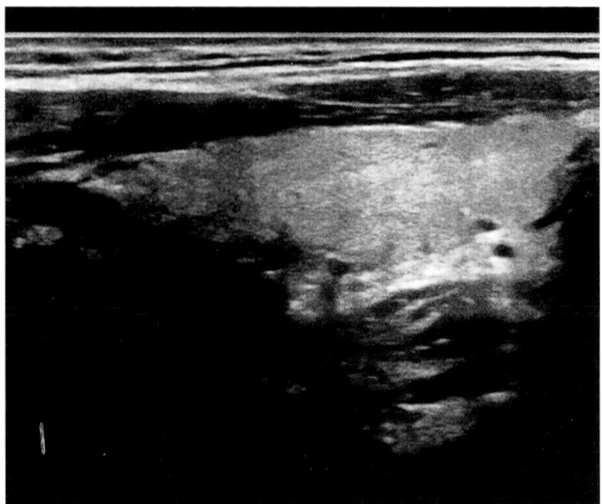

▶ **267** Left lobe of thyroid gland, sternohyoid muscle, sternothyroid muscle

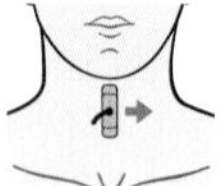

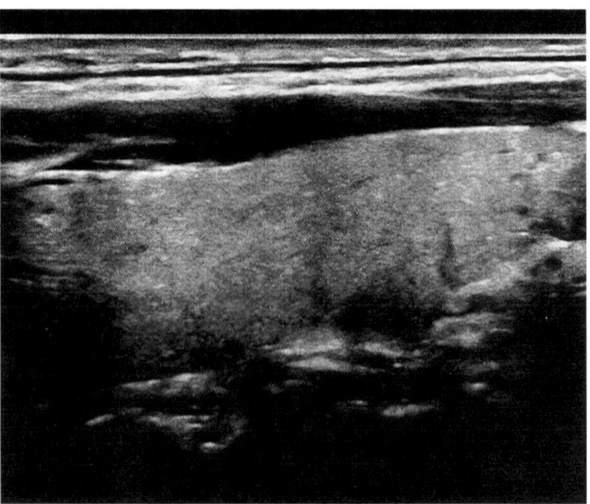

▶ **268** Left lobe of thyroid gland, sternohyoid muscle, sternothyroid muscle

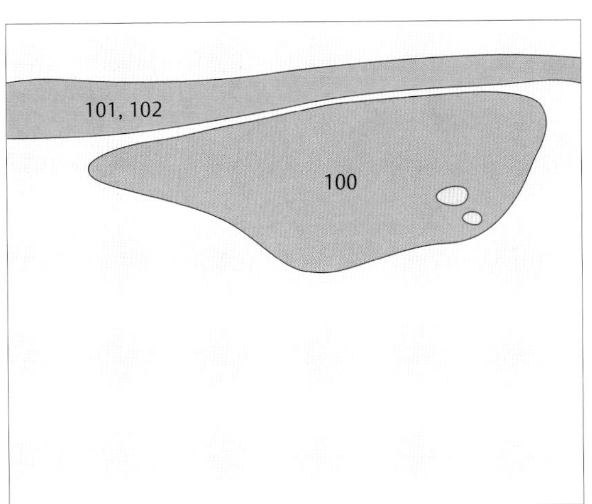

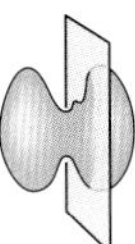

Scant vascularity is seen in the normal thyroid parenchyma.

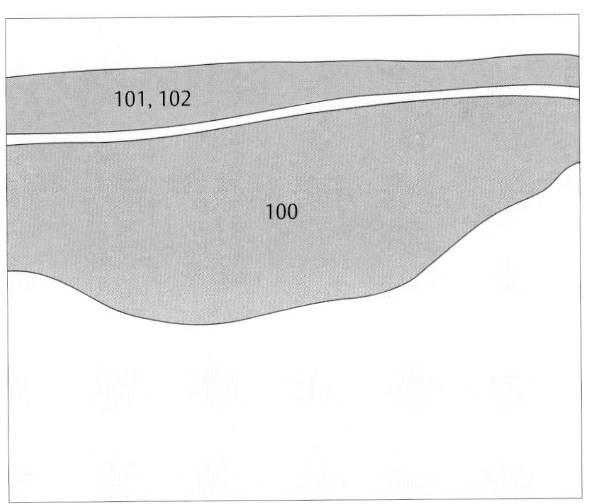

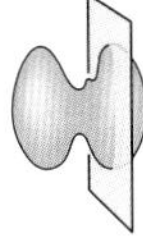

The sternohyoid and sternothyroid muscles are anterior to the thyroid gland.

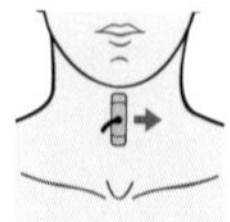

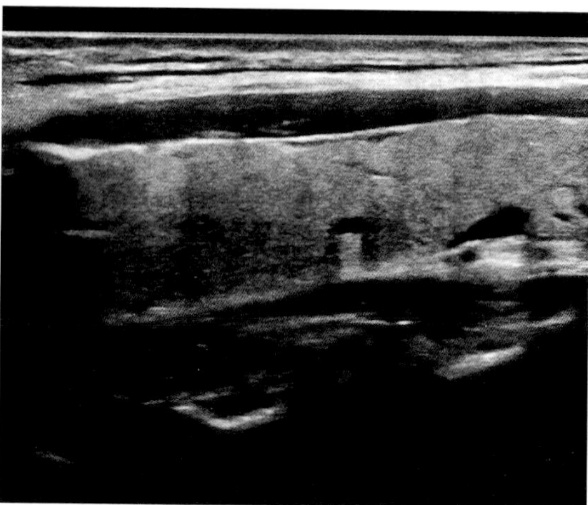

▶ **269** Left lobe of thyroid gland, sternohyoid muscle, sternothyroid muscle

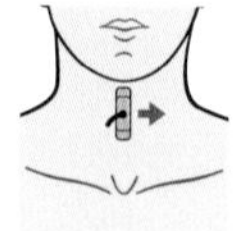

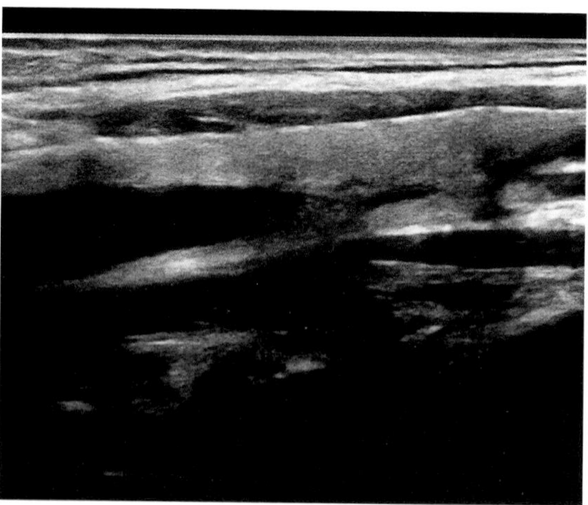

▶ **270** Left lobe of thyroid gland, common carotid artery

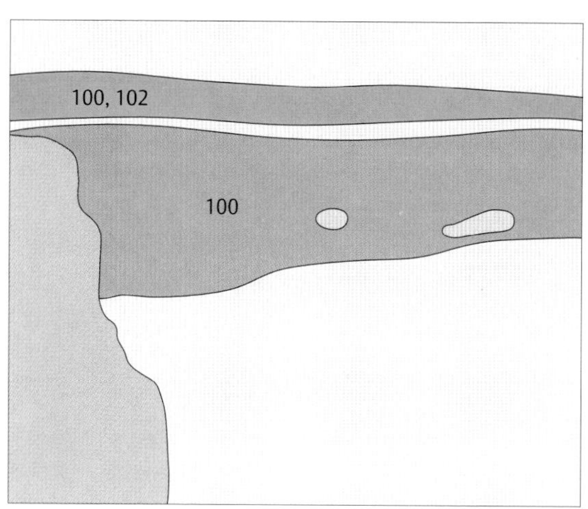

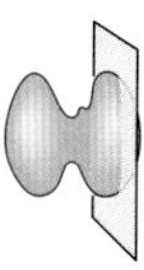

Normal thyroid parenchyma has a homogeneous echo pattern.

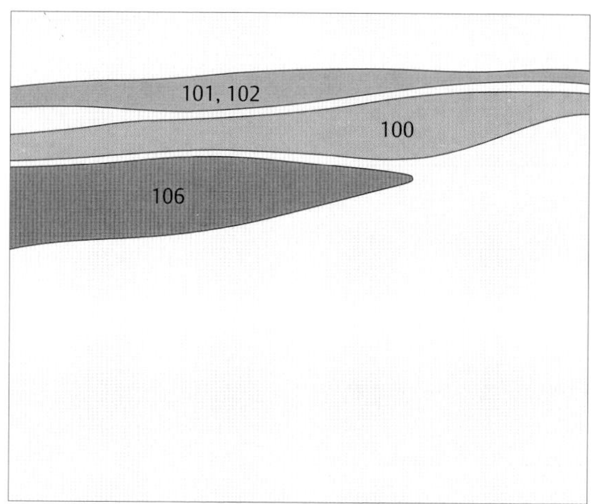

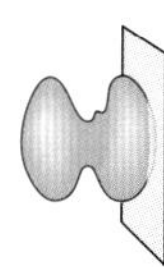

The thyroid gland narrows markedly in the lateral direction.

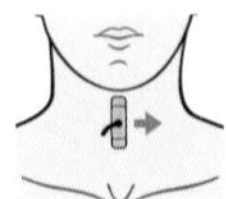

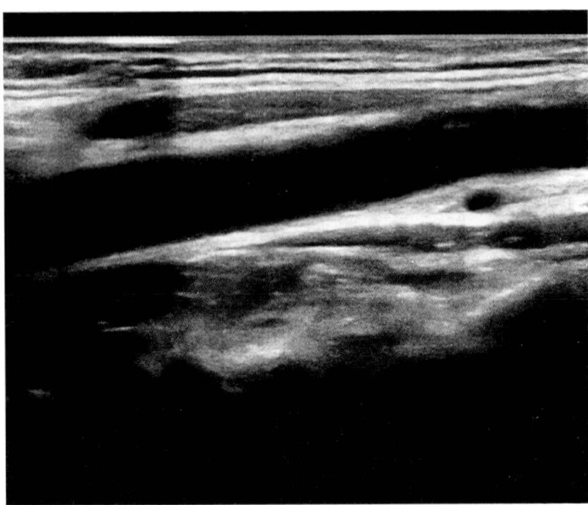

▶ **271** Internal jugular vein, sternocleidomastoid muscle

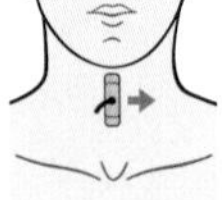

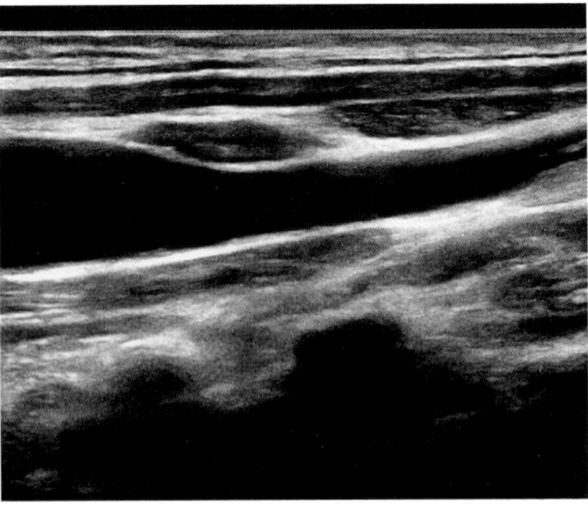

▶ **272** Internal jugular vein, sternocleidomastoid muscle

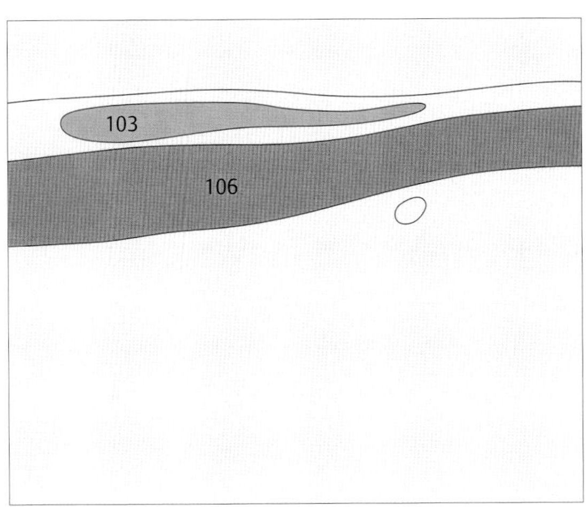

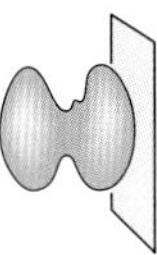

The common carotid artery is in contact with the lateral aspect of the thyroid gland.

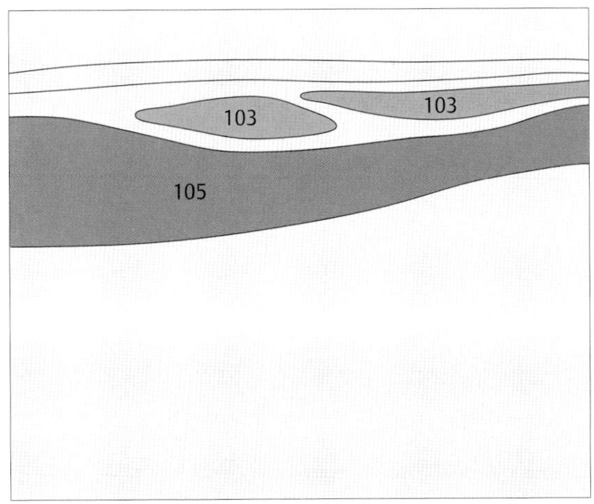

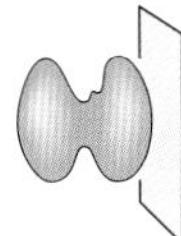

The large jugular vein appears lateral to the common carotid artery.

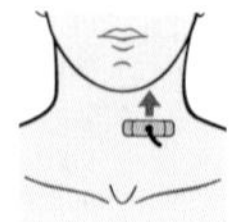

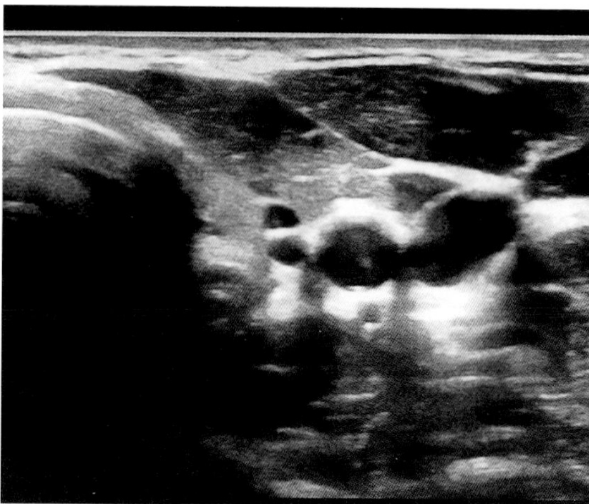

▶ **273** Left lobe of thyroid gland, common carotid artery, internal jugular vein

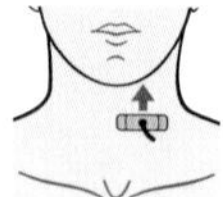

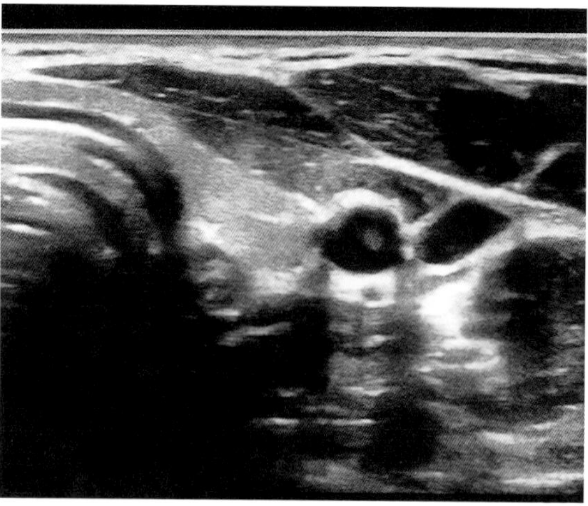

▶ **274** Left lobe of thyroid gland, common carotid artery, internal jugular vein

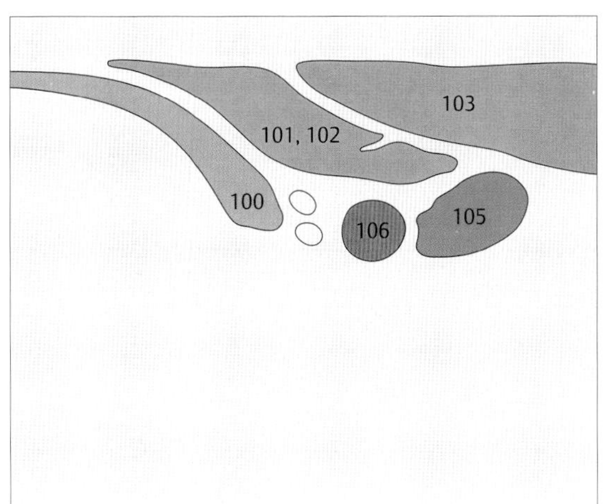

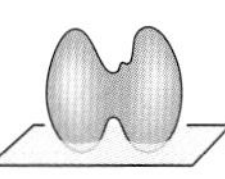

The large vessels in the neck run just lateral to the thyroid gland.

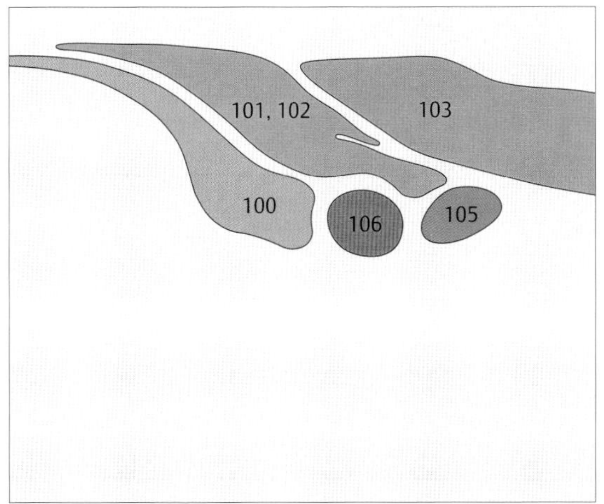

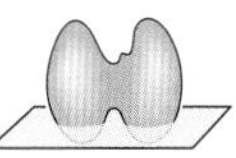

The common carotid artery appears just lateral to the thyroid gland in a transverse scan.

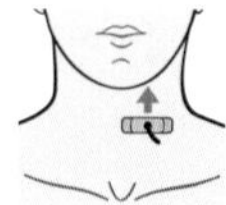

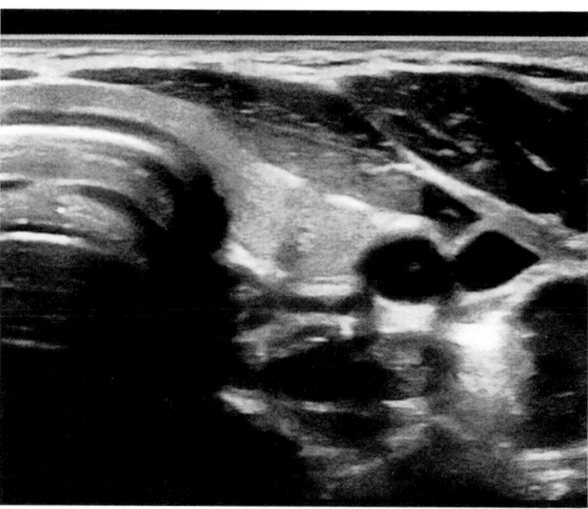

▶ **275** Left lobe of thyroid gland, common carotid artery, internal jugular vein

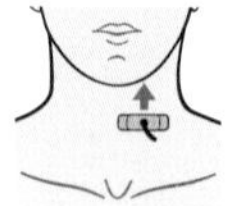

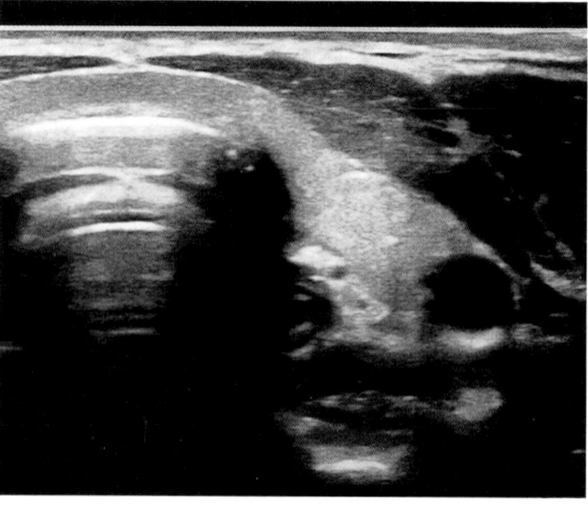

▶ **276** Left lobe of thyroid gland, common carotid artery, internal jugular vein

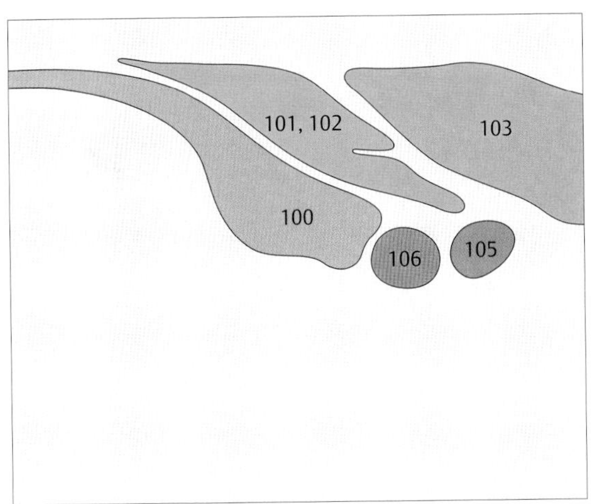

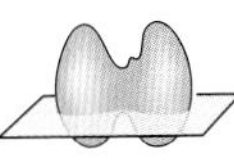

The jugular vein appears as a hypoechoic structure, not completely circular, located adjacent to the common carotid artery.

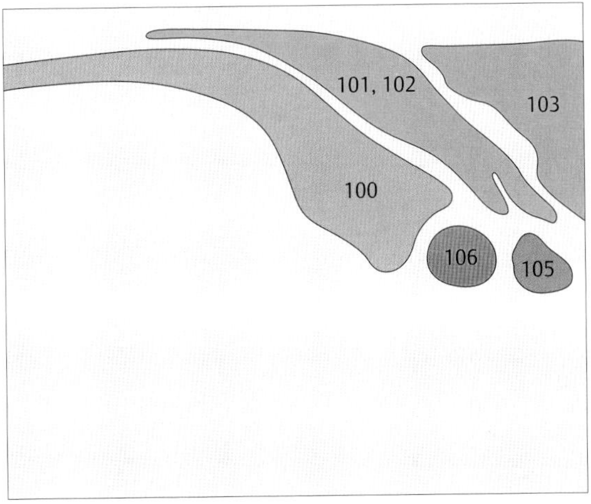

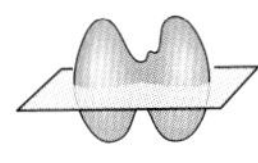

The sternocleidomastoid is a powerful muscle located anterior and lateral to the thyroid gland.

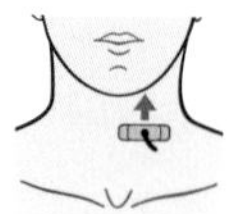

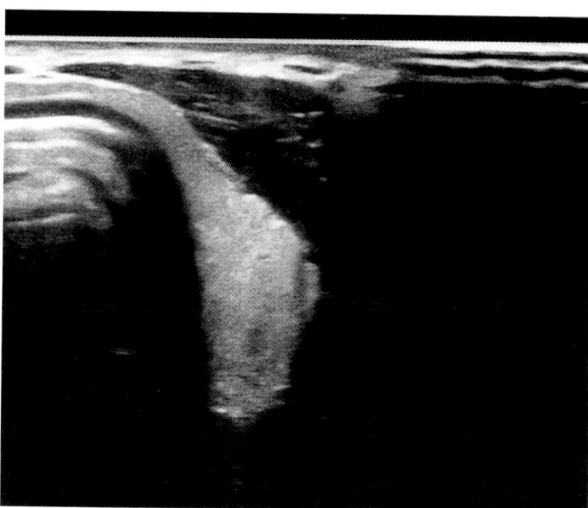

► **277** Left lobe of thyroid gland

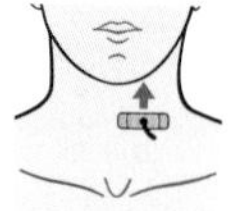

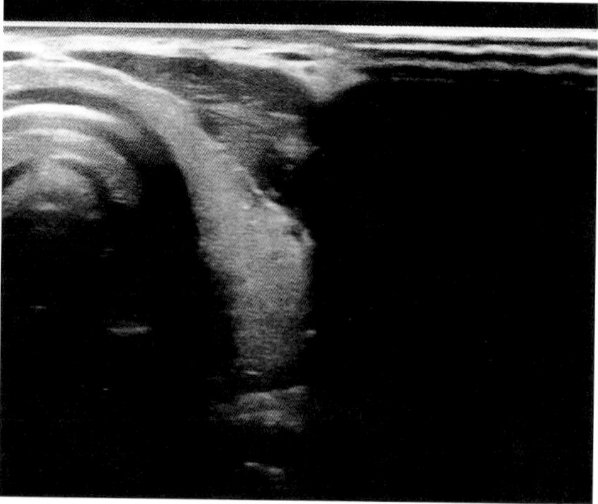

► **278** Left lobe of thyroid gland

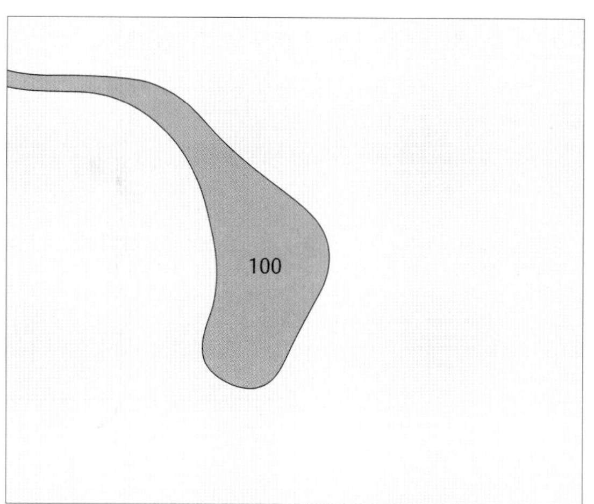

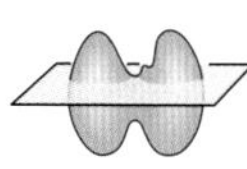

The thyroid gland is a butterfly-shaped organ with smooth borders and high-level internal echoes.

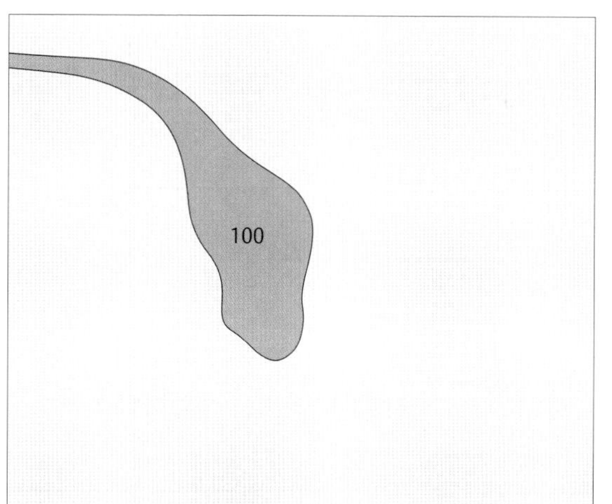

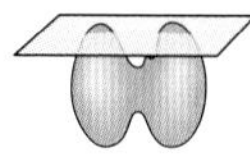

The parathyroid glands are located posterior to the lateral and superior poles of the thyroid gland. They may not be visible at ultrasound unless they are enlarged.

Normal Sonographic Dimensions of the Pancreas, Spleen, and Kidneys

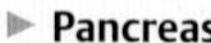

▶ Pancreas

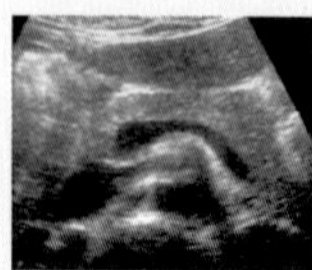

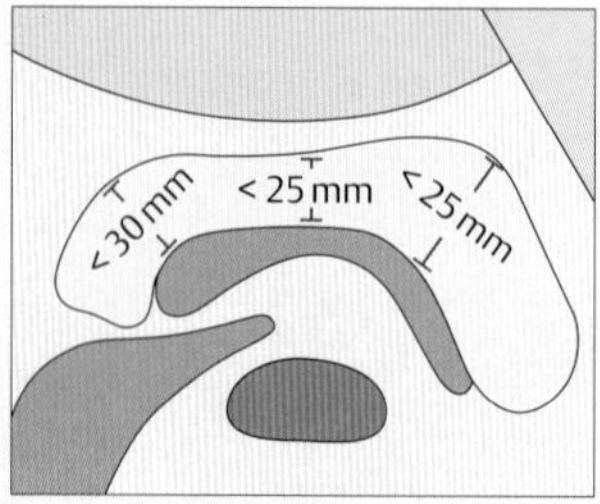

Head < 30 mm

Body < 25 mm

Tail < 25 mm

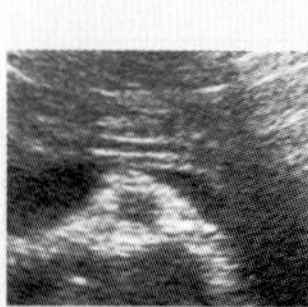

Pancreatic duct

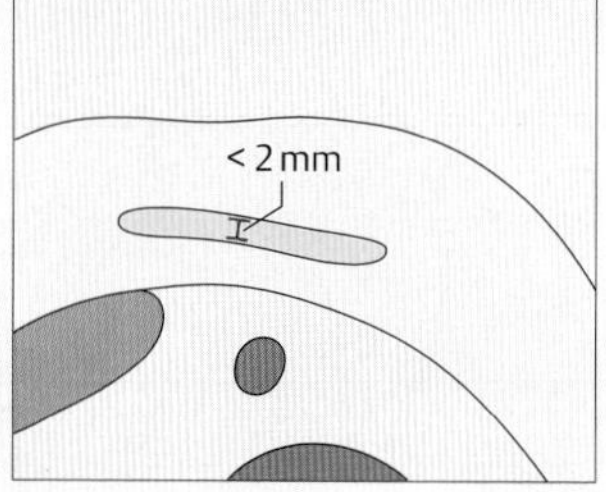

Pancreatic duct
< 2 mm

▶ Spleen

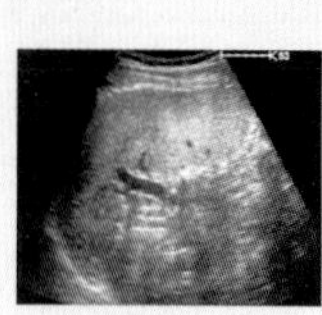

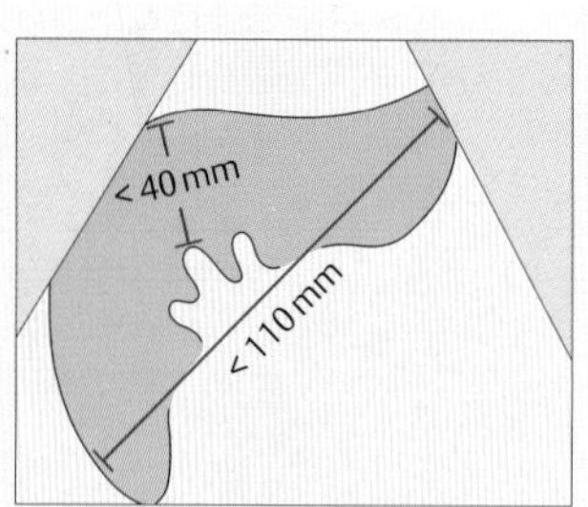

In longitudinal flank scan:
Length < 110 mm
Thickness < 40 mm

▶ Kidneys

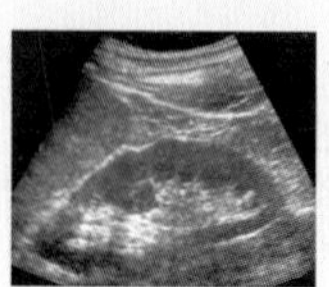

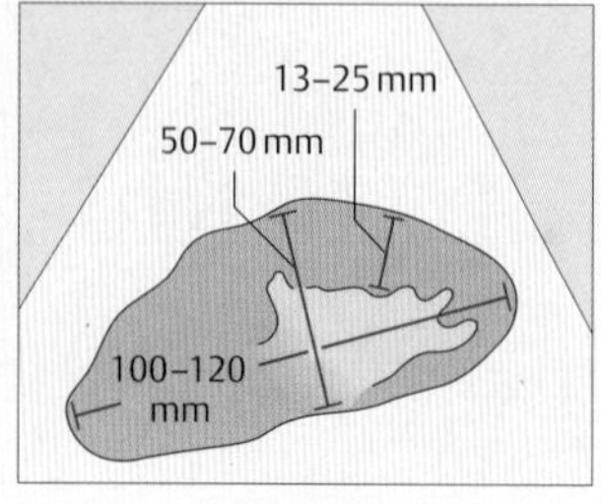

length 100–120 mm

width 50–70 mm

Width of parenchyma: 13–25 mm

Parenchymal-pelvic ratio:
60 years or younger 1.6 : 1
Over 60 years 1.1 : 1